Analytical Techniques for Decision Making in Agriculture

I0005649

The Editors

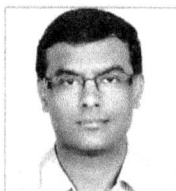

Dr. S. S. Raju is currently working as a Principal Scientist (Agricultural Economics) at ICAR-National Institute of Agricultural Economics and Policy Research (NIAP), New Delhi, India. Prior to this he has been Scientist (SS) at ICAR-National Institute of Animal Nutrition and Physiology, Bangalore. Dr. Raju has been awarded APAU Agro-economic Research Gold Medals at M.Sc (Ag) and PhD (Ag) levels for obtaining highest OGPA in the discipline of Agricultural Economics at University level. He is also recipient of Team Research award of ICAR for biennium 1999-2000. At present Dr. Raju is engaged in research on Regional Crop Planning, Agricultural Risk and Insurance, Biofuels and energy use in agriculture, livestock and growth and development. Dr. Raju is author of one book and 35 research papers published in reputed national and international journals. He was associated with 10 national and international research projects. Besides, he has organized many capacity building programmes for the researches in national agricultural research system. He can be reached at rajuss67@yahoo.co.in.

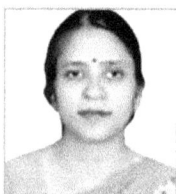

Dr. Rajni Jain is currently working as a Principal Scientist (Computer Application) at ICAR-National Institute of Agricultural Economics and Policy Research (NIAP) since 1996. She was awarded Ph.D. degree in Computer Science from Jawaharlal Nehru University in 2005 in the area of data mining and M.Sc. degree in the discipline of Computer Application from P.G. School, Indian Agricultural Research Institute in 1991 with a gold medal for her outstanding academic performance. Dr. Jain made important and useful contributions to the discipline of agricultural economics by planning, design and development of many online software and data mining base for agriculture. Her research interests include development of decision support systems for agriculture domain using data mining techniques. Dr. Jain has contributed nearly 80 research papers in journals, conferences, workshops and seminars. Besides she has organized many training programmes for the researches in national agricultural research system. She can be reached at rajni@ncap.res.in.

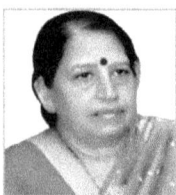

Dr.Usha Ahuja is Principal Scientist at the National Institute for Agricultural Economics and Policy Research (NIAP), New Delhi. She did her Ph.D. and M.Sc. in the discipline of Dairy Economics from National Dairy Research Institute Karnal (Haryana) in India. Usha joined as Scientist (Agricultural Economics) in April 1986 at Central Arid Zone Research Institute (CAZRI) Jodhpur (Raj.) and worked there for more than 21years (from 24th April 1986 to 25th May 2007). During her stay at CAZRI she conducted research on agricultural issues related to arid zone through internally (institutional) and externally (Indo-Australian & NATP) funded projects. She joined National Centre for Agricultural Economics and Policy Research (NCAP) New Delhi, India on 26th May, 2007. Usha in her initial period in NCAP worked on Gender Budgeting in agriculture, Conservation Agriculture and Diversified Farming Systems. Now she is pursuing research on mainstreaming gender in agriculture. Usha has contributed several research papers in national/international journals/conferences/workshops/seminars. She can be reached at usha@ncap.res.in.

Analytical Techniques for Decision Making in Agriculture

— *Editors* —

S.S. Raju

Rajni Jain

Usha Ahuja

2016

Daya Publishing House®

A Division of

Astral International Pvt. Ltd.

New Delhi – 110 002

Cataloging in Publication Data--DK
Courtesy: D.K. Agencies (P) Ltd. <docinfo@dkagencies.com>

Analytical techniques for decision making in agriculture /
editors, S.S. Raju, Rajni Jain, Usha Ahuja.

pages cm
Includes index.

ISBN 978-93-5130-976-5 (International Edition)

1. Agriculture--India--Decision making. 2. Agriculture--India--Data processing.   I. Raju, S. S., editor. II. Jain, Rajni (Computer scientist), editor. III. Ahuja, Usha, editor.

S494.5.D3A53 2016   DDC 630.954   23

Published by   : **Daya Publishing House®**
                         A Division of
                         Astral International Pvt. Ltd.
                         – ISO 9001:2008 Certified Company –
                         4760-61/23, Ansari Road, Darya Ganj
                         New Delhi-110 002
                         Ph. 011-43549197, 23278134
                         E-mail: info@astralint.com
                         Website: www.astralint.com

Laser Typesetting   : **Classic Computer Services**, Delhi - 110 035

Printed at   : **Replika Press Pvt. Ltd.**

Preface

The book titled "Analytical Techniques for Decision Making in Agriculture" provides a summary of analytical techniques used by the professionals for Decision Making in Agriculture. The book is divided in 25 chapters. Each chapter has been developed based on the presentations by the respective authors in training programme to the faculty working in the areas of agricultural research. However, the analytical techniques covered are useful for the scholars working in other domains also.

The book is different from other books on analytical techniques in many aspects. Some books cover analytical techniques in theoretical sense. Some other books cover practical aspects of a single issue without the emphasis on quantitative analysis. However, the application of analytical techniques presented in the book is based on actual research, several years of experience of the authors and the actual datasets rather than hypothetical ones. Hence, the chapters offer real problems and the solutions while using the specified analytical technique. Further, the book provides a comprehensive overview of bioinformatics, ICT, GIS *etc.*, in modern research.

We take this opportunity to gratefully acknowledge the contribution made by the authors of various chapters in the preparation of this book. We warmly acknowledge the various sources and publications from which valuable materials for this book has been drawn.

We sincerely acknowledge the help received from Dr P S Birthal, Acting Director, ICAR-National Institute of Agricultural Economics and Policy Research, New Delhi who encouraged and provided institutional facilities in preparation of the book. We acknowledge the financial assistance received from Education Division, ICAR in organizing the Summer School on "Analytical Techniques for Decision Making in Agriculture".

We also take this opportunity to express our sincere thanks and gratitude to all who have made valuable suggestions to enhance the utility of the book and also wish to acknowledge and express our sincere thanks and gratitude to Astral International (P) Ltd, New Delhi for providing the necessary encouragement to publish this book.

S.S. Raju
Rajni Jain
Usha Ahuja

Contents

Chapter 1

Estimating Performance of Agriculture in India

Ramesh Chand

Member,
NITI Aayog, New Delhi-110 001

1. Introduction

Agriculture sector in India and in many other countries faced several tough challenges for couple of years after implementation of the WTO agreement on agriculture in year 1995, primarily due to sharp fall in prices of agricultural commodities. The fall in prices led to perceptible decline in growth of agricultural output after the mid 1990's which had several consequences including widespread agrarian distress. It was a great challenge and formidable task to arrest the decline and to reverse the slowing growth of agriculture sector. Several initiatives were taken by the central and state governments to address this challenge. The last nine years (2004-05 to 2012-13) have witnessed impressive revival of agriculture growth rate eventhough growth rate of non agriculture sector decelerated in recent years. Besides growth per se the quality of growth has also seen considerable improvement and there has been progress relating to inclusiveness, regional equity, and nutrition security. Though these achievements are highly significant and unique in many respects, there is not adequate appreciation or realization about these in the country. Many of us seem to be obsessed with achievement of green revolution and not willing to acknowledge the recent accomplishments as these are not concentrated on revolution around one or two crops, or, concentrated in a particular geographic region. Second, high food inflation has overshadowed progress on production front. Proper understanding of the decline and improvement in performance of agriculture since the mid 1990s is very important for shaping the future of Indian agriculture.

This chapter compares the performance of agriculture in the recent years with the preceding decade and provides an update on the achievements of the agriculture sector in recent 10 years or so. It also discusses, with evidence, how and when the turnaround in agriculture took place, for developing proper understanding of India's agriculture growth story.

2. Growth Trend and Composition

The country achieved close to 5 per cent average annual rate of growth in agriculture during 8th Plan (1992-93 to 1996-97) and fixed a target of 4.5 per cent growth for the 9th Plan (1997-2002). Against this target, the actual growth rate turned out to be 2.48 per cent during the 9th as well as 10th Plan. The target growth rate was fixed at 4 per cent for 11th Plan and the same has been kept for the 12th Plan. Unlike the previous two Five Year Plans, the 11th Plan recorded an average growth rate of 4.06 per cent in the agricultural GDP. The growth rate during 2012-13, which is the first year of the 12th Plan has been 1.4 per cent and the advance estimate for 2013-14, which is the second year of 12th Plan, puts the growth rate at 4.6 per cent. The growth rates reveal that after growing at 2.5 per cent for 10 years, during 9th and 10th Plan, agriculture growth in the subsequent period has accelerated to 3.5 per cent level. It is interesting to find out precisely in which year the turnaround in growth rate took place, and how the period after turnaround compares with the corresponding period before turnaround.

According to a study done by Ramesh Chand and Parappurathu (2012) agriculture GDP witnessed a structural break in the year 1995-96, which brought down the growth trajectory, followed by another break in the year 2004-05, which turned the growth path upward. The same can also be seen from the decadal trend growth rates in the agricultural GDP beginning with the decade 1971-72 to 1980-81and ending with the decade 2003-04 to 2012-13 (Figure 1.1). When ten years period is used to estimate trend growth rates two clear breaks are observed, one in 1996-97 and another in 2005-06.

The above evidence clearly points out that the performance of agriculture during the last two decades can be divided in two phases: phase I from 1995-96 to 2005-06 representing a period of slowdown in agriculture, and, phase II beginning with year 2005-06 representing a period of recovery and acceleration in growth. Further, a comparison of growth rates achieved during the decade beginning from 2004-05 is made with the previous two decades. The data on GDP of the sector (agriculture and allied) after 2004-05 is available till year 2012-13 *i.e.* for nine years. The trend growth rates in GDP during recent decade (nine years only) at constant prices and for similar two previous periods is presented in Figure 1.2. This shows that Indian agriculture moved on a growth trajectory of 3.15 per cent per annum during 1988-89 to 1996-97 which plummeted to 1.92 per cent in the next nine years. This was a very low growth having several adverse effects on farm economy and livelihood of farming community and posed a serious threat to the national food security.

Some initiatives were taken towards the end of 10th Plan and during 11th Plan to revive the sector. Consequently, the growth rate accelerated to 3.75 per cent

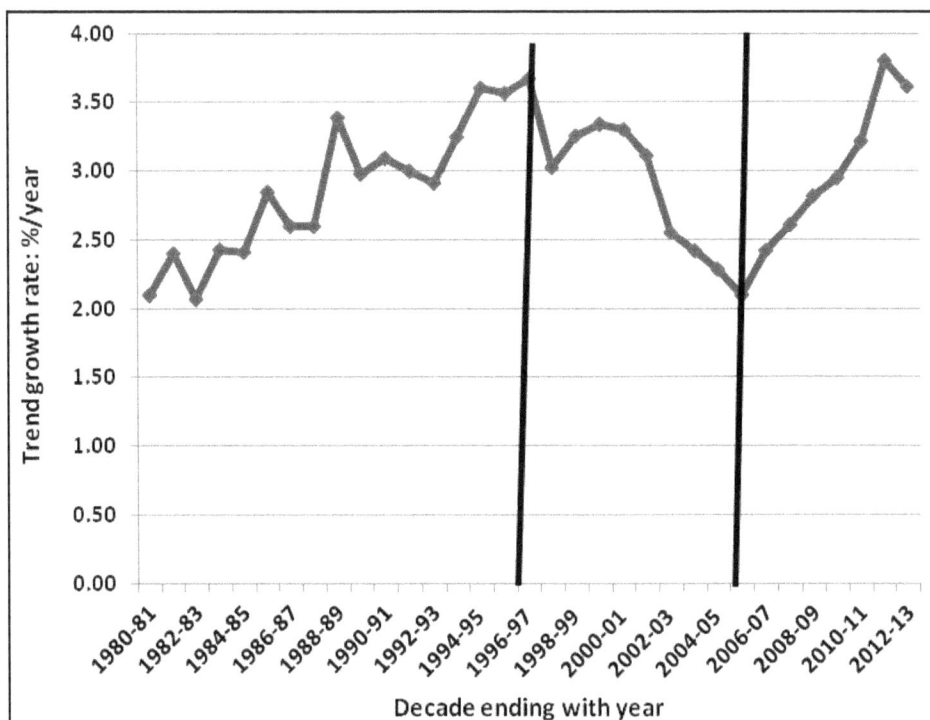

Figure 1.1: Growth Trajectory of GDP Agriculture in Various Decades
from 1971-72/1980-81 to 2003-04/2012/13.

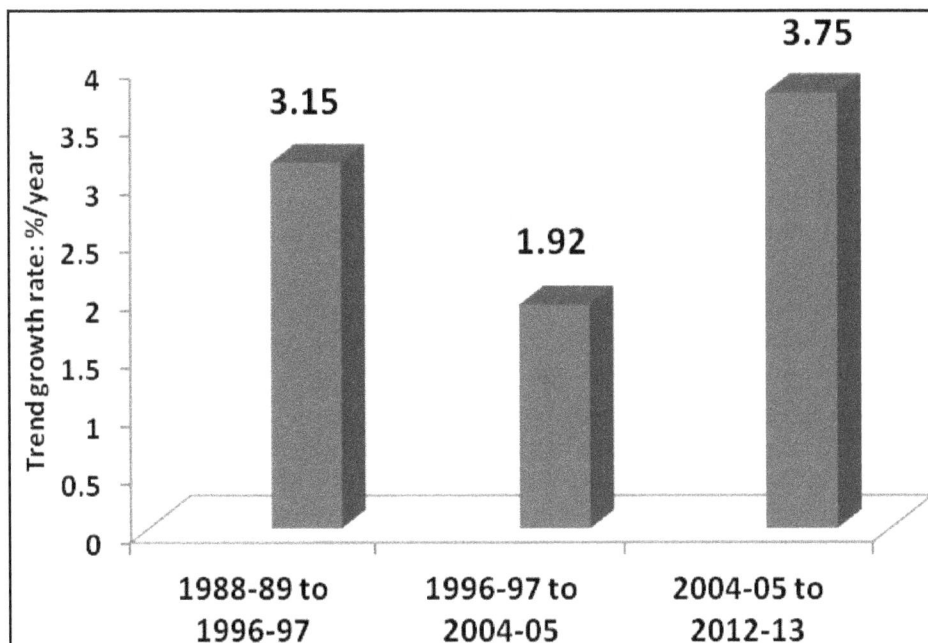

Figure 1.2: Growth Rate in GDP Agriculture and Allied Sector at 2004-05 Prices.

during 2004-05 to 2012-13. It is a matter of pride for the country that agriculture sector moved back on long term growth trajectory and now approaching targeted growth rate of 4 per cent.

2.1 Broad Based Growth

The increase in growth rate of agricultural output was not confined to a few segments or commodity groups or to dominant products. Rather, the growth has been experienced across the board. Within the subsectors, crop sector recorded 3.3 per cent and fruits and vegetables recorded 5.3 per cent annual rate of growth. Livestock output increased at 4.8 per cent per annum while fishery sector recorded 4.5 per cent growth rate. The rate of growth in the recent decade has been historical in most cases. Growth rate of crop sector in recent nine years (2003-04 to 2011-12) has been 75 per cent higher than the previous decade (Table 1.1). The growth rate in livestock and horticulture growth was higher by 41 per cent and fisheries by 48 per cent over the preceding nine years period.

Table 1.1: Trend Growth Rate in Output of Various Sub Sectors of Agriculture: Per cent

Sub-sector	1987-88 to 1995-96	1995-96 to 2003-04	2003-04 to 2011-12
Crop sector	2.97	1.87	3.28
Livestock	4.10	3.43	4.84
Fruits and vegetables	4.29	3.79	5.33
Fishery sector	7.22	3.02	4.48

2.2 Performance of Various Crops

Foodgrain production in India increased from 190 to 206 million tonne (mt) between 1995-97 and 2003-05 registering an increase of 16 mt in 8 years. In the next 8 years foodgrain production increased by more than 50 mt and reached 257 mt by 2011-13. Rice, wheat and maize witnessed a record increase in their production after 2003-05. Maize production in the country was below 10 mt till 1995-96 and crossed level of 21 mt in year 2010-11. Thus, maize production in the country doubled in 15 years.

Pulse production in India stagnated around 13 mt for 15 years from 1990-91 to 2005-06. It showed record growth in year 2010-11 with output climbing up by 25 per cent in one year, from 14.6 mt to 18.2 mt.

Soybean and cotton have shown miraculous growth with doubling of output in about 8 years. India now produces 13.4 mt of soybean and 34.6 million bales of cotton as against the production of 7.3 mt of soybean and 15.1 million bales of cotton in 2003-5. Indian agriculture made another very noteworthy achievement by raising output of sugarcane. Sugarcane production in India reached close to 300 million tonne in year 1999-2000 and faced decline thereafter, cane production recovered in year 2006-07 in a big way. Current level of sugarcane output is 350 mt and India is having large surplus of sugar.

India produced 114 mt of fruits and vegetables in the mid 1990's. In next 8 years production increased to 143 mt. Between 2003-05 and 2011-13 production of fruits and vegetables increased to 235mt. Both vegetable as well fruit production increased by more than 60 per cent in 8 years after 2003-05 which is much higher than the growth in the previous period. These growth rates have taken fruit production to 77 mt and vegetable production to 158 mt during 2011-13.

The increase in production of onion and potato has been remarkable. Onion production increased from 6.18 mt in 2003-5 to 16.9 mt in 2011-13. Production of potato, which increased by less than 2 mt in 8 years before 2003-5 showed an increase of nearly 20 mt in recent 8 years.

Trend growth rates in production of various crops are presented in Table 1.2. The growth rate in many crops was negative during 1994-95 to 2003-04, which has been reversed in the recent decade. In other cases there has been sharp acceleration. It is worth mentioning that cotton production followed double digit growth in last 10 years while soybean, maize and gram experienced more than 5 per cent annual growth. Output of pulses, which was stagnating for quite some time, also moved on a rising trend with growth rate of more than 3 per cent.

Table 1.2: Trend Growth Rate in Physical Output of Selected Crops/Groups: Per cent

Crop/Group	1994-95 to 2003-04	2003-04 to 2012-13
Foodgrains	0.71	2.66
Cereals	0.81	2.61
Pulses	−0.64	3.31
Rice	0.62	1.99
Wheat	1.03	3.60
Maize	4.43	5.51
Gram	−2.37	5.59
Pigeonpea	0.14	2.05
Oilseeds	−1.65	2.47
Soybean	3.35	7.61
Sugarcane	−0.47	4.01
Cotton	−2.23	10.46
Fruits and vegetables	2.64	6.26
Vegetables	3.24	6.37
Fruits	1.53	6.04
Banana	0.92	7.57
Mango	0.96	4.44
Citrus	4.50	5.34
Onion	3.07	12.98
Potato	2.90	8.94

The growth rates in output of horticultural crops during the decade 1994-95 to 2003-04 and 2003-04 to 2012-13 reveal grand success of the horticulture in the second decade. Growth rate in fruits as well as vegetables accelerated from 2.64 per cent during 1994-95 and 2003-04 to 6.26 per cent during 2003-04 to 2012-13. Among vegetables, onion production recorded 13 per cent annual growth while potato production increased by 8.9 per cent per year. Among various fruits, highest growth is observed in banana, 7.57 per cent.

2.3 Performance of Livestock and Fishery Produce

All livestock and fishery products showed higher growth after 2003-04 compared to 1994-95 to 2003-04 (Table 1.3). Milk production growth accelerated after 2003-04, from 3.78 per cent per annum to 4.72 per cent per annum. Growth in production of egg accelerated from 5.69 to 6.2 per cent. After 2003-04, growth rate in marine as well as inland fishery witnessed acceleration. Output of marine fish increased by less than 1 per cent a year during the 10 years period before 2003-04. The growth rate picked up to 2 per cent in the recent decade. Inland fish experienced more than 5.5 per cent annual increase during 1995-96 to 2003-04 which further increased to close to 6 per cent.

Table 1.3: Trend Growth Rate in Production of Livestock and Fish: Per cent/year

Product	1994-95 to 2003-04	2003-04 to 2011-12
Milk	3.78	4.72
Egg	5.69	6.20
Marine fish	0.71	2.01
Inland fish	5.55	5.99
Total fish	3.04	4.30

3. Agricultural Growth at State Level

The growth rate in NSDP agriculture across states varies from (-) 1.15 per cent in Kerala to 5.91 per cent in Chattisgarh (Table 1.4). The states like Madhya Pradesh, Karnataka, Rajasthan, Jharkhand and Chattisgarh achieved more than 5 per cent annual growth rate in agriculture, and Gujarat, Tamil Nadu, Maharashtra and Andhra Pradesh, exceeded the national target of agriculture growth. Haryana, recorded close to 4 per cent annual growth in NSDP agriculture even with high level of productivity. In east India, both Assam and Bihar recorded more than 3 per cent annual growth.

Uttar Pradesh and Odisha are still stuck in low growth trap. The state of Punjab comes at the bottom in the list of states which recorded positive growth in agriculture, with only 1.5 per cent annual growth. In the North West Himalayan region, agriculture growth rate in Jammu and Kashmir and Uttarakhand was around 2 per cent whereas agriculture was stagnant in the state of Himachal Pradesh. In West Bengal, agriculture sector was growing at about 2 per cent per annum. Agriculture sector was found to be shrinking in the state of Kerala.

Table 1.4: Growth Rate in NSDP Agriculture during 2004-05 to 2011-12 at 2004-05 Prices in Major States Per cent

State	Trend Growth Rate	State	Trend Growth Rate
Chhatisgarh	5.91	Haryana	3.94
Jharkhand	5.76	Assam	3.84
Rajasthan	5.63	Bihar	3.32
Karnataka	5.59	Odisha	2.67
Madhya Pradesh	5.22	Uttar Pradesh	2.33
		Jammu and Kashmir	2.04
Andhra Pradesh	4.94	West Bengal	1.98
Maharashtra	4.84	Uttarakhand	1.95
Tamil Nadu	4.21	Punjab	1.49
Gujarat	4.08		
		Himachal Pradesh	**−0.09**
All India	**3.70**	**Kerala**	**−1.15**

4. Initiatives and Factors Underlying the Achievements

Performance of agriculture improved in in the last decade as a result of strong policy and institutional support provided to the sector. The major contributing factors are:

☆ Improvement in terms of trade for agriculture in the last 10 years and remunerative prices for farm produce.

☆ Higher use of productivity enhancing inputs like fertilizer and quality seed.

☆ Expansion of irrigation and increase in agricultural investments supported by public sector capital formation.

☆ Substantial increase in the supply of institutional credit to agriculture.

☆ Achievements in technology and strengthening of extension.

☆ Initiatives like NFSM, RKVY and BGREI and other missions and programmes.

4.1 Better Prices

Terms of trade between agriculture and non-agriculture, represented by ratio of implicit price deflators of agriculture GDP to non-agriculture GDP, followed a decline of 7 per cent between 1997-98 and 2004-05. Thereafter, agricultural prices received by farmers increased at a faster rate under the influence of the substantial hike in the minimum support prices, higher level of foodgrain procurement by government agencies, strong domestic demand and rise in international prices. Between 2004-5 and 2011-12, agricultural prices relative to non-agricultural prices have risen by about 30 percent (Figure 1.3). Thus, better pricing environment provided incentive to farmers to use more and better input and adopt modern technology.

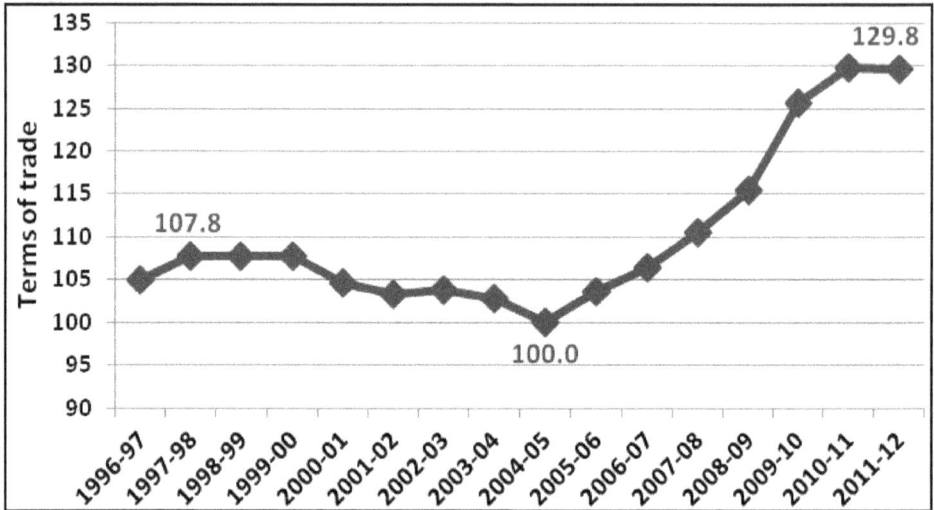

Figure 1.3: Terms of Trade between Agriculture and Non-agriculture.

4.2 Higher Use of Material Inputs

Supply of certified or quality seed in the country increased by about 50 per cent between 1997-98 and 2004-05 (Figure 1.4). In the next 8 years seed supply increased by more than 100 per cent. As seed is the carrier of technology, the growth in supply of quality seed has been a major factor for increase in agriculture production in recent years. Similarly, use of fertilizer which showed a meager increase of 14 per

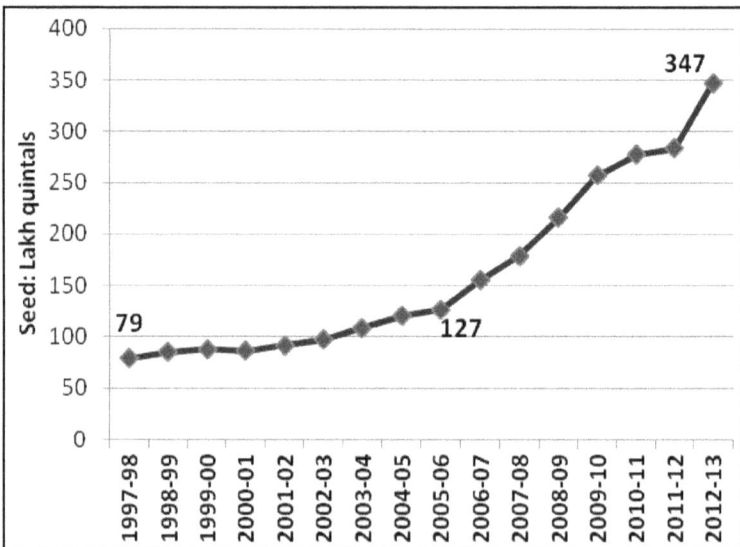

Figure 1.4: Supply of Certified or Quality Seed: Lakh Quintal.

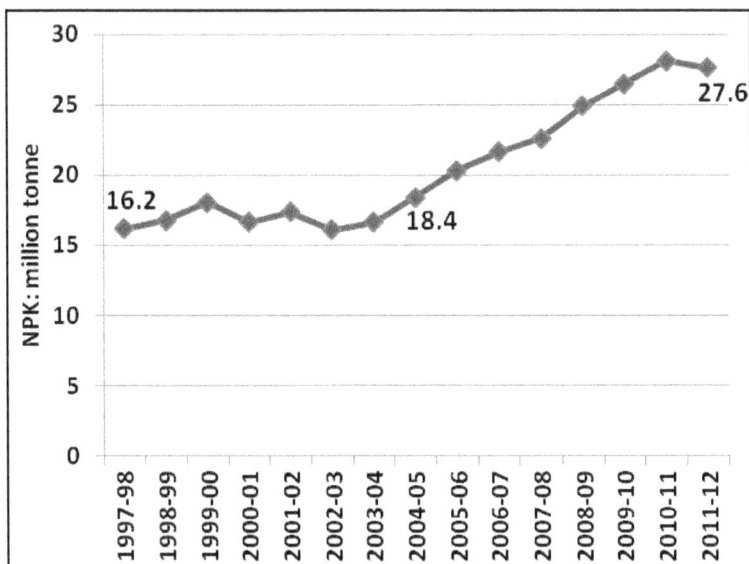

Figure 1.5: Use of Fertilizer in India: NPK: Million Tonne.

cent during 1997-98 to 2004-05 increased by 50 per cent in next 7 years, from 18.4 million tonne (mt) of NPK in 2004-05 to close to 28 mt in year 2011-12 (Figure 1.5).

4.3 Electricity Consumption and Irrigation Expansion

Consumption of electricity for agriculture purposes and expansion of gross irrigated area are closely linked (Figure 1.6). Electricity consumption in agriculture sector was 85.7 thousand GWh in year 1995-96. The consumption increased to 97.2 thousand GWh by the year 1998-99 and sharply declined thereafter. It reached bottom level in year 2001-2 and then started increasing slowly. The consumption of electricity in agriculture picked up in year 2006-07 and the upward trend continued thereafter. The electricity consumption reached 129 thousand GWh in year 2010-11. Between 1998-99 and 2005-06 electricity consumption in agriculture declined by 7 per cent and in next 5 years it increased by as much as 43 per cent.

Expansion in gross irrigated area showed somewhat similar pattern as seen in electricity consumption in agriculture. During the ten years period from 1995-96 and 2004-05 gross irrigated are increased by 10 million hectare from 71.4 million hectare to 81.1 million hectare. The provisional data available for the recent years shows an increase of 8.3 million hectare in the next six years.

5. Recent Scenario

India had unseasonal rains in March and April 2015 after an adverse monsoon in 2014. While the poor monsoon caused a decline in the kharif output, prolonged and heavy unseasonal rains and hail damaged wheat and other rabi crops in many parts of the country when they were ready for harvest. Two consecutive seasons of poor harvest and apprehensions about the Land Acquisition Bill have led to a

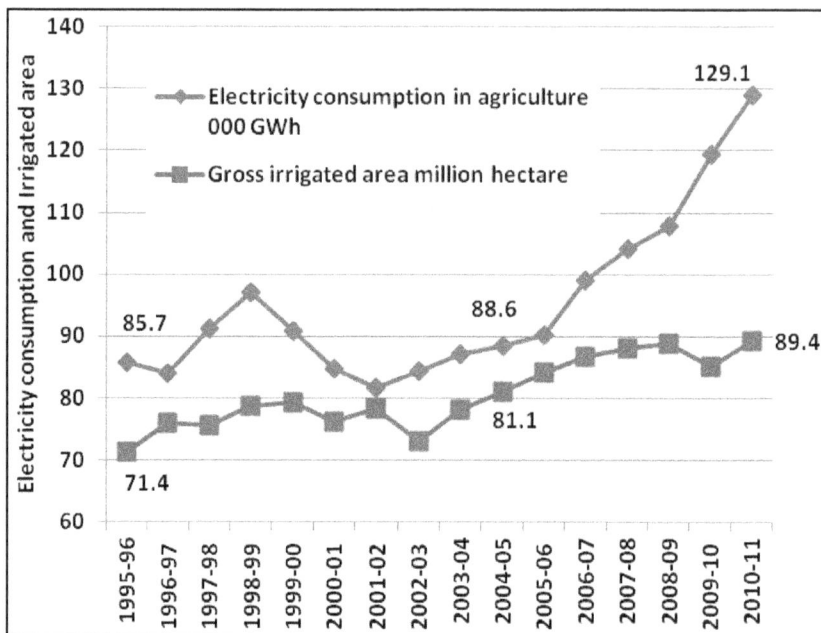

Figure 1.6: Progress in Electricity Consumed in Agriculture and Expansion of Irrigation.

spate of protests by farmers on the neglect of agriculture and the injustice to them. This has again brought the issue of famers' distress to the centre stage, though there have been signs of improvement since the mid-2000s. It is ironical that a country that boasted of record production, a large export surplus and other achievements in agriculture a year ago (2013–14) is suddenly haunted by farmers' distress and suicides attributed to low and stagnant farm income.

The value added in agriculture shows a growth of 1.19 per cent in 2013–14 and 3.8 per cent in 2013–14. As per the advance estimates of GDP for 2014-15 released by the CSO, the gross value added in agriculture and allied sectors was expected to increase by 1.1 per cent in 2014–15. However, the revised estimate show that the growth rate will drop from ealier anticipated level of 1.1 per cent to 0.2 per cent due to crop losses caused by the freak weather in recent months. Thus, the average growth in value added or GDP agriculture during the three years after 2011–12 drops to 1.7 per cent, which is less than half the growth rate achieved from 2004–05 to 2011–12. Excluding 2002–03, this is the lowest growth in GDP agriculture in any three consecutive years since 1991–92. The reasons for this decline are obvious. The use of productivity-enhancing inputs has dropped sharply in the last three years. Between 2011–12 and 2013–14, consumption of NPK declined from 27.7 million tonnes to 24.48 million tonnes and production of breeder seeds and foundation seeds declined from 145,000 tonnes to 99,700 tonnes.

Another important factor for lower use of inputs and resulting fall in growth rate is the change in the real prices of agricultural commodities. The index of wholesale prices shows that even after 2011–12, wholesale agricultural prices increased at a faster rate than non-agricultural prices. However, the CPIAL, which is considered a relevant deflator for farm income, shows a higher increase than the increase in the wholesale price index (WPI) for agricultural commodities and farm gate prices. As producers, farmers get wholesale prices, and as consumers, they pay retail or consumer prices. The WPI for agriculture and farm gate price index deflated by the CPIAL shows a negative growth of around 1 per cent per year from 2011–12 to 2014–15. Thus the value added in agriculture deflated by the CPIAL increased by about 1 per cent a year after 2011–12. Such a low growth in value added in agriculture is a strong factor for the increase in distress among farmers.

6. Conclusions and Lessons

During the last two decades, since mid 1990s, Indian agriculture has moved through two distinct phases. The period from mid 1990s to mid 2000s witnessed slowdown of agriculture growth from above 3.5 per cent to below 2 per cent. This has been followed by a sharp turnaround in year 2005-06 which took agriculture back to above 3.5 per cent growth. The most important factor for improved and impressive performance of agriculture, post 2004-05, has been the increase in the prices received by the farmers. This was a result of hike given to MSP, increase in foodgrain procurement, increase in global agricultural prices and strong domestic demand for food. Favourable prices induced farmers to use better seed, apply higher doses of inputs, take better care of crops and livestock, adopt improved technology and methods of production. This process was further aided by liberal supply of institutional credit, and irrigation expansion. Slowdown of agriculture growth and its recovery in response to changes in price and non price factors clearly establish that Indian farmers respond rather strongly to various types of incentives. It also refutes to some extent the argument that the interest in farming is diminishing. We find the interest depends on profitability from farming.

State level comparison of agriculture growth offers useful lessons. With the same set of national policies and macro environment some states achieved more than 5 per cent growth and some could not grow even at 3 per cent. Low growth states, particularly Uttar Pradesh and Odisha, can learn a lot from the experience of the states like Chhatisgarh, Jharkhand, Rajasthan, Karnataka, Madhya Pradesh, Andhra Pradesh and Maharashtra.

It is a challenge to maintain the growth tempo achieved during 2004-05 to 2013-14. As no country can afford to keep real agricultural prices rising for a very long time, therefore, ways and means have to be devised to sustain profitability incentive. One way to maintain price or profitability incentive for farmers is to increase their share in final prices paid by consumers and other end users. The second source is technology either through resource saving or through increase in productivity. The agricultural development strategy in the last ten years has focused on production and MSPs. For a long time, significant progress has not been made in agricultural markets like reforms in market regulation, development of infrastructure, entry of modern capital, and development of new models of marketing. Thus, agricultural marketing has not moved to the next stage of development (Ramesh Chand, 2012).

Agricultural development strategy should be expanded to bring marketing in its fold to improve competition, reduce efficiency and harness market innovations. This should enable famers to get better prices and higher share in prices paid by end users without adding to inflation. Without this, it will be very difficult to sustain the agricultural achievements of the last decade in the coming years.

References

Ramesh Chand (2012). Development Policies and Agricultural Markets, *Economic and Political Weekly*, Vol. XLVII, No. 52, 53-63, December 29.

Ramesh Chand and Shinoj Parapppurathu (2012). Temporal and Spatial Variations in Agricultural Growth and its Determinants. *Economic and Political Weekly*, Vol. XLVII No. 26 and 27: 55-64. June, 30.

Chapter 2

Total Factor Productivity using Data Envelopment Analysis: A Case Study of District Level Analysis in Bihar Agriculture

Rajni Jain[1] and Ashok Mittal[2]

[1]*Principal Scientist, ICAR-NIAP, New Delhi-110 012*
[2]*Retired Principal Scientist, ICAR-IASRI, New Delhi-110 012*

ABSTRACT

Agriculture sector in Bihar contributes about 16 per cent to SGDP and provides employment to about 70 per cent of rural working force. Recognizing this critical role of agricultural sector in the economy of Bihar, attempt has been made to examine the status of total factor productivity (TFP) growth at district level for the period 2001-2009 based on Malmquist Index estimated using Data Envelopment Analysis approach. TFP growth was decomposed into efficiency and technological growth. Study shows that TFP change was positive in 23 districts out of total 37 districts in Bihar. One district showed no change. Average total factor productivity increased at the rate of 3.06 per cent in Bihar during this period 2001-2009. Technical efficiency was positive in 26 districts and no change was observed in four districts. Average technical efficiency in Bihar increased at the rate of 2.24 per cent. Technological change was positive in 20 districts and no change was observed in one district. Average technological change has increased at the rate of 0.63 per cent. Thus, the contribution of technical efficiency change was more in the growth of TFP while the change due to technological adoption was quite slow in most of the districts. Out of 37 districts, the TFP was negative in 14 districts and the reason was low growth in both use of input mix efficiency as well as technology adoption in agriculture. Based on TFP values, districts were classified into three categories namely 'above average', 'average' and 'below average'. Analysis revealed that application of inputs like irrigation, fertilizer and credit were significantly different between the 'above average' and 'below average' categories. The study concludes that TFP can be improved in the districts of Bihar by improving availability of irrigation, fertilizer and credit.

Keywords: Malmquist index, TFP, Data envelopment analysis, District level TFP, Bihar agriculture.

Introduction

Agriculture is an important sector in Bihar since it contributes about 16 per cent to State Gross Domestic Product and provides employment to about 70 per cent of working force in rural area. More than 90 per cent of farm households belong to marginal farm category (less than 1 ha land) but own about 44 per cent of cultivated land in Bihar. During the period 2004-11, the state AgGDP grew at the annual growth rate of 2.7 per cent. Bihar ranks sixth among major states of India with respect to per hectare State Net Agricultural Domestic Product (SNAgGDP) but at the lowest ladder with respect to per capita SNAgGDP. The population density of the state stands at 1102 persons per sq km, which is the highest in the country, as against an All-India population density of 382 per sq km. Characterized by low and stagnant economic growth, the state has high levels of poverty and the lowest levels of per capita income among major states in the country. Recognizing this critical role of agricultural sector in the overall growth as well as development performance of Bihar, it is imperative to estimate the status of total factor productivity (TFP) growth in the state. An attempt has been made to estimate the TFP using Malmquist Index for different districts of Bihar.

The basic objective of this paper is to estimate total factor productivity growth in agriculture for districts of Bihar and to decompose TFP growth into technical change, technical efficiency change and scale efficiency change for understanding the source of productivity for Bihar agriculture sector. From agriculture sector perspective, this study could help decision makers to assess the district wise agriculture performance and facilitate policy formulations to increase the productivity and efficiency.

Review of Literature

A number of studies are available in the literature using different methods along Malmquist index at country level. Fulginiti and Perrin (1998) used a parametric meta-production function and a non-parametric Malmquist index to examine the performance of the agricultural sectors in 18 less developed countries. They found that productivity has regressed in many of them. Trueblood (1996) used non-parametric Malmquist index and also estimated Cobb-Douglas production function for 117 countries and he found that there was a negative productivity growth in a significant number of developing countries. Arnade (1998) estimated agricultural productivity indices using non-parametric Malmquist index approach for 70 countries during the years 1961-1993. The study revealed that thirty six out of forty seven developing countries had negative rates of technical change. Nin *et al.*

(2003) estimated TFP growth for 20 countries for the period 1961-1994 using non-parametric Malmquist TFP index and found that most of the developing countries experienced productivity growth. Coelli *et al.* (2003) estimated TFP for Bangladesh crop agriculture sector for the period 1961-1992 using stochastic frontier approach and found a decline in TFP over the period while Rahman (2004) applies sequential Malmquist index approach to same dataset and finds TFP rising at the annual rate of 0.9 per cent and this growth is primarily led by those regions where high levels of green revolution technology was experienced.

In Indian context, a number of studies for agriculture sector and crop-specific on measurement of TFP have been carried out at national as well as state level. Rosegrant and Evenson (1992) use Tornqvist-Theil index to estimate TFP change for Indian crop sector. They find rate of growth of TFP to be one per cent for the entire period 1957-1985, 0.81 per cent for the period 1957-1965, 1.22 per cent during 1965-1975 and 0.98 per cent during 1975-1985. Kumar and Rosegrant (1994) estimated TFP growth for rice crop in different states classifying in four regions and they found that the TFP index increased by about 1.85 per cent p.a. in southern region, 0.76 per cent in the northern region and 0.36 per cent in the eastern region while in the western region TFP growth was found to be negative but insignificant. Bhushan (2005) uses DEA to estimate Malmquist TFP index for major wheat producing states in India, he found that TFP growth rate was highest in Punjab and Haryana which is attributed to technical progress in these two states. Rajasthan (with no efficiency change) and Uttar Pradesh (with improvement in efficiency and negative growth in technological progress) had positive TFP growth rate while Madhya Pradesh (with no change in efficiency and negative growth of technical progress) reported to record negative TFP growth rate. As compared to 1980s, mean growth of TFP is found to be higher in 1990s and the primary source of TFP growth is technical progress and not efficiency improvements. Shilpa Chaudhary (2012) estimates total factor productivity (TFP) in Indian agriculture at state-level. Using Index of Agricultural Production as the measure of output, changes in TFP are estimated using non-parametric Sequential Malmquist TFP index. The TFP change is decomposed into efficiency change and technical change. It is found that productivity improvements are marked in very few states, and so is technical change. The improvements in efficiency are observed to be low for most of the states and efficiency decline is observed in several states implying huge gains in production possible even with existing technology. Despite the importance and need for improving TFP in Bihar, no disaggregated level study is observed for Bihar. The present study aims to fill the gap by analysing district level data for the period 2000-2009.

Data and Methodology

The data was collected from various authentic government websites including Department of Economics and Statistics (www.dacnet.nic.in) for the period 2000 to 2009. Regarding the production data, output of four major crop groups *viz.*, cereals, pulses, oilseeds and sugarcane produced in each district of Bihar was considered. The input variables include net sown area, gross irrigated area, agricultural workers (cultivators plus agricultural labour), fertilizer consumption (NPK) and annual rainfall. Data regarding fertilizer consumption in terms of N, P and K was computed from different fertilizers consumed in each district. In this study annual production and input consumption data pertaining to 37 major districts of Bihar was analysed. Data pertaining to districts Arwal and Jehanabad was merged because Arwal was part of Jehanabad district prior to August 2001.

Malmquist TFP Index

The Malmquist Total Factor Productivity Index (MTFPI) was first introduced by Caves, Christensen and Diewert (1982). They defined the TFP index using Malmquist input and output distance functions, and thus the resulting index came to be known as MTFPI. Malmquist productivity index for a period t is given by

$$M^t = \frac{d_0^t(x^{t+1}, y^{t+1})}{d_0^t(x^t, y^t)}$$

(1)

i.e., they define the productivity index as the ratio of two output distance functions taking technology at time t as the reference technology. Instead of using period t's technology as the reference technology it is possible to construct output distance functions based on period $(t+1)$'s technology and thus another Malmquist productivity index can be laid down as:

$$M^{t+1} = \frac{d_0^{t+1}(x^{t+1}, y^{t+1})}{d_0^{t+1}(x^t, y^t)}$$

(2)

Fare *et al.* (1994) attempt to remove the arbitrariness in the choice of benchmark technology by specifying their Malmquist productivity change index as the geometric mean of the two-period indices, that is

$$M_0 = \left(x^{t+1}, y^{t+1}, x^t, y^t\right) = \left[\left(\frac{d_0^t(x^{t+1}, y^{t+1})}{d_0^t(x^t, y^t)}\right)\left(\frac{d_0^{t+1}(x^{t+1}, y^{t+1})}{d_0^{t+1}(x^t, y^t)}\right)\right]^{\frac{1}{2}}$$

(3)

Using simple arithmetic manipulation, the equation (3) can be written as the product of two distinct components- technical change and efficiency change (Fare *et al.* (1994)).

$$M_0 = \left(x^{t+1}, y^{t+1}, x^t, y^t\right) = \frac{d_0^{t+1}(x^{t+1}, y^{t+1})}{d_0^t(x^t, y^t)}\left[\left(\frac{d_0^t(x^{t+1}, y^{t+1})}{d_0^{t+1}(x^{t+1}, y^{t+1})}\right)\left(\frac{d_0^t(x^t, y^t)}{d_0^{t+1}(x^t, y^t)}\right)\right]^{\frac{1}{2}}$$

(4)

where the ratio outside the bracket in equation (4) measures technical efficiency change between period t and $t+1$ and other part measures the technical change which is geometric mean of the shift in technology between two periods evaluated at x^{t+1} and x^t.

The Malmquist productivity index is simply the product of the change in relative efficiency that occurred between periods t and $t+1$, and the change in technology that occurred between periods t and $t+1$. A value of Malmquist TFP index equal to one implies there has been no change in total factor productivity across the two time periods, greater than one implies a rise/improvement in TFP and a value less than one is interpreted as a regress in TFP. A similar interpretation applies to the two components as well.

We can decompose the total factor productivity growth in following way as well.

$$\text{Technical Efficiency Change} = \frac{d_0^{t+1}(x^{t+1}, y^{t+1})}{d_0^t(x^t, y^t)} \quad \text{(Catching up effect)} \tag{5}$$

$$\text{Technical change} = \left[\left(\frac{d_0^t(x^{t+1}, y^{t+1})}{d_0^{t+1}(x^{t+1}, y^{t+1})} \right) \left(\frac{d_0^{t+1}(x^t, y^t)}{d_0^{t+1}(x^t, y^t)} \right) \right] \quad \text{(Frontier Effect)} \tag{6}$$

MTFPI is the product of measure of efficiency change (catching up effect) at current period t+1 and previous period t (average geometrically) and a technical change (frontier effect) as measured by shift in a frontier over the same period. The catching up effect measures that a district is how much close to the frontier by capturing extent of diffusion of technology or knowledge of technology use. On the other side frontier effect measures the movement of frontier between two periods with regards to rate of technology adoption.

Measuring productivity change is an important exercise. Decomposing measured productivity change into its sources is an equally important exercise, since the enhancement of productivity growth requires knowledge of the relative importance of its sources. In this regard the Malmquist productivity index is particularly enlightening, since it decomposes naturally into a technical efficiency change index and a technical change index. Building on this elementary decomposition, Fare *et al.* (1994) obtained a further decomposition of the technical efficiency change index into a "pure" technical efficiency change index, a scale efficiency change index, and a congestion change index.

Further all districts were divided into three categories on the basis of TFP change *viz.*, districts having TFP above average, average and below average. The districts of average TFP were defined as mean TFP±0.25. To examine the determinants of TFP change the data of variables like, agricultural productivity, cropping intensity, labour productivity, proportionate irrigated area, fertilizer consumption, agricultural credit by commercial banks and literacy rate in districts were considered. Two tailed, two sample t-test for inequality of sample sizes was applied to test the difference of means for all three categories separately.

Results and Discussions

The TFP Index technique is used to construct a production frontier using the input output data from 37 districts of Bihar. Technical efficiency means that how much closer a district to the production frontier while technical change means that how much this frontier shift at each district observed input mix.

Table 2.1: District-wise Mean Malmquist Index and its Components
Over Years (2001-2009)

Sl.No.	District	Technical Efficiency Change	Technical Change	Pure Tech. Efficiency Change	Scale Efficiency Change	TFP Change
1.	Muzaffarpur	0.9686	1.0158	0.9703	1.0067	0.9852
2.	Darbhanga	1.0009	0.9844	0.9923	1.0154	0.9821
3.	Saharsa	1.0088	0.9753	1.0014	1.0070	0.9964
4.	Purnea	0.9793	0.9662	0.9782	1.0027	0.9488
5.	Saran	0.9942	1.0006	0.9924	1.0004	1.0019
6.	Patna	1.0203	1.0266	1.0158	1.0003	1.0117
7.	Mungair	1.0327	0.9453	1.0000	1.0327	0.9972
8.	Bhagalpur	1.0104	1.0058	1.0093	1.0007	1.0116
9.	Gaya	1.1141	1.0318	1.1844	1.0576	1.1180
10.	Nalanda	1.0322	0.9966	1.0427	1.0086	1.0394
11.	Nawada	1.1306	0.9743	1.1199	1.0610	1.1120
12.	Aurangabad	1.0041	1.0253	1.0001	1.0038	1.0401
13.	Bhojpur	1.0557	1.0340	1.0488	1.0006	1.0937
14.	Rohtas	1.0000	1.0239	1.0000	1.0000	1.0239
15.	Siwan	1.0163	0.9851	1.0146	1.0004	0.9844
16.	Gopalganj	1.0000	1.0202	1.0000	1.0000	1.0202
17.	Champaran (East)	0.9484	1.0149	0.9691	0.9959	0.9962
18.	Champaran (West)	1.0000	1.0878	1.0000	1.0000	1.0878
19.	Vaishali	1.0284	1.0226	1.0256	1.0041	1.0062
20.	Sitamarhi	1.0262	1.0392	1.0060	1.0080	1.0428
21.	Madhubani	1.0463	0.9806	1.0462	1.0038	1.0296
22.	Samastipur	1.0196	1.0249	1.0186	1.0012	1.0492
23.	Begusarai	1.0214	1.0630	1.0210	1.0000	1.0692
24.	Katihar	1.0181	0.9696	1.0152	1.0053	0.9832
25.	Jehanabad	1.0790	1.0000	1.1044	0.9994	1.0939
26.	Madhepura	0.9854	0.9211	0.9854	0.9993	0.9028
27.	Khagaria	1.0176	1.0136	1.0146	1.0028	1.0409
28.	Aarreya	1.0057	1.0057	1.0050	1.0008	1.0113
29.	Kishanganj	1.0000	0.9898	1.0000	1.0000	0.9898
30.	Buxar	0.9959	0.9768	1.0000	0.9959	0.9713
31.	Bhabhua	0.9904	0.9464	1.0000	0.9904	0.9370
32.	Banka	1.0897	1.0279	1.0852	1.0033	1.1144
33.	Jamui	1.0976	1.1000	1.0250	1.0679	1.2477
34.	Supaul	1.0007	0.9997	1.0006	1.0000	1.0043
35.	Lakhisarai	1.0104	0.9892	1.0002	1.0090	0.9990
36.	Sheikhpura	1.0506	1.0853	1.0000	1.0506	1.2058
37.	Sheohar	1.0292	0.9649	1.0000	1.0292	0.9759
	Mean	**1.0224**	**1.0063**	**1.0187**	**1.0099**	**1.0304**

Productivity Growth in District of Bihar

The agriculture sector in the state experienced an overall TFP growth of 3 per cent during the period 2001-2009 (Table 2.1). The analysis shows that 23 districts out of 37 districts of Bihar had positive TFP growth. Among these 23 districts, almost all districts had positive TFP due to improvement in technical efficiency as well as Technical change. This means that in these districts improvement is due to their productivity based catching up capability. In Saran district the TFP was found more than 1 due to the improvement in technical change while in Nalanda, Nawada, Madhubani and Supaul districts TFP change was more than 1 due to improvement in technical efficiency.

The combined effect of both pure technical efficiency change and scale efficiency change contributes to technical efficiency change. Technical efficiency change less than one indicates that the districts are operating far away from the production frontier. Thus from the policy point of view these districts need to make judicious and efficient use of inputs. On the other hand technical change is less than one indicates that the production frontier shift at each district observed improper input mix. The results show that the efficiency of farmers regarding input mix is getting better while the improvement in technological adoption is quite slow in most of the districts (Figure 2.1).

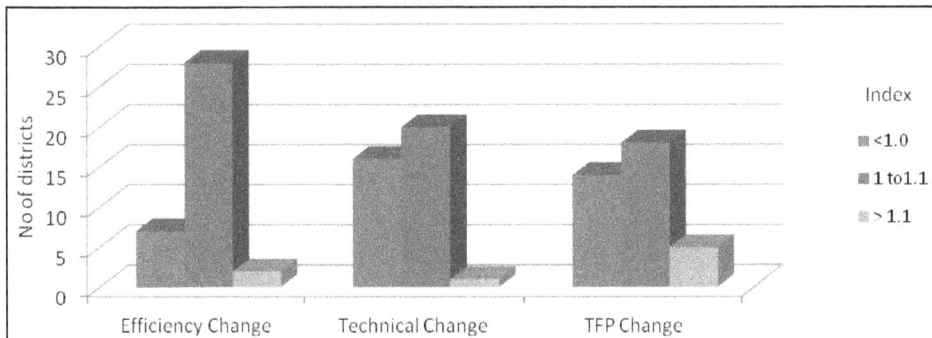

**Figure 2.1: Efficiency, Technical and TFP Changes in Districts
of Bihar during Years 2001-2009.**

Total Factor Productivity (TFP)

The comparative results of total factor productivity change for all districts of Bihar in each year during the period 2001-2009 provides performance of each district over the years (Table 2.2).

During the nine years period, TFP growth was positive during six years in seven districts (Gaya, Bhojpur, Gopalganj, Vaishali, Samastipur,Begusarai and Banka), five years in eleven districts (Muzaffarpur, Saran, Bhagalpur, Nawada, Rohtas, East and West Chmparan, Madhubani, Jehanabad, Lekhisarai and Seohar), four year in twelve districts (Darbhanga, Patna, Nalanda, Aurangabad, Sitamarhi, Katihar, Khagaria, Aarreya, Buxar, Jamui, Supaul and Sheikhpura) three years in five districts (Saharsa, Mungair, Siwan, Madhepura and Kishanganj) and two

Table 2.2: Total Factor Productivity of all Districts of Bihar during 2001 to 2009

Sl.No.	District	2001	2002	2003	2004	2005	2006	2007	2008	2009	Mean
1.	Muzaffarpur	1.0040	0.9710	1.0110	0.7840	1.1310	1.0510	0.7990	1.2470	0.8690	0.9852
2.	Darbhanga	0.6640	1.2410	0.9590	0.8550	1.0230	1.1960	0.9300	1.0140	0.9570	0.9821
3.	Saharsa	0.8230	1.1390	0.9600	0.9420	0.6760	1.6160	0.9020	1.1740	0.7360	0.9964
4.	Purnea	0.6940	1.4580	0.9160	0.9150	0.8850	1.3350	0.7540	0.7410	0.8410	0.9488
5.	Saran	0.8730	0.9540	1.2150	0.8560	1.0130	1.0250	1.4180	0.6400	1.0230	1.0019
6.	Patna	0.7780	1.1250	0.9830	0.9170	1.0350	0.7520	0.7610	1.6820	1.0720	1.0117
7.	Mungair	0.8750	0.7980	1.6490	0.8820	0.8770	1.5000	0.4050	1.1570	0.8320	0.9972
8.	Bhagalpur	0.9700	0.7810	1.2090	0.7910	1.3140	1.2030	0.6720	1.0710	1.0930	1.0116
9.	Gaya	1.1380	1.0750	0.8390	0.6290	1.1960	1.0410	1.7240	0.9380	1.4820	1.1180
10.	Nalanda	0.9780	0.8650	0.9920	0.6000	1.0680	1.8350	0.7830	1.1980	1.0360	1.0394
11.	Nawada	1.3120	1.0210	1.0180	0.5340	0.9320	2.1990	0.7990	1.3070	0.8860	1.1120
12.	Aurangabad	1.1750	0.7250	1.3810	0.8990	0.8740	1.5830	0.6760	0.8970	1.1510	1.0401
13.	Bhojpur	1.0110	0.8570	1.0280	0.5570	2.0150	0.9090	1.1020	1.2820	1.0820	1.0937
14.	Rohtas	1.0290	0.9890	1.0920	1.0760	0.8940	0.9930	0.8030	1.2660	1.0730	1.0239
15.	Siwan	0.9170	0.9350	1.1300	0.8770	0.8690	1.2690	0.7850	1.0830	0.9950	0.9844
16.	Gopalganj	1.3060	0.7700	1.1400	0.7980	1.1590	1.1910	0.6170	1.0390	1.1620	1.0202
17.	Champaran (East)	1.0310	1.0210	1.0130	0.7570	0.9870	1.1100	0.6830	0.9600	0.4040	0.9962
18.	Champaran (West)	1.2850	0.8920	0.9910	0.9050	1.2170	1.4310	0.6000	1.3550	1.1140	1.0878
19.	Vaishali	0.7520	1.1280	0.5960	1.2280	1.0390	1.0610	0.9220	1.2180	1.1120	1.0062
20.	Sitamarhi	1.9170	0.4850	0.9890	0.6930	0.9240	1.3130	1.1140	0.8600	1.0900	1.0428
21.	Madhubani	0.7710	1.0060	1.4590	0.5770	0.8780	1.4250	0.6410	1.4080	1.1010	1.0296
22.	Samastipur	1.0900	0.7370	0.7300	1.1490	1.3740	1.1380	0.8040	1.2340	1.1870	1.0492
23.	Begusarai	0.7780	1.3420	0.7610	1.1200	1.1650	1.0320	0.8110	1.4060	1.2080	1.0692

Contd...

Table 2.2–Contd...

Sl.No.	District	2001	2002	2003	2004	2005	2006	2007	2008	2009	Mean
24.	Katihar	1.0070	0.8390	1.0960	0.8980	1.0400	1.2020	0.9510	0.8620	0.9540	0.9832
25.	Jehanabad	1.2560	1.0920	0.9220	0.8360	0.9410	1.6950	0.2900	1.2490	1.5640	1.0939
26.	Madhepura	0.8760	0.7760	1.0710	1.0570	1.0590	0.9280	0.9860	0.6880	0.6840	0.9028
27.	Khagaria	1.2820	0.6910	1.3790	0.8190	0.9280	1.4710	1.1100	0.8180	0.8700	1.0409
28.	Aarreya	0.9160	1.0150	1.0560	0.9560	1.4410	0.9000	1.1020	0.7180	0.9980	1.0113
29.	Kishanganj	0.9080	0.7810	1.4690	0.9630	0.8070	0.9750	1.3310	0.6110	1.0630	0.9898
30.	Buxar	1.1180	0.8670	1.1150	0.6980	1.0810	0.8980	1.2040	0.8790	0.8820	0.9713
31.	Bhabhua	0.9450	0.9810	0.9460	0.6920	1.1610	1.0430	0.9010	0.8690	0.8950	0.9370
32.	Banka	1.1490	1.1900	1.6780	0.5080	1.8300	0.8360	0.5580	1.0460	1.2350	1.1144
33.	Jamui	0.8890	0.4150	1.7360	0.5780	0.8450	2.9220	1.5280	1.6190	0.6970	1.2477
34.	Supaul	0.8620	0.8930	1.4180	1.2980	0.7990	1.7640	0.3650	0.4860	1.1540	1.0043
35.	Lakhisarai	1.0670	1.0950	0.8460	0.5590	1.7120	1.3080	0.5190	1.0700	0.8150	0.9990
36.	Sheikhpura	0.7690	3.0470	0.3700	1.1390	1.3520	1.5110	0.5140	1.3190	0.8310	1.2058
37.	Sheohar	1.0390	0.8380	1.7200	0.5650	1.1450	0.5120	1.0670	0.8970	1.0000	0.9759
	Mean	**0.9840**	**0.9430**	**1.0610**	**0.8100**	**1.0690**	**1.2130**	**0.8060**	**1.0450**	**0.9800**	**0.9901**

years in two districts (Purnea and Bhabhua). Looking during individual years, 2006 was found to be the most favourable for TFP growth, as maximum 28 (76 per cent districts) out of 37 districts showed positive TFP growth and it was followed by year 2008 (62 per cent districts), 2003 and 2005 (59 per cent districts), 2009 (54 per cent districts), 2001(49 per cent districts), 2002 (38 per cent districts) 2007 (27 per cent districts) and the worst year was 2004 (19 per cent districts).

Resource Use Efficiency

Technical efficiency shows the extent of efficient use of existing inputs to produce more. Technical efficiency is an important contributor to TFP. It is observed that 26 districts have used the available inputs efficiently during the period 2001-2009 as the technical efficiency growth was positive ranging from 0.067 per cent in Supaul to 13.056 per cent in Nawada district (Table 2.3).

In districts Rohtas, Gopalganj, Champaran(W) and Kishanganj the technical efficiency was consistently without any change during the entire study period (2001-2009). The districts with negative technical efficiency growth like Buxar, Saran, Bhabhua, Madhepura, Purnea, Muzaffarpur and Champaran (East) were not up to the mark in use of inputs. It was also observed that the average technical efficiency in overall Bihar districts has maximum increase of 4.7 per cent during the year 2009 followed by 3.8 per cent in 2008, 2.2 per cent in 2006, 1.8 per cent in 2002 and 0.20 per cent in 2005 while it was negative during 2001, 2003, 2004 and 2007.

Technological Adoption

Technological Change is the second important source of TPF change. Technological change refers to adoption of new technology to improve or shift the production frontier upward. Out of 37 districts, 21 districts have the positive growth while 16 have the negative growth in technological change (Table 2.4).

The maximum growth in technological change was observed in the Jamui district (10 per cent) and minimum in Saran district (0.056 per cent) while Jehanabad district showed no change in the growth of technological change. The maximum growth in technological change was observed as 18.7 per cent in the year 2006 followed by 6.80 per cent in year 2003, 6.7 per cent in 2005, 0.60 per cent in 2008 and 0.10 per cent in 2001. The ranking of districts is presented in Table 2.5.

TFP is the multiplicative effect of efficiency change (resource efficiency) and the technological Change (technology adoption). It can be observed from the table that out of 37 districts TFP growth was positive in 23 districts ranging from 0.2 per cent in Saran to 24.7 per cent in Jamui district while in Lakhisarai it was almost zero percent. The growth in TFP component-efficiency change was positive in 26 districts ranging from 0.07 per cent in Supaul to 13.06 per cent in Nawada, while no change was observed in Rohtas, Gopalganj, Champaran (West) and Kishanganj districts. The growth in TFP component -technological change was positive in 20 districts ranging from 0.06 per cent in Saran to 10.00 per cent in Jamui with no change in Jahanabad district.

Table 2.3: Technical Efficiency Change in all Districts of Bihar during 2001-2009

Sl.No.	District	2001	2002	2003	2004	2005	2006	2007	2008	2009	Mean
1.	Muzaffarpur	1.0600	0.9040	1.0800	0.9080	1.0050	0.9030	0.8580	1.0900	0.9090	0.9686
2.	Darbhanga	0.7110	1.1810	1.0140	0.9780	0.9520	1.0040	0.8780	1.0750	1.2150	1.0009
3.	Saharsa	0.9270	1.0790	0.9320	1.0730	0.7670	1.2700	0.9510	1.0800	1.0000	1.0088
4.	Purnea	0.8080	1.2900	0.9830	0.8060	0.8160	1.2700	1.0920	0.7900	0.9590	0.9793
5.	Saran	0.9460	0.9650	1.0960	1.0000	1.0000	0.9320	1.0730	0.8430	1.0930	0.9942
6.	Patna	1.0000	1.0000	1.0000	1.0000	1.0000	0.6550	1.5280	1.0000	1.0000	1.0203
7.	Mungair	0.9250	0.8970	1.3880	1.1720	0.8770	1.1180	0.5910	1.3230	1.0030	1.0327
8.	Bhagalpur	1.0000	0.7460	1.3410	0.9670	1.0340	1.0000	1.0000	0.9260	1.0800	1.0104
9.	Gaya	1.1330	1.1340	0.8090	0.6500	1.1110	0.8320	2.0010	0.7810	1.5760	1.1141
10.	Nalanda	0.9810	0.8720	0.9600	0.8090	1.0800	1.5880	0.9950	0.8930	1.1120	1.0322
11.	Nawada	1.5340	1.0710	0.9030	0.6460	0.9810	1.9470	0.7540	1.3710	0.9680	1.1306
12.	Aurangabad	1.0000	0.8930	1.1200	1.0000	0.8530	1.1540	1.0170	1.0000	1.0000	1.0041
13.	Bhojpur	1.0150	0.8680	0.9500	0.6780	1.9420	0.8050	1.2430	1.0000	1.0000	1.0557
14.	Rohtas	1.0000	1.0000	1.0000	1.0000	1.0000	1.0000	1.0000	1.0000	1.0000	1.0000
15.	Siwan	0.8700	1.1400	0.9790	1.0290	0.9320	1.0730	0.6980	1.4110	1.0150	1.0163
16.	Gopalganj	1.0000	1.0000	1.0000	1.0000	1.0000	1.0000	1.0000	1.0000	1.0000	1.0000
17.	Champaran (East)	1.0660	1.0300	0.9900	0.9190	0.9840	0.9220	0.7460	1.3320	0.5470	0.9484
18.	Champaran (West)	1.0000	1.0000	1.0000	1.0000	1.0000	1.0000	1.0000	1.0000	1.0000	1.0000
19.	Vaishali	0.6860	1.3830	0.5870	1.4630	1.0000	0.9000	0.6970	1.0630	1.4770	1.0284
20.	Sitamarhi	1.1390	1.0000	0.9240	0.8420	0.8770	1.0500	1.0790	0.6610	1.6640	1.0262
21.	Madhubani	0.7640	0.9710	1.2750	0.9610	0.9110	1.1960	0.6950	1.6440	1.0000	1.0463
22.	Samastipur	1.0730	0.9600	0.7120	1.2060	1.2130	0.9930	0.9000	1.1190	1.0000	1.0196
23.	Begusarai	1.0000	1.0000	1.0000	1.0000	1.0000	0.9700	0.6590	1.5640	1.0000	1.0214

Contd...

Table 2.3–Contd...

Sl.No.	District	2001	2002	2003	2004	2005	2006	2007	2008	2009	Mean
24.	Katihar	1.0450	1.0610	0.9070	1.0520	0.9990	1.0540	1.0570	0.9390	1.0490	1.0181
25.	Jehanabad	1.2140	1.1640	0.8500	1.1280	0.8310	1.2090	0.5560	0.9870	1.7720	1.0790
26.	Madhepura	1.0000	1.0000	1.0000	1.0000	1.0000	0.8230	1.2150	1.0000	0.8310	0.9854
27.	Khagaria	1.1450	0.9020	1.1090	1.0000	0.9510	1.0510	1.0000	1.0000	1.0000	1.0176
28.	Aarreya	0.9920	1.1090	0.8870	1.0110	1.1150	0.8900	1.1240	0.9880	0.9350	1.0057
29.	Kishanganj	1.0000	1.0000	1.0000	1.0000	1.0000	1.0000	1.0000	1.0000	1.0000	1.0000
30.	Buxar	1.0000	1.0000	1.0000	0.9640	1.0370	0.8090	1.2350	1.0000	0.9180	0.9959
31.	Bhabhua	1.0000	1.0000	1.0000	1.0000	1.0000	1.0000	1.0000	1.0000	0.9140	0.9904
32.	Banka	0.9000	1.6530	1.0000	0.7120	1.4040	1.0000	0.6220	1.3250	1.1910	1.0897
33.	Jamui	1.0000	0.5330	1.7680	0.7380	0.6600	2.1790	1.0000	1.0000	1.0000	1.0976
34.	Supaul	0.9420	0.9690	1.0950	1.0000	1.0000	1.0000	1.0000	1.0000	1.0000	1.0007
35.	Lakhisarai	1.0000	1.0000	1.0000	0.7670	1.3040	0.8590	1.1640	1.0000	1.0000	1.0104
36.	Sheikhpura	0.8470	1.5210	0.7370	1.3260	1.0240	1.0000	1.0000	1.0000	1.0000	1.0506
37.	Sheohar	1.0000	1.0000	1.0000	1.0000	1.0000	0.5770	1.4770	0.8880	1.3210	1.0292
	Mean	0.9830	1.0180	0.9940	0.9530	1.0020	1.0220	0.9630	1.0380	1.0470	1.0022

Table 2.4: Technological Change in all Districts of Bihar during 2001-2009

Sl.No.	District	2001	2002	2003	2004	2005	2006	2007	2008	2009	Mean
1.	Muzaffarpur	0.9470	1.0740	0.9360	0.8640	1.1260	1.1640	0.9310	1.1440	0.9560	1.0158
2.	Darbhanga	0.9330	1.0510	0.9460	0.8740	1.0750	1.1910	1.0580	0.9440	0.7880	0.9844
3.	Saharsa	0.8890	1.0550	1.0300	0.8780	0.8820	1.2720	0.9490	1.0870	0.7360	0.9753
4.	Purnea	0.8580	1.1300	0.9320	1.1340	1.0850	1.0510	0.6900	0.9380	0.8780	0.9662
5.	Saran	0.9230	0.9880	1.1090	0.8560	1.0130	1.0990	1.3220	0.7590	0.9360	1.0006
6.	Patna	0.7780	1.1250	0.9830	0.9170	1.0350	1.1490	0.4980	1.6820	1.0720	1.0266
7.	Mungair	0.9460	0.8900	1.1880	0.7530	0.9990	1.3420	0.6850	0.8750	0.8300	0.9453
8.	Bhagalpur	0.9700	1.0480	0.9020	0.8180	1.2700	1.2030	0.6720	1.1570	1.0120	1.0058
9.	Gaya	1.0040	0.9480	1.0360	0.9670	1.0760	1.2520	0.8620	1.2010	0.9400	1.0318
10.	Nalanda	0.9980	0.9920	1.0330	0.7410	0.9890	1.1550	0.7870	1.3420	0.9320	0.9966
11.	Nawada	0.8550	0.9530	1.1270	0.8270	0.9500	1.1290	1.0600	0.9530	0.9150	0.9743
12.	Aurangabad	1.1740	0.8110	1.2330	0.8990	1.0250	1.3730	0.6650	0.8970	1.1510	1.0253
13.	Bhojpur	0.9960	0.9860	1.0830	0.8220	1.0380	1.1300	0.8870	1.2820	1.0820	1.0340
14.	Rohtas	1.0290	0.9890	1.0920	1.0760	0.8940	0.9930	0.8030	1.2660	1.0730	1.0239
15.	Siwan	1.0530	0.8200	1.1540	0.8520	0.9320	1.1830	1.1250	0.7670	0.9800	0.9851
16.	Gopalganj	1.3060	0.7700	1.1400	0.7980	1.1590	1.1910	0.6170	1.0390	1.1620	1.0202
17.	Champaran (East)	0.9670	0.9910	1.0230	0.8230	1.0030	1.2050	0.9140	1.4710	0.7370	1.0149
18.	Champaran (West)	1.2850	0.8920	0.9910	0.9050	1.2170	1.4310	0.6000	1.3550	1.1140	1.0878
19.	Vaishali	1.0960	0.8150	1.0150	0.8390	1.0390	1.1790	1.3220	1.1450	0.7530	1.0226
20.	Sitamarhi	1.6830	0.4850	1.0700	0.8230	1.0540	1.2500	1.0320	1.3010	0.6550	1.0392
21.	Madhubani	1.0090	1.0360	1.1450	0.6000	0.9630	1.1920	0.9230	0.8560	1.1010	0.9806
22.	Samastipur	1.0170	0.7670	1.0250	0.9530	1.1330	1.1460	0.8930	1.1030	1.1870	1.0249

Contd...

Table 2.4—Contd...

Sl.No.	District	2001	2002	2003	2004	2005	2006	2007	2008	2009	Mean
23.	Begusarai	0.7780	1.3420	0.7610	1.1200	1.1650	1.0630	1.2310	0.8990	1.2080	1.0630
24.	Katihar	0.9640	0.7910	1.2090	0.8530	1.0410	1.1410	0.8990	0.9180	0.9100	0.9696
25.	Jehanabad	1.0340	0.9380	1.0840	0.7410	1.1320	1.4020	0.5220	1.2650	0.8820	1.0000
26.	Madhepura	0.8760	0.7760	1.0710	1.0570	1.0590	1.1270	0.8120	0.6880	0.8240	0.9211
27.	Khagaria	1.1200	0.7660	1.2440	0.8190	0.9760	1.3990	1.1100	0.8180	0.8700	1.0136
28.	Aarreya	0.9230	0.9150	1.1900	0.9450	1.2920	1.0110	0.9810	0.7270	1.0670	1.0057
29.	Kishanganj	0.9080	0.7810	1.4690	0.9630	0.8070	0.9750	1.3310	0.6110	1.0630	0.9898
30.	Buxar	1.1180	0.8670	1.1150	0.7240	1.0430	1.1090	0.9750	0.8790	0.9610	0.9768
31.	Bhabhua	0.9450	0.9810	0.9460	0.6920	1.1610	1.0430	0.9010	0.8690	0.9800	0.9464
32.	Banka	1.2770	0.7200	1.6780	0.7130	1.3040	0.8360	0.8970	0.7890	1.0370	1.0279
33.	Jamui	0.8890	0.7790	0.9820	0.7840	1.2810	1.3410	1.5280	1.6190	0.6970	1.1000
34.	Supaul	0.9150	0.9210	1.2950	1.2980	0.7990	1.7640	0.3650	0.4860	1.1540	0.9997
35.	Lakhisarai	1.0670	1.0950	0.8460	0.7290	1.3130	1.5220	0.4460	1.0700	0.8150	0.9892
36.	Sheikhpura	0.9080	2.0030	0.5030	0.8590	1.3200	1.5110	0.5140	1.3190	0.8310	1.0853
37.	Sheohar	1.0390	0.8380	1.7200	0.5650	1.1450	0.8870	0.7220	1.0110	0.7570	0.9649
	Mean	**1.0010**	**0.9270**	**1.0680**	**0.8500**	**1.0670**	**1.1870**	**0.8380**	**1.0060**	**0.9350**	**0.9866**

Table 2.5: Ranking of Districts Based on Malmquist TFP Index and its Components

Rank	District	Efficiency Change	District	Technological Change	District	TFP Change
1.	Nawada	1.1306	Jamui	1.1000	Jamui	1.2477
2.	Gaya	1.1141	Champaran (W)	1.0878	Sheikhpura	1.2058
3.	Jamui	1.0976	Sheikhpura	1.0853	Gaya	1.1180
4.	Banka	1.0897	Begusarai	1.0630	Banka	1.1144
5.	Jehanabad	1.0790	Sitamarhi	1.0392	Nawada	1.1120
6.	Bhojpur	1.0557	Bhojpur	1.0340	Jehanabad	1.0939
7.	Sheikhpura	1.0506	Gaya	1.0318	Bhojpur	1.0937
8.	Madhubani	1.0463	Banka	1.0279	Champaran (W)	1.0878
9.	Mungair	1.0327	Patna	1.0266	Begusarai	1.0692
10.	Nalanda	1.0322	Aurangabad	1.0253	Samastipur	1.0492
11.	Sheohar	1.0292	Samastipur	1.0249	Sitamarhi	1.0428
12.	Vaishali	1.0284	Rohtas	1.0239	Khagaria	1.0409
13.	Sitamarhi	1.0262	Vaishali	1.0226	Aurangabad	1.0401
14.	Begusarai	1.0214	Gopalganj	1.0202	Nalanda	1.0394
15.	Patna	1.0203	Muzaffarpur	1.0158	Madhubani	1.0296
16.	Samastipur	1.0196	Champaran (E)	1.0149	Rohtas	1.0239
17.	Katihar	1.0181	Khagaria	1.0136	Gopalganj	1.0202
18.	Khagaria	1.0176	Bhagalpur	1.0058	Patna	1.0117
19.	Siwan	1.0163	Aarreya	1.0057	Bhagalpur	1.0116
20.	Bhagalpur	1.0104	Saran	1.0006	Aarreya	1.0113
21.	Lakhisarai	1.0104	Jehanabad	1.0000	Vaishali	1.0062
22.	Saharsa	1.0088	Supaul	0.9997	Supaul	1.0043
23.	Aarreya	1.0057	Nalanda	0.9966	Saran	1.0019
24.	Aurangabad	1.0041	Kishanganj	0.9898	Lakhisarai	0.9990
25.	Darbhanga	1.0009	Lakhisarai	0.9892	Mungair	0.9972
26.	Supaul	1.0007	Siwan	0.9851	Saharsa	0.9964
27.	Rohtas	1.0000	Darbhanga	0.9844	Champaran (E)	0.9962
28.	Gopalganj	1.0000	Madhubani	0.9806	Kishanganj	0.9898
29.	Champaran (W)	1.0000	Buxar	0.9768	Muzaffarpur	0.9852
30.	Kishanganj	1.0000	Saharsa	0.9753	Siwan	0.9844
31.	Buxar	0.9959	Nawada	0.9743	Katihar	0.9832
32.	Saran	0.9942	Katihar	0.9696	Darbhanga	0.9821
33.	Bhabhua	0.9904	Purnea	0.9662	Sheohar	0.9759
34.	Madhepura	0.9854	Sheohar	0.9649	Buxar	0.9713
35.	Purnea	0.9793	Bhabhua	0.9464	Purnea	0.9488
36.	Muzaffarpur	0.9686	Mungair	0.9453	Bhabhua	0.9370
37.	Champaran (E)	0.9484	Madhepura	0.9211	Madhepura	0.9028

Table 2.6: Two Tailed, Two Sample t-test for Inequality of Variances and Sample Sizes

Variable	Districts Above Average and Average (Case-I)			Districts Average and Below Average (Case-II)			Districts Above Average and Below Average (Case-III)		
	Pooled SD	p-value	Mean Diff.	Pooled SD	p-value	Mean Diff.	Pooled SD	p-value	Mean Diff.
Tech Efficiency Change	0.040	0.144	0.036	0.022	0.118	0.019	0.033	0.001	0.0546***
Technology Change	0.030	0.177	0.025	0.028	0.205	0.019	0.032	0.005	0.0433***
TFP Change	0.023	0.003	0.049***	0.025	0.002	0.047***	0.028	0.000	0.0961***
Productivity	4149.3	0.970	-91.000	3464.0	0.154	2660.0	3312.27	0.091	2568.0*
Cropping Intensity	12.479	0.560	-4.270	16.098	0.903	-1.020	16.013	0.458	-5.3000
Labour Productivity	2650.0	0.722	554.000	1456.7	0.885	110.000	1956.7	0.448	662.0000
Irrigation	20.052	0.828	2.500	13.224	0.089	12.280	14.636	0.031	14.82**
Fertiliser	90.403	0.633	25.300	72.432	0.611	19.400	48.231	0.046	44.70**
Credit	2802.3	0.579	-914.000	2009.5	0.018	2705.0**	1910.3	0.044	1791.0**
Literacy	6.471	0.607	-1.960	6.695	0.100	6.000*	6.367	0.162	4.040

***, ** and * indicate significant at 1 per cent, 5 per cent and 10 per cent, respectively.

Determinants of TFP

Based on the TFP growth values, the Bihar districts were categorised as average, above average and below average and the differences were analysed among the three categories. Table 2.6 shows the results obtained from t-test for different cases *viz.*, between districts above average and average (case-I), average and below average (case-II) and above average and below average (case-III).

It was observed that the means of change in technical efficiency and technology were significantly different only in case-III while mean difference of TFP change were significant at 1 per cent level of significance in all three cases. The mean difference of productivity was significant at 10 per cent while for irrigation and fertilizer at 5 per cent in case-III. Mean difference of credit was significant at 5 per cent for case-II and at case-III. The mean difference of literacy was significant at 10 per cent in case-II only. The significant mean difference of irrigation, fertilizer and credit in case-III indicates that in the districts where TFP was below average require an increase in the application of these inputs to improve the TFP.

Conclusion

In this paper Data Envelopment Analysis approach is used to estimate the total factor productivity change, technical efficiency change and technological change in districts of Bihar state for the period 2001-2009 using the Malmquist productivity index. It was found that the overall agriculture in Bihar state has improved during 2001-2009 as average total factor productivity increased at the rate of 3.04 percent during this period where 2.24 per cent is contributed by technical efficiency and a meagre 0.63 per cent by technological change. It is also observed from the analysis that change in technical efficiency was positive in 30 while technological change was positive only in 21 districts out of total 37 districts. Thus, farmers are efficient in judicious use of input mix but the improvement in technological adoption is quite slow in most of the districts. There was divergence in all districts in TFP and its components during the study period and also among each other in any selected year. This divergent trend is expected as Bihar agriculture has been victim of frequent natural vagaries. The study clearly suggests that emphasis must be laid on technological adoption at district level in Bihar state.

Based on significant mean difference of irrigation, fertilizer and credit between districts having TFP above average and below average, it is recommended to formulate and implement appropriate policies for improvement in irrigation, fertilizer and access to credit.

References

1. Arnade C. (1998). "Using a programming approachto measure international agricultural efficiency and productivity", *Journal of Agricultural Economics*, Vol. 49, pp. 67-84.

2. Bhushan Surya (2005). "Total Factor Productivity Growth of Wheat in India: A Malmquist Approach", *Indian Journal of Agricultural Economics*, Vol 60, No.1 Jan-March 2005.

3. Caves D.W., Christensen L.R., Diewert W.E. (1982). "The economic theory of index numbers and the measurement of input, output and productivity", *Econometrica* 50, pp. 1393-1414.

4. Coelli Tim J., Rao D.S. Prasada (2003). "Total Factor Productivity Growth in Agriculture: A Malmquist Index Analysis of 93 Countries1980-2000", Centre for Efficiency and Productivity Analysis, Working Paper Series, No. 02/2003, School of Economics, University of Queensland Australia.

5. Coelli Tim J., Rao D.S. Prasada, O'Donnell Christopher J., Battesse George E. (2005). "An Introduction to Efficiency and Productivity Analysis (Second Edition)", Springer.

6. Coelli Tim. "A Data Envelopment Analysis (Computer) Program", Centre for Efficiency and Productivity Analysis, Department of Econometrics, University of New England, Australia.

7. Coelli Tim, Rahman Sanzidur, Thirtle Colin (2003). "A Stochastic Frontier Approach to Total Factor Productivity measurement in Bangladesh crop agriculture", *Journal of International Development*, 15, 321-333.

8. Fare, R., Grosskopf, S., Norris, M., and Zhang, Z. (1994). Productivity Growth, Technical Progress, and Efficiency Change in Industrialized Countries. *The American Economic Review*, 84, 66-83.

9. Fulginiti L. E., and Perrin R.K. (1993). "Prices and Productivity in Agriculture", *Review of Economics and Statistics*, Vol. 75, pp. 471-482.

10. Fulginiti L. E., and Perrin R.K. (1997). "LDC Agriculture: Non-parametric Malmquist Productivity Indices", *Journal of Development Economics*, Vol.53, pp. 373-390.

11. Fulginiti L. E., and Perrin R.K. (1998). "Agricultural Productivity in Developing Countries", *Agricultural Economics*, Vol. 19, pp. 45-51.

12. Kumar Praduman, Rosegrant Mark W (1994). "Productivity and Sources of Growth for Rice in India", *Economic and Political Weekly*, December 31, 1994, p. A-183 to A-188.

13. Nin Alejandro, Arndt Channing, Preckel Paul V. (2003). "Is agricultural productivity in developing countries really shrinking? New evidence using a modified nonparametric approach", *Journal of Development Economics* 71, pp. 395-415.

14. Rahman Sanzidur (2004). "Regional Productivity and Convergence in Bangladesh Agriculture", Paper presented at the Annual Meeting of the American Agricultural Economics Association held in Aug 1-4, 2004, *Project MUSE Scholarly Journals Online*.

15. Rosegrant Mark W, Evenson (1992). "The rate of growth of Total Factor Productivity in Indian crop sector 1957-1985", *American Journal of Agricultural Economics*, August 1992, 757-763.

16. Statistical Abstract, India and of individual states, various issues.

17. Trueblood M.A. (1996). "An intercountry comparison of agricultural efficiency and productivity", Ph.D dissertation, University of Minnesota.

18. Shilpa Chaudhary (2012). Trends in Total Factor productivity in Indian Agriculture: State-level Evidence Using Non-Parametric Sequential Malmquist Index, Working Paper No. 215, CDE, Delhi School of Economics, University of Delhi.

Chapter 3

Assessing Performance of Various Crops Based on Alternative Approaches: A Case of Punjab

S.S. Raju[1], Ramesh Chand[2], S.K. Srivastava[3],
Amrit Pal Kaur[4], Jaspal Singh[4], Rajni Jain[1],
and Kingsly Immaneulraj[3]

[1]Principal Scientist, [3]Scientist, [4]Research Associate
ICAR-NIAP, New Delhi-110 012
[2]Member, NITI Aayog , New Delhi-110 001

ABSTRACT

The present study assesses the performance of different crops and cropping pattern in the state of Punjab using alternative scenarios like market prices; economic prices (net out effect of subsidy) and Natural Resource Valuation (NRV) considering environmental benefits like biological nitrogen fixation and greenhouse gas costs. The study uses unit-level cost of cultivation data for the triennium ending with 2010-11. It also analyses crop wise use of fertilizers and ground and surface water and subsidies. The paper provide insights into relative profitability of various crops with and without state support in the form of subsidies and by reckoning positive and negative environmental externalities. This study shows that even after netting out the effect of input subsidies and effect on environment and natural resource the relative profitability of various crops doesn't change. Under the present set of marketing infrastructure, minimum support price, and agricultural technological know-how, rice-

wheat cropping pattern produces the highest and more stable incomes. Farmer may not move towards diversification until incentivized by economically attractive alternatives.

Keywords: *Market prices, Economic prices, NRV, Sustainability, Punjab.*

Introduction

Growth in agricultural output in Punjab, since the onset of green revolution, has played a vital role in achieving and sustaining food security in India. In the recent years the strategic importance of the state has begun to decline. Punjab today stands at a critical juncture, with ecological thresholds for soil fertility and water availability nearing their tipping points (Jasdev Singh *et al.*, 2012; Kulkarni and Shah, 2013) and fiscal burden of support to agriculture becoming unsustainable. This has raised serious questions about the future of agriculture in the state. The crisis manifests itself in a number of ways: stagnating growth rates in agricultural production and productivity, rising average cost of production, falling profitability in farming, swelling input subsidy bill, over-exploitation of water and land resources, resulting into degradation of the environment and ecology. A large number of studies point out that sustainability in agricultural production and the natural resource base are under threat in Punjab (Sidhu, *et al.*, 2010).

The three pillars of the agricultural revolution in Punjab- high-yield crop intensification, subsidized access to electricity for drawing water for irrigation and increased chemical fertilizer use under favorable output price policy regime resulted in the tremendous increase in area under cereals, namely wheat and rice, cultivation. The state has reached cropping intensity of more than 189 per cent as against 140 per cent in the country as a whole, and consumption of fertilizer (NPK) is 250.19 kilogram per hectare as compared to the Indian average of 128.34 kilogram per hectare in 2012-13. About 18 per cent of the total tractors in India are in Punjab and the production is supported by about 98 per cent irrigation coverage. However, these three pillars of the agricultural revolution in Punjab have culminated in several negative ecological externalities. Thus rising stress on water availability, rice-wheat monocultures, higher use of energy and fertilizers in agriculture necessitates optimum use of resources and reallocation of production choices without price distortions.

Many studies have raised issues regarding sustainability of agriculture production in Punjab (Shergill, 2007, Sidhu, *et al.*, 2010, Kaur and Vatta, 2010), deterioration of water, land and natural resources (Sidhu *et al.*, 1997; Kaur *et al.*, 2015), profitability of cropping patterns (Sukhwinder *et al.*, 2011, World Bank, 2003) but no systematic study is there which link crop profitability with social cost *i.e.* subsidy and natural resource accounting. The available literature compares performance and profitability of various crops by using market prices of inputs which are highly distorted because of subsidy. For instance, electric power used for agriculture (irrigation) is free to farmers but it has a cost for the society. Similarly, a farmer pay Rs. 276 for one bag of urea weighing 50 kg and society pays Rs. 480 as subsidy and total cost of one bag to society is Rs. 480 whereas it's cost to the country is Rs. 756. Thus, computing cost and return at market prices of inputs represent income to the producer but not to the society. The return to the society must consider subsidy as a cost while deriving figure of net return or value added. The present study attempts to fill this gap by assessing the performance of various crops and crop sequences in the region of Punjab in terms of market prices, economic prices and natural resource valuation and it will help to gain insight into suitability of various crops in the state of Punjab from long term prospects of society. It will show the extent to which crop profitability changes based on alternative criteria for assessment. The study further estimates crop wise fertilizer consumption, groundwater extraction, surface water use and their respective subsidies in the state.

Data and Methodology

Data for this study were taken from the "Comprehensive Scheme for Studying the Cost of Cultivation (CoC) of Principal Crops in Punjab", Directorate of Economics and Statistics, Ministry of Agriculture, GoI. Under this scheme, data are collected from a sample of 300 farm households in 30 tehsils spread across three agro-climatic zones for the block year ending 2011. The data on per unit fertilizer subsidy was derived from annual reports of Department of Fertilizers, Ministry of Chemicals and Fertilizers, GoI and data on per unit power subsidy was taken from Punjab state electricity regulatory commission (website: http://www.pserc.nic.in/). For estimating groundwater subsidies, total volume of groundwater extraction was estimating using the data from CoC survey as well as ground water level data of Central Ground Water Board (CGWB), Ministry of Water Resources, GoI. District wise average ground water level data was compiled for the corresponding years of 2008, 2009 and 2010. For estimating canal water subsidies, data on financial aspects of irrigation projects was collected from Central Water Commission during 2008 to 2011.

The data on canal irrigation expenditure and receipts was collected from Central Water Commission. The study covers the triennium ending 2010-11.

Net return at market prices was defined as the gross return (value of main product and by product) less variable Costs (Cost A1 + imputed value of family labour) at market prices actually paid and received by the farmer or imputed in some cases.

Net return at economic prices was defined as the net return or income at market prices less subsidies on inputs like fertilizers and irrigation used in crop production.

The subsidy component was internalized into the estimation by covering two aspects *viz.*, fertilizer subsidy and irrigation subsidy. Fertilizer subsidy consists of subsidy on nitrogen (N) and combination of Phosphorus (P) and Potassium (K). The total irrigation subsidy includes canal, electricity and diesel subsidy and has been distributed over selected crops based on area under irrigation under each crop.

Crop wise irrigation subsidy has two components: Surface water subsidy and Ground water subsidy. Ground water subsidy was estimated by initially calculating the crop-wise ground water use, *i.e.*

Groundwater use (cubic meter) = Irrigation hours (hrs/ha) * Groundwater draft (cum/hr)

The irrigation hours (hrs/ha) for each crop were taken from plot-wise CCS data. Groundwater draft was estimated using the following formula,

$$\text{Ground water draft (lit/sec)} = \frac{HP \times 75 \times \text{Pump efficiency}}{\text{Total head (m)}}$$

The information on horse power (Hp) of the pumps owned by the farmers is available in CCS data set. For the households purchasing groundwater, average HP of the pumps (estimated separately for electric and diesel) in respective tehsil was taken as proxy. Pump efficiency was assumed to be 40 percent. The total head was obtained as:

Total head =water level (mbgl*) + friction loss (10 per cent of water level) + draw down (m)

For submersible pumps which are installed underground, additional 10 M height (after discussion with experts) was added to total head.

The summation of groundwater draft from each category of pumps gave total groundwater use (cum/ha) for each crop cultivated by the farmer. Further the GW cost has been estimated separately for diesel pump, electric pump and submersible pumps, which are the summation of depreciation (tube well and pump set), interest (tube well and pump set) and upkeep costs. The subsidy per hectare of groundwater use has been estimated separately for electric (product of per kilo-watt groundwater volume (cum/kwhr) and subsidy rate (Rs/kwhr) and diesel pumps (product of diesel use in extraction of groundwater and per litre subsidy rate during 2008-11).

Surface/Canal water irrigation subsidy was estimated using the data of Central Water Commission. For this, first total expenditure on major, medium and minor irrigation projects was estimated as sum of capital expenditure and working expenses for triennium ending 2010-11. Then gross receipts out of irrigation projects were subtracted from the total expenditure to get the gross subsidy.

Gross Subsidy = Total Expenditure – Gross Receipts

The canal subsidy for each crop was estimated by allocating gross subsidy across different crops on the basis of proportion of their area under canal irrigation.

Net return based on natural resource valuation technique has taken care of nitrogen fixation by legume crops and GHG emission from crop production. As such NRNRV is computed by adding value of nitrogen fixation by crops at economic price of nitrogen (Value of N) and deducting the imputed value of increase in greenhouse gas (GHG) emission cost to the atmosphere.

The value of GHG emissions in terms of CO_2 kg equivalent was taken at the rate of US$ 10 per tonne of CO_2. The data on contribution of pulses by biological nitrogen fixation and emission of greenhouse gases of different crops were collected from the published scientific literature, (Peoples *et al.*, 1995, IIPR, 2003, IARI, 2014) and has been calculated by taking the average value of nitrogen fixed by various legumes and then multiplied with the price of nitrogen prevailed during TE 2010-11.

Results and Discussion

Cost and Returns based on Market Prices

The comparative returns or profitability is affected by factors as yield levels, input use in production and their respective prices, and output price. The comparative returns at market prices along with variable cost for various crops in Punjab are shown in Table 3.1. The variable costs included the cost incurred on different inputs such as seed, fertilizer, manure, insecticides, human labour charges (including family labour), machine labour charges and irrigation charges.

Table 3.1: Comparative Costs and Returns of different Crops in Punjab Based on Market Prices (Rs/ha), TE 2010-11

Crops	Variable Cost (Cost A1+FL)	Gross Returns	Net Returns Over Variable Costs
Wheat	17413	53657	36244
Paddy –non Basmati	21372	67570	46198
Paddy Basmati	23853	77230	53377
Maize	19529	33321	13792
S. Cane (Planted)	58028	156412	98384
S. Cane (Ratoon)	34798	153474	118676
Rapeseed and Mustard	16694	31144	14450
Cotton	29046	71233	42187
Potato	42256	69394	27138
Peas	30391	74940	44549
Vegetables	37745	74243	36497
Fodder	30764	35903	5139

Source: Estimated using unit level CoC data of Punjab (TE 2010-11).

Among various crops, per hectare variable cost was highest in sugarcane planted (Rs. 58028 per hectare) during TE 2010-11. Sugarcane was followed by potato with variable cost of cultivation of Rs. 42256 per hectare. The lowest per hectare cost of cultivation was observed in the case of rapeseed and mustard (Rs. 16694 per hectare).

Structure of cost varied across different crops. Among kharif crops, cotton cultivation is on the higher end with variable cost of Rs. 29046 per hectare followed by paddy and maize. Variable cost incurred in production of Basmati rice was Rs. 23853 per hectare which was 11.6 per cent higher than the cost of cultivation of non-basmati paddy. While in rabi season, variable costs were higher for potato as compared to its competing crops such as wheat and rapeseed and mustard.

The return depends on cost of cultivation as well as on productivity of crop and its price. Among the crops, sugarcane accrued highest net return (Rs./ha) over the variable costs. As this crop occupies land for the whole year therefore its net returns need to be compared with crop rotation or crop sequence in the year like paddy-wheat. Interestingly, net return from sugarcane at market prices turned out to be the highest even compared to sum of the net returns from paddy and wheat. The combination of wheat-rice generated net returns of Rs. 83927 per hectare which is lower as compared to sugarcane cultivation. However lack of marketing infrastructure for crops other than wheat and rice, high transport costs and inadequate agro-processing units in the rural areas are the constraints in the spread of sugarcane cultivation in Punjab. The combination of wheat-rice (basmati), due to its lower costs of cultivation turns out to be the best combination as the net profits from other combinations are less as wheat- maize (Rs. 50036 per hectare) and wheat- cotton (Rs. 78431 per hectare). Wheat-cotton yields less profit due to high cost of cultivation and it also involves higher risk due to price instability of cotton.

Among kharif crops, paddy-basmati has the highest gross returns (Rs. 77230 per hectare) while rapeseed and mustard has reported the lowest per hectare value of output (Rs. 31144 per hectare) among all selected crops in TE 2010-11. Among all other crops basmati rice reaps the highest net returns of Rs. 53377 per hectare followed by non-basmati. Cotton comes next in the kharif season with net income of Rs. 42187 per hectare, while maize gives the lowest net income of Rs. 13792 per hectare. As can be observed from the Table 3.4, cultivation of basmati paddy in Punjab required higher costs than non-basmati paddy but provides much higher gross returns and net income.

At market prices basmati rice is found most superior and it also involves lower use of irrigation water and other inputs especially fertilizers when compared to non-basmati paddy.

Among rabi crops, pea gives highest net returns of Rs. 44549 per hectare, although this commodity does not have required marketing infrastructure in Punjab. Wheat and potato on an average yielded net returns of around Rs. 36244 per hectare and Rs. 27138 per hectare respectively.

It can be concluded that the wheat-rice (basmati) cropping pattern is producing higher financial returns with relatively low risks. From the comparative cost and return analysis for different crops in Punjab in TE 2010-11 sugarcane and paddy-basmati comes out with the most efficient crops in financial aspects. Sugarcane and cotton seem to be the potential substitutes of rice. As such the wheat- rice cropping pattern offered the best returns to the farmers in the given framework of productivity and marketing criteria.

Net Returns based on Economic Prices

Net returns at economic prices from different crops were computed by subtracting input subsidies as shown in Table 3.2. Potato is receiving the highest subsidy Rs. 18929 per hectare, because of higher fertilizer component followed by sugarcane (Rs. 13231per hectare), being an annual crop, closely followed by paddy-non basmati (Rs. 13007 per hectare). In the total subsidy in paddy- non basmati,

Table 3.2: Crop-wise Net Returns Based on Economic Prices (Rs./ha) in Punjab TE 2010-11

Crop Name	Irrigation Subsidy		NPK# Subsidy	Total Subsidy	Net Returns by Economic Prices
	Ground Water (Diesel* and Electricity$)	Canal Water			
Paddy-non Basmati	5051	1059	6897	13007	33191
Paddy-Basmati	5031	583	5974	11588	41789
Wheat	1122	1454	8036	10612	25747
Maize	823	28	7547	8398	5394
Potato	1113	348	17468	18929	8209
Pea	754	0	10441	11195	33354
Sugarcane(Planted)	2559	352	10320	13231	85153
Sugarcane (Ratoon)	2446	144	8010	10600	108077
Rapeseed and Mustard	1005	1285	4707	6997	7556
Cotton-Medium Staple	1074	4405	6178	11657	30530
Vegetables	2417	97	7440	9954	26543
Fodder	2441	1293	6234	9968	-4829

Source: Estimated using unit level CoC data of Punjab (TE 2010-11)

Notes: # Subsidy Rate @ Rs. 19.35/kg of N; Rs. 42.56/kg of P and K combine for TE 2010-11

*Diesel Subsidy rate @ 12.95 per litre.

$ Electricity subsidy rate @ Rs. 2.40, Rs. 2.85 and Rs. 3.20 per unit in 2008-09, 2009-10 and 2010-11 respectively.

irrigation has a higher share with subsidy of Rs. 6110 per hectare. Cotton received the highest canal water subsidy of Rs. 4405 per hectare. Among the selected crops the minimum subsidy is used in rapeseed and mustard (Rs. 6997 per hectare).

The Table 3.2 also reveals that the net returns based on economic prices are highest in sugarcane crop. Apart from the annual crop, the paddy-basmati remains the most remunerative crop with net income of Rs. 41789 per hectare at economic prices, followed by peas that offer the net returns of Rs. 33354 per hectare after deducting the subsidies. Potato ranks first in terms of inputs subsidy but still not able to compete with the other important crops in terms of net income. Rice, cotton and wheat provide net income of Rs. 33191, Rs. 30530 and Rs. 25747 per hectare respectively. After removing subsidies the net returns from fodder became negative (Rs. 4829 per hectare) and also maize has become the least profitable crop in terms of economic prices.

Net Returns based on Natural Resource Valuation (NRV)

Agriculture produces significant effects on climate change, primarily through the production and release of greenhouse gases such as carbon dioxide, methane, and nitrous oxide (Environment Statistics of Punjab, 2012). Further, open field burning of straw after combine harvesting is a common practice in the state in order to ensure early preparation of fields for the next crop. On the contrary, legumes are environment friendly crops and are different from other food plants in having the property of synthesizing atmospheric nitrogen into plant nutrients. As such the economic valuation has been done by taking into account the positive impact of legume crops by biological nitrogen fixation and the negative impact of GHG emissions, and has been presented in the Table 3.3.

Table 3.3: Economic Valuation of Nitrogen Fixation and GHG by Various Crops in Punjab

Crop	Valuation (Rs/ha)	
	Nitrogen Fixation	GHG
Paddy	0	1838
Wheat	0	183
Maize	0	159
Sugarcane	0	3798
Rape and Mustard	0	115
Cotton	0	51
Potato	0	235
Peas	1389	97
Vegetables	0	235
Fodder	4187	97

Source: Calculated by using Peoples *et al.* (1995); IIPR (2003) and IARI (2012).

Required data was available only for two legume crops peas and fodder. Fodder grown in Punjab fixed nitrogen equivalent to the economic contribution of Rs. 4187 per hectare while peas are fixing nitrogen worth Rs. 1389 per hectare (Table 3.3). Paddy causes highest negative externality by producing GHG emissions costing Rs. 1838 per hectare, whereas the minimum GHG costs were incurred by peas and fodder valued at Rs. 97 per hectare.

When these benefits are added and the costs are deducted from net returns based on economic prices then we get over-all returns of cultivation of different crops to society and natural resource system. The information in Table 3.4 based on NRV indicates highest net income in sugarcane ratoon (Rs. 104279 per hectare) followed by sugarcane planted (Rs. 81355 per hectare). Paddy-basmati still stands at the top in seasonal crops in terms of gross and net income. In rabi season peas with Rs. 34646 per hectare net returns based on NRV comes at the top. Paddy-non-basmati, cotton, vegetables and wheat are giving net returns of Rs. 31353, Rs. 30479, Rs. 26308 and Rs. 25564 per hectare respectively on the basis of NRV.

Table 3.4: Net Returns Based on Natural Resource Evaluation (Rs/ha) in Punjab TE 2010-11

Crops	Returns by Adding Economic Value of Nitrogen	Returns by Deducting Cost of GHG Emissions	Net Returns Based on NRV
Paddy- non Basmati	33191	31353	31353
Paddy Basmati	41789	39951	39951
Wheat	25747	25564	25564
Maize	5394	5235	5235
Sugarcane (Planted)	85153	81355	81355
Sugarcane (Ratoon)	108077	104279	104279
Rapeseed and Mustard	7556	7441	7441
Cotton	30530	30479	30479
Potato	8209	7974	7974
Peas	34743	33257	34646
Vegetables	26543	26308	26308
Fodder	–642	–4926	–739

Source: Estimated by using unit level CoC data of Punjab (TE 2010-11) and based on Peoples *et al.* (1995); IIPR (2003) and IARI (2014).

Comparative Returns of Crops Using Various Approaches of Valuation

A comparative picture of net income from various crops based on market prices, economic prices (net of subsidies) and natural resource valuation is presented in Table 3.5. As it is obvious there is moderate to high decline in net income from different crops after netting out subsidies on fertilizer, power, canal and diesel. The impact of subsidy is so large that in some cases net income turned negative (fodder) and in some cases it reduced to one third (potato). Removal of subsidy reduced net income from maize to 40 per cent and in rapeseed and mustard to close to half. Due to high rate of profitability in sugarcane, paddy and wheat the removal of subsidy lowered net income moderately even though subsidy level in paddy was much higher compared to maize. Placing economic value on environmental effect further reduced profitability of various crops except peas and fodder. However, this effect was mild.

Table 3.5: Net Returns from different Crops in Punjab Using Various Approaches of Valuation (Rs./ha), TE 2010-11

Crops	Based on Market Prices	Based on Economic Prices	Based on NRV
Paddy- NB	46198	33191	31353
Paddy Basmati	53377	41789	39951
Wheat	36244	25747	25564
Maize	13792	5394	5235
S. Cane (Planted)	98384	85153	81355
S. Cane (Ratoon)	118676	108077	104279
Rapeseed and Mustard	14450	7556	7441
Cotton	42187	30530	30479
Potato	27138	8209	7974
Peas	44549	33354	34646
Vegetables	36497	26543	26308
Fodder	5139	−4829	−739

Source: Estimated using unit level CoC data of Punjab (TE 2010-11).

It is often felt that free power supply in the state of Punjab is keeping profitability of paddy artificially high and thus discouraging diversification of crop pattern away from paddy. Our study shows that under the present set of marketing infrastructure, minimum support price, and agricultural technological know-how, rice-wheat cropping pattern produces the highest and more stable incomes. Farmer may not move towards diversification until incentivized by economically attractive alternatives.

Conclusions

The study reveals that sugarcane and paddy, both basmati as well as non-basmati, remain the most rewarding crops in terms of market prices, economic prices and natural resource valuation. Sugarcane and peas offer scope for competing with rice –wheat rotation but their prospects are marred by lack of marketing infrastructure, government incentives for crops other than wheat and rice. Thus under the present set of marketing infrastructure and agricultural technological know-how rice-wheat cropping pattern are likely to produce the highest and more stable incomes. Farmer may not move towards diversification until incentivized by economically attractive alternatives.

The factors which are not captured by the market like subsidies- that is the direct cost to the society; factors affecting the natural resources and environment as nitrogen fixation and greenhouse gas costs, need to be considered and should be internalized through appropriate policies. Reckoning such costs and return alters level of net income from various crops.

This study shows that even after netting out the effect of input subsidies and effect on environment and natural resource the relative profitability of various crops doesn't change. Among seasonal crops paddy remains the most profitable crop in *kharif* and wheat remains the second most profitable crop after peas in *Rabi*. The reason is that technological superiority of paddy and wheat in Punjab is much higher than the difference in input support given to various crops. However, these findings should not be taken to interpret that removal of subsidies on water or fertilizers will not affect use of these inputs. Use of fertilizers and irrigation will be definitely much lower without subsidy than what it is with subsidy. Thus, over-exploitation of water and indiscriminate use of fertilizer can be checked by reducing level of subsidies but shift in crop pattern require developing superior alternative which are not there at present.

Acknowledgements

This chapter is an output of the Social Science Network Project on "Regional Crop Planning for Improving Resource Use Efficiency" awarded to National Institute of Agricultural Economics and Policy Research by the Indian Council of Agricultural Research and is largely drawn from the paper published in the AERA Conference issue 2015.

References

Agricultural Statistics at a Glance (2014). Directorate of Economics and Statistics, Department of Agriculture and Cooperation, Ministry of Agriculture, Government of India.

Central Water Commission (Various Issues). Report on "Financial aspects of irrigation projects in India" Information technology directorate information system organization, Water planning and projects wing.

GoI (2011). Central Ground Water Board (CGWB), Ministry of Water Resources, Govt. of India. Website: http://cgwb.gov.in/

GoI (Various Issues). Annual Report of Ministry of Chemicals and Fertilizers, Department of Fertilizers, Government of India

GoPb (Various Issues). Statistical Abstracts of Punjab, Government of Punjab, Chandigarh.

GoPb, (2011). Report on "Environment Statistics of Punjab", *Economic and Statistical Organisation,* Government of Punjab, Chandigarh

GoPb, Punjab State Electricity Regulatory Commission, Website: http://www.pserc.nic.in/

IARI (2014). "GHG emission from Indian Agriculture: Trends, Mitigation and Policy Needs" Centre for Environment Science and Climate Resilient Agriculture, IARI, p.16.

IIPR (2003). "Pulses in New Perspective", Proceedings of the National Symposium on Crop Diversification and Natural Resource Management, pp. 20 - 22 December 2003, IIPR, Kanpur.

Jasdev Singh, D.K. Grover and Tejinder K. Dhaliwal (2012). "State agricultural profile-Punjab"Agro-Economic Research Centre, Department of Economics and Sociology, PAU.

Kaur, B., Sidhu, R.S., and K. Vatta (2010). " Optimal crop plans for sustainable water use in Punjab" *Agricultural Economic Research Review*, Vol. 23, July-December, pp. 273-284.

Kaur, S. and K. Vatta (2015). "Groundwater Depletion in Central Punjab: Pattern, Access and Adaptations", *Current Science*, Vol.108 (4), pp. 485-490.

Kulkarni H, and M. Shah (2013). "Punjab Water Syndrome-Diagnostics and Prescriptions" *Economic and Political Weekly*, XLVIII (52).

M. B. Peoples, J. K. Ladha, D. F. Herridge (1995). "Enhancing legume N_2 fixation through plant and soil management" Developments in Plant and Soil Sciences, Vol. 174, pp. 83-101.

Shergill, H.S (2007). "Sustainability of wheat-rice production in Punjab: A re-examination" *Economic and Political Weekly*, Dec 29, pp. 81-85.

Sidhu R.S., Vatta, Kamal and Dhaliwal, H. S. (2010). "Conservation agriculture in Punjab: economic implications of technologies and practices" *Indian Journal of Agricultural Economics*, Vol. 53, 3, pp. 1413- 27.

Sidhu, R. S. and Dhillion M. S. (1997). "Land and Water Resources in Punjab: Their Degradation and Technologies for Sustainable Use" *Indian Journal of Agricultural Economics*, Vol. 52, No 3, July-September, pp. 508-518.

Sukhwinder Singh, Julian Park and Jennie Litten-Brown (2011). "The economic sustainability of cropping systems in Indian Punjab: A farmers' perspective" Paper prepared for presentation at the International Congress, EAAE 2011.

World Bank (2003). "Resuming Punjab's Prosperity: The opportunities and Challenges ahead" Poverty Reduction and Economic Management Sector Unit, South Asia Region, World Bank, Washington. D.C., U.S.A.

Chapter 4
Agricultural Risk and Insurance in India

S.S. Raju, Ramesh Chand and Sonia Chauhan

Principal Scientist, Director and Senior Technical Officer respectively
ICAR- NIAP, New Delhi – 110 012

Introduction

Despite progress in irrigation and technology, the agricultural production and income are subject to large year-to-year fluctuations, playing havoc with farmers' income from farming. These fluctuations discourage investments in farming and also undermine the viability of agriculture sector and its potential to contribute to economic growth as well as food and nutritional security. Most of the studies on Indian agriculture have looked at the instability in agricultural production at aggregate level and have focused mainly on production (Hazell, 1982; Dev, 1987; Sharma *et al.,* 2006). These studies suffer from major limitation *i.e.* conceal the instability at disaggregate level when different parts forming the aggregate follow different distributions.

Agriculture production everywhere is vulnerable to natural forces like rainfall and temperature. As a result agricultural production deviates from normal trend. This instability in agricultural production imparts considerable risk to production and farm income and directly affects livelihood of farmers. It also affects the prevailing prices in the markets, which in turn affects the economy of the country as a whole. Instability in production is a major factor in causing price volatility which in turn has serious implications for food management, food security and economic stability of a country. The interest of researchers in instability analysis stems mainly from the fact that degree of vulnerability in production can be considerably reduced through technological intervention, infrastructure like irrigation, farm investments, choice of method of production, input use and management, and right set of policies. In order to develop effective strategy to deal with instability and its effects there is a need to have a clear picture of degree of instability at various levels and how it moved over time.

The paper estimates instability in major crops grown in the country and major states for the period of 1950-51 to 2010-11. The paper also analyses the progress and problems of national agricultural insurance scheme in country, examines the progress of various insurance schemes launched in the country from 1999-2000 onwards. Major issues and problems faced in implementing agricultural insurance in the country are discussed in detail.

Data and Methodology

The study estimates risk associated with crop production at state level by estimating instability index earlier used widely by Chand and Raju (Chand and Raju 2009; Chand *et al.,* 2011, Raju *et al.,* 2014) as under:

Instability index = Standard deviation of natural logarithm (Y_{t+1}/Y_t).

Where, Y_t is the crop area/production/yield in the current year and, Y_{t+1} represent the same in the next year. This index is unit free and very robust and it measures deviations from the underlying trend (log linear in this case). When there are no deviations from trend, the ratio Y_{t+1}/Y_t is constant, and thus standard deviation in it is zero. As the series fluctuates more, the ratio of Y_{t+1}/Y_t also fluctuates more, and standard deviation increases.

Data on important variables like area, production and yield of all major food crops and groups were compiled for the period 1950-51 to 2010-11 from Directorate of Economics and Statistics, Ministry of Agriculture, Government of India, New Delhi. In order to capture the impact of green revolution on stability of agriculture, we have divided the entire selected period into three phases and termed them as Pre-green revolution phase, Period of green revolution and post green revolution phase with wider dissemination of technology. Pre-green revolution is taken from 1950-51 to 1964-65. The food grains production seems to be abnormal for the years 1965-66 and 1966-67, so the next period is taken from 1967-68 to 1987-88, which we referred as green revolution phase. Post green revolution period is taken from 1988-89 to 2010-11. Detailed information about crop insurance was collected from the Agriculture Insurance Company of India Limited (AICL), New Delhi.

Results and Discussions

Inter year variation in area, production and yield of individual crops is presented in Table 4.1. It can be inferred from the Table 4.1 that green revolution has impacted the instability in desired direction. The instability of wheat, which is one of the most important staple food shows decline in instability after 1968 in all three respects. Area instability reduced by 27 per cent and almost same reduction is observed in yield instability after adoption of green revolution technology. Wider dissemination of technology and irrigation facility brought down the instability

Table 4.1: Instability in Area, Production, Yield and Irrigated Area of Selected Crops in different Periods from 1950–51 to 2010-11 at all India Level (Percent)

Crop	Area			Production			Yield			Area under Irrigation		
	1951-1966	1968-1988	1989-2011	1951-1966	1968-1988	1989-2011	1951-1966	1968-1988	1989-2011	1951-1966	1968-1988	1989-2011
Paddy	2.13	3.38	3.20	12.18	13.62	9.16	10.96	11.05	6.64	35.65	40.63	52.55
Wheat	6.61	4.59	3.34	12.93	8.97	6.67	10.56	6.58	4.75	34.29	65.99	87.12
Jowar	3.93	3.80	4.96	16.11	13.32	18.47	14.84	11.32	16.14	3.54	4.46	7.25
Bajra	5.89	10.10	10.61	18.30	39.54	38.67	15.32	32.55	29.88	2.97	5.02	7.15
Maize	3.44	3.06	2.62	10.81	18.44	12.99	9.19	16.74	11.52	12.49	18.49	21.83
Gram	8.05	10.42	14.29	20.14	21.68	20.19	17.95	16.94	10.66	13.21	16.62	27.09
Red gram	3.71	5.31	6.43	18.81	14.34	18.42	18.97	14.28	16.41	0.49	1.84	4.81
Groundnut	9.52	4.12	7.00	14.07	23.00	32.93	15.19	20.18	29.51	2.39	10.71	18.87
R/Mustard	7.97	9.66	13.69	20.31	21.26	21.07	20.98	18.20	15.33	10.34	41.68	66.86
Coconut	3.12	3.11	2.93	7.21	6.87	12.87	5.82	5.81	12.85	–	–	–
Cotton	5.71	4.76	7.12	17.25	16.51	17.92	15.31	14.52	15.57	12.21	24.94	34.75
Sugarcane	10.90	9.27	8.94	14.67	11.64	10.86	9.47	6.78	4.85	68.25	79.19	90.89
Potato	3.70	6.95	5.84	16.24	14.00	13.43	13.81	10.72	11.39	–	–	–
Tobacco	11.17	10.48	14.95	15.24	13.29	19.16	9.35	7.29	8.08	16.23	29.86	45.64

of paddy after 1988 onwards. Maize shows lowest instability in area, whereas, Bajra shows the maximum among all the selected cereals. Instability in production and yield of Bajra remained almost double as compared to pre green revolution period. Maize production variability registered sharp decline after 1988 because of reduction in yield instability. Instability in jowar yield, production and area showed decline during second phase but a big increase is registered in third period of wider dissemination of technology.

Among pulses, instability in area under gram increased over time whereas yield instability declined over time. The yield instability was reduced by 37 per cent after 1988. Because of these counteracting factors instability in production of gram in all the three phases remained around 21 per cent. Area under red gram also shows increase in instability over time but its yield instability show decline during green revolution period which again increased in post green revolution period. The variability in Red gram output came down from 18.8 during 1951-1966 to 14.34 during 1968-1988 which again increased to 18.42 during 1989–2011.

Within oilseeds group of crops, area instability in the case of groundnut declined to less than half during second phase and then increased by almost 70 per cent after 1988. Variability in its productivity increased by 33 per cent between first and second period which further increased by 46 per cent between second and third phase. Almost similar trend was observed for production instability. In the case rapeseed and mustard area instability experienced substantial increase over time but yield instability registered decline in all the phases and production shows inter year variability of about 21 per cent.

Coconut registers decline in inter year variation in area but instability in output and productivity increased in the recent period. Sugarcane is another crop which shows decline in instability in all respects over all time periods. Yet production and productivity of sugarcane appears to be more stable than area. Area under cotton witnessing decline during green revolution period as compared to pre green revolution but after that it registered increase of 50 per cent. Variability in cotton productivity varied around 15 per cent and output around 18 per cent with little change between different periods.

In case of potato, area instability is much higher in green revolution period as compared to pre green revolution period. Modern technology has some impact on the cultivation of potato and its area instability come down during post green revolution period. However, its production shows decline in instability over time and productivity register marginal increase in post green revolution period. Variability in area and production of tobacco followed a small decline in the phase of green revolution, but it increased sharply during post green revolution period.

It may be concluded here that crops which are grown under irrigated conditions register low instability in their production. Sugarcane and wheat area covered under irrigation is nearly 90 per cent and for paddy it is around 53 per cent. Whereas, area under irrigation is 7-16 per cent for the coarse cereals. Among pulses, 27 per cent area is irrigated under gram and for red gram it is around 5 per cent (Table 4.1).

Instability at State Level

Different types of agricultural conditions are prevailing in different states of India. Therefore variation in instability and growth in crop production is expected across states. State level analysis focuses on instability and growth in area, production and yield for foodgrains. The entire period 1967-68 to 2010-11 is divided into two sub period. First period of green revolution 1967-68 to 1987-88 and second 1988-89 to 2010-11 as post green revolution period with wider dissemination of technology respectively. The results are presented in Table 4.2.

Table 4.2: State-wise Instability in Food Grains Production during 1968-2011 (Per cent)

State	Period	Instability			Growth Rates		
		Area	Production	Yield	Area	Production	Yield
Andhra Pradesh	I	5.99	12.94	8.87	−0.86	2.48	3.37
	II	8.14	17.75	10.96	−0.14	2.27	2.42
Assam	I	4.91	12.16	9.65	0.96	1.57	0.61
	II	3.68	8.95	5.84	−0.20	1.13	1.33
Bihar	I	5.33	16.43	12.57	−0.32	1.30	1.63
	II	3.78	15.77	13.53	−1.17	0.69	1.88
Gujarat	I	14.29	40.47	28.53	−0.92	0.73	1.66
	II	15.93	42.59	28.35	−0.25	2.38	2.64
Haryana	I	9.91	17.54	12.38	0.22	4.22	3.99
	II	7.75	11.11	6.76	0.84	2.72	1.86
Himachal Pradesh	I	2.27	13.73	12.86	0.43	0.63	0.20
	II	1.98	19.29	18.40	−0.43	−0.01	0.43
Jammu and Kashmir	I	1.60	12.20	11.78	0.63	1.38	0.74
	II	1.59	10.29	10.74	0.19	0.58	0.39
Karnataka	I	10.74	22.32	13.41	0.32	1.13	0.81
	II	4.82	18.83	16.11	0.44	2.33	1.88
Kerala	I	3.28	6.07	4.39	−1.96	−0.91	1.07
	II	3.82	8.15	5.48	−4.98	−3.65	1.40
Madhya Pradesh	I	2.49	19.84	18.55	0.42	2.21	1.79
	II	4.59	20.17	16.27	−0.12	0.80	0.92
Maharashtra	I	8.18	27.44	20.08	0.62	3.28	2.64
	II	5.38	21.60	18.65	−0.66	0.37	1.03
Odisha	I	4.50	21.92	18.14	1.11	1.40	0.29
	II	6.66	28.82	24.73	−0.99	0.27	1.28
Punjab	I	3.58	5.00	5.11	2.16	5.59	3.35
	II	1.81	4.92	4.10	0.75	1.83	1.07

Contd...

Table 4.2–Contd...

State	Period	Instability			Growth Rates		
		Area	Production	Yield	Area	Production	Yield
Rajasthan	I	10.92	27.89	21.34	–0.08	2.00	2.08
	II	17.54	38.88	23.88	0.50	2.69	2.18
Tamil Nadu	I	10.17	22.76	15.03	–1.17	–0.32	0.86
	II	7.70	18.98	14.24	–1.48	–1.02	0.47
Uttar Pradesh	I	2.18	14.78	13.73	0.34	3.78	3.42
	II	2.84	8.34	6.59	0.08	1.38	1.30
West Bengal	I	4.69	15.83	12.94	–0.08	1.49	1.58
	II	4.44	6.51	5.21	–0.18	1.51	1.69
India	I	3.49	9.90	7.56	0.19	2.57	2.38
	II	3.30	8.80	5.83	–0.08	1.42	1.50

Source: Agricultural Statistics at a Glance, various issues, Directorate of Economics and Statistics, Ministry of Agriculture, GoI.

Note: Period I is 1968-88 and Period II is 1989-2011.

As already discussed instability in food grains area, production and productivity declined in second phase as compared to first phase at Country level. At state level, 10 out of 17 major states exhibit similar pattern. Gujarat registered highest instability in area under food grains during green revolution period. Rajasthan, Karnataka and Tamil Nadu are the next states in order according to area under food grains instability. During post green revolution period, Gujarat and Rajasthan exchanged their ranks and witnessed increase in instability, whereas, Karnataka and Tamil Nadu followed decline in year to year variation. Andhra Pradesh, Kerala, Madhya Pradesh, Orissa, Rajasthan and Uttar Pradesh are the other states which register increase in variation in area under food grains during 1988-89 to 2010-11. Andhra Pradesh, Kerala, Orissa and Rajasthan are the states, which witnessed increase in area instability in second period as compared to first period also witnessed increase in instability in production and productivity of food grains.

Punjab witnessed highest growth in the food grains production in green revolution period, whereas, Haryana registered highest growth in the food grains production in the post green revolution period. Haryana witnessed significant decline in the production instability over the first period. Karnataka and West Bengal are the states which showed increase in growth rates of food grains production and decline in instability in second period as compared to first period. Andhra Pradesh, Himachal Pradesh, Kerala, Madhya Pradesh and Orissa states are registering decline in growth and increase in instability of food grains production in post green revolution period over green revolution period.

Most of the selected states registered decline in instability of production of food grains over time but Andhra Pradesh, Himachal Pradesh, Kerala, Odisha and Rajasthan are the states which showed more than 30 per cent increase in instability in production of food grains in second period as compared to first period. Production of Punjab seems to be most stable followed by Madhya Pradesh. Production of food grains in Assam, Haryana, Uttar Pradesh and West Bengal turned more stable in the second period. Instability in production remained very high - to the tune of 40 per cent in Gujarat and Rajasthan. Karnataka, Maharashtra, Orissa, Rajasthan and Tamil Nadu are the states which exceeded scale of 20 in instability. Orissa, which is located in high rainfall eastern region, shows high instability like dry-land arid region states.

Himachal Pradesh witnessed highest increase in yield variability over the time followed by Odisha. Karnataka, Kerala and Andhra Pradesh are the other states which registered increase in instability more than 20 per cent over pre green revolution period. West Bengal, Uttar Pradesh and Haryana were able to bring down yield instability to less than half after 1988.

Adoption of new agricultural technology of green revolution period and its wider dissemination after 1987-88 have affected instability in area and production differently. In the case of cereals, pulses and food grains, there is a clear evidence of decline in inter year variation in yield in the green revolution period which gained momentum in the post green revolution period. However, spread and progress in agricultural technology did not help in reducing instability in area under cereals and pulses at country level. Even irrigation expansion, which helped in reducing yield variability, did not reduce instability in area. One reason for this could be increase in cropping intensity which is more sensitive to weather aberrations than net cultivated area. In the case of oilseeds, area as well as productivity witnessed increase in inter year variation throughout. Thus, none of the factors like irrigation, technology could help in reducing risk in oil seed production in the country.

At the level of individual crops both technology as well as irrigation has played a vital role in determining the level of instability. Paddy and wheat which benefitted most from green revolution technology and state support have turned least risky. Instability in crops like jowar and bajra remained very high. Maize shows decline in inter year deviations from the underlying trend in all respects, after 1988, matching with spread of improved technology. This again demonstrate big role of technology particularly hybrids and irrigation in stabilization of production. Groundnut shows worst performance with big increase in production instability. Even in the case of cotton there was no improvement in production risk.

Among states Gujarat faced highest instability in food grain production closely followed by Rajasthan and Odisha. Andhra Pradesh, Himachal Pradesh and Odisha also show big increase in production instability after 1987-88. The state level data doesn't reveal clear pattern of association between instability and growth.

The states which were well endowed with irrigation facility adopted new technology faster and achieved higher growth in output. At the same time convincing evidence on the impact of green revolution technology in reducing instability in total agricultural production has been lacking though productivity of some crops became very stable. It is inferred that the spread of improved technology, over wider area, brings stability to agriculture production. As the fluctuations in agricultural output remain high in most of the crops, there is a need to strengthen and develop effective instruments of crop insurance to help farmers cope up with production risk. Country also needs stabilization strategy to deal with consequences of high instability in production.

Crop Insurance in India

National Agricultural Insurance Scheme (NAIS) 1999-DATE

The National Agricultural Insurance Scheme (NAIS) was introduced in the country from the *rabi* season of 1999-2000. Agricultural Insurance Company of India Ltd (AIC) which was incorporated in December, 2002, and started operating from April, 2003, took over the implementation of NAIS. This scheme is available to both loanees and non-loanees. It covers all food grains, oilseeds and annual horticultural/ commercial crops for which past yield data are available for an adequate number of years. Among the annual commercial and horticultural crops, sugarcane, potato, cotton, ginger, onion, turmeric, chillies, coriander, cumin, jute, tapioca, banana and pineapple, are covered under the scheme. The scheme is operating on the basis of both *'area approach'*, for widespread calamities, and *'individual approach'*, for localized calamities such as cyclone and floods.

The premium rates applicable on the sum insured are:

Bajra and oilseeds   : 3.5 per cent

Other *kharif* crops   : 2.5 per cent

Wheat   : 1.5 per cent

Other *rabi* crops   : 2.0 per cent

Annual commercial/horticultural crops: Actuarial rate

Initially, the premium in the case of small and marginal farmers was subsidized @ 50 per cent, which was shared equally by the Government of India and the concerned State/UT. The premium subsidy was to be phased out over a period of five years, at present 10 per cent subsidy was provided on the premium payable by small and marginal farmers. At present, the NAIS is being implemented by all the states except Arunachal Pradesh, Manipur, Mizoram, Nagaland and Punjab. These 5 states did not join the NAIS and extend different reasons for not joining the scheme. For example, NEH region states were interested in covering perennial horticultural crops under NAIS. Similarly, Punjab was not interested in multi-peril crop insurance and wanted insurance cover against hailstorm only with higher indemnity limits.

During the last 13 years of its implementation, the scheme covered 9-18 per cent farmers, 8-18 per cent crop area and 2.22 -4.49 per cent of crop output in value terms in different years (Table 4.3). The amount of claims was much higher than the premium paid, indicating a loss in the operation of this scheme. During 2000-01 and 2002-03, the claims were more than five times of the premium paid. During 2003-04 to 2007-08, the amount of claims was more than double the amount of premium collected. As claims exceeded premiums, there was a net loss in the scheme, even without considering administrative cost. The magnitude of loss can also be seen by comparing the ratio of 'claims to sum assured' with ratio of 'premium to sum assured'. During the year 2012-13, claims constituted 10.85 per cent as against 3.07 per cent premium on the sum assured. This implies a loss of 7.78 per cent of the assured value of output. The scheme is not financially viable, as it depends on government for subsidization. The claim to premium ratio is still very high. The question is posed that if disaster strikes how the government will manage the claims? Second, though the area yield approach minimizes or eliminates the problem of moral hazards, but problem of adverse selection seems to be affecting the existing NAIS as indicated by higher claim ratio or loss ratio for non loanee farmers. Third, there is inordinate delay in settling the claims in the event of crop failures.

Table 4.3: Performance of National Agricultural Insurance Scheme

Year	Farmers Covered Per cent	Area Covered (Per cent GCA)	Sum Assured as Per cent of Value of Crop Output	Claims Ratio (Claims/ Premium)	Premium/ Sum Assured (Per cent)	Claims/ Sum Assured (Per cent)
1999-00 (*Rabi*)	0.50	0.41	0.09	1.60	1.40	2.25
2000-01	9.09	8.73	2.28	5.45	2.76	15.06
2001-02	9.23	8.42	2.22	1.91	3.24	6.20
2002-03	10.48	11.12	2.92	5.52	3.23	17.84
2003-04	10.73	9.88	2.46	3.29	3.11	10.22
2004-05	14.04	15.53	3.70	2.24	3.16	7.06
2005-06	14.45	14.56	3.55	2.53	2.97	7.52
2006-07	15.51	14.32	3.72	2.98	3.03	8.53
2007-08	13.90	14.42	3.59	2.53	2.79	7.05
2008-09	14.29	13.56	3.53	4.81	3.01	14.50
2009-10	17.57	17.52	4.49	4.46	2.99	13.34
2010-11	12.81	16.98	3.30	2.24	2.94	6.57
2011-12	12.19	16.52	3.00	2.17	2.80	6.07
2012-13	11.96	16.97	3.27	3.54	3.07	10.85

Source: Authors' calculation based on data taken from Economic Survey 2013-14.

National Accounts Statistics 2014 and AICL 2015.

The Scheme was continued till *Kharif* 2013, however, some States are allowed to implement NAIS during *Rabi* 2013-14 also.

Pilot Modified National Agricultural Insurance Scheme (MNAIS)

(Being implemented on full-fledged basis from *Rabi* 2013-14)

With a view to make the scheme simpler and more farmer friendly, a Joint Group was constituted in 2004 under the Chairmanship of Additional Secretary in the Department of Agriculture and Cooperation to study the improvements required in the then existing NAIS. Based on the recommendations of the Joint Group and views/comments of various stake-holders, a pilot proposal on MNAIS was prepared which was approved by Government of India for implementation on pilot basis in 50 districts from Rabi 2010-11 season. The major improved provisions/features of MNAIS over NAIS are as under:

☆ Reduction in unit area of Insurance for major crops to village/village panchayat,

☆ Actuarial premium rates for insuring crops and hence claims liability is on Insurance Company, private insurance companies have also been involved for implementation to provide competitive service to the farmers.

☆ Higher subsidy in premium ranging upto 75 per cent to all farmers,

☆ More proficient basis for calculation of threshold yield (average yield of last 7 years excluding up to two years of declared natural calamity)

☆ Higher minimum indemnity level of 70 per cent instead of 60 per cent in NAIS,

☆ Indemnity amount for prevented sowing/planting risks and for post-harvest losses due to cyclones.

☆ On account payment up to 25 per cent of likely claims as advance for providing immediate relief to farmers during adverse season,

☆ An individual assessment of claims in case of specified localized calamity *viz.* hailstorm, landslide,

☆ Uniform seasonality norms for both loanee and non loanee farmers,

Weather Based Crop Insurance Scheme (WBCIS)

During the year 2003-04 the private sector came out with some insurance products in agriculture based on weather parameters. The insurance losses due to vagaries of weather, *i.e.* excess or deficit rainfall, aberrations in sunshine, temperature and humidity, etc. could be covered on the basis of weather index. If the actual index of a specific weather event is less than the threshold, the claim becomes payable as a percentage of deviation of actual index. One such product, namely Rainfall Insurance was developed by ICICI-Lombard General Insurance Company. This move was followed by IFFCO-Tokio General Insurance Company and by public sector Agricultural Insurance Company of India (AIC). Under the scheme, coverage for deviation in the rainfall index is extended and compensations for economic losses due to less or more than normal rainfall are paid.

Agricultural Insurance Company of India (AIC) introduced rainfall insurance (VarshaBima) during 2004 South-West Monsoon period. Varsha Bima provided for five different options suiting varied requirements of farming community. These are (1) seasonal rainfall insurance based on aggregate rainfall from June to September, (2) sowing failure insurance based on rainfall between 15th June and 15th August, (3) rainfall distribution insurance with the weight assigned to different weeks between June and September, (4) agronomic index constructed based on water requirement of crops at different pheno-phases and (5) catastrophic option, covering extremely adverse deviations of 50 per cent and above in rainfall during the season.

With the objective to bring more farmers under the fold of Crop Insurance, a Pilot Weather Based Crop Insurance Scheme (WBCIS) was launched in 20 States in 2007. Apart from Agricultural Insurance Company of India, some private companies have also been allowed to implement the Scheme. The WBCIS is intended to provide insurance protection to the farmers against adverse weather incidences, such as deficit and excess rainfall, high or low temperature, humidity etc. which are deemed to impact adversely the crop production. It has the advantage to settle the claims within shortest possible time. The WBCIS is based on actuarial rates of premium but to make the Scheme attractive, premium actually charged from farmers has been restricted at par with NAIS.

The Weather Based Crop Insurance Scheme (WBCIS) of AIC is a unique weather based insurance product designed to provide insurance protection against losses in crop yield resulting from adverse weather incidences. It provides payout against adverse rainfall incidence (both deficit and excess) during *kharif* and adverse incidence in weather parameters like frost, heat, relative humidity, un-seasonal rainfall etc., during *rabi*. It operates on the concept of area approach *i.e.*, for the purpose of compensation, a reference unit area shall be linked to a reference weather station on the basis of which weather data and claims would be processed. This scheme is available to both loanees (compulsory) and non-loanees (voluntary). The NAIS is not available for the locations and crops selected for WBCIS pilot. It has the advantage to settle the claims with the shortest possible time. Though, weather insurance coverage was limited, it holds lessons for future programmes. Important distinguishing features of weather insurance scheme and yield insurance scheme are presented in Table 4.4.

National Crop Insurance Programme (NCIP)

In order to serve farmers' needs in still better ways and to make crop insurance schemes more farmers' friendly, three pilot schemes of MNAIS, WBCIS and Coconut Palm Insurance Scheme (CPIS) have recently been evaluated. Based on the recommendations of evaluation studies, experience gained through implementation of crop insurance schemes and views of the stakeholders, states and appraisal agencies, various improvements/changes have been incorporated in these schemes and a Central Sector Scheme in the name of National Crop Insurance Programme (NCIP) has been formulated by merging MNAIS, WBCIS and CPIS (as its components) and rolling back NAIS.

Issues Related to Crop Insurance

The farming community at large does not seem to be satisfied with the partial expansion of scope and content of crop insurance scheme in the form of NAIS. There are issues relating to its operation, governance and financial sustainability. After extensive reviewing, gathering perceptions of the farming community and discussion with experts from AIC, agricultural department, bankers, academicians

Table 4.4: Comparison of Yield and Weather Insurance

Parameter	Yield Insurance	Weather Insurance
Scope of insurance cover	Covers yield shortfall	Covers anticipated shortfall in yield due to adverse weather parameters
Scope of perils covered	All natural and non-preventable perils	Rainfall, minimum and maximum temperature, soil moisture, relative humidity, sunlight, day length etc.
Target Group	All farmers growing insured crops	Farmers and others
Crops	All crops for which past yield data is available	All crops for which correlation is established between yield and weather parameters
Scheme Approach	Homogeneous area approach (Taluk/block/mandal)	Homogeneous area approach(Jurisdiction of rain gauge)
Scope for introduction of insurance	Can be introduced for all crops with yield data	Can be introduced successfully for crops with good sensitivity to weather parameters
Premium Rates	High	Relatively lower and flexible
Sum Insured	Loan amount/150 per cent of value of production	Flexible. Can range from input cost to value of production
Control on adverse selection/ moral hazard	Relatively less control	Almost complete control
Time taken for settlement of Claims	May range from 6-9 months from occurrence of loss	Within two weeks from close of indemnity period
Administrative set up	Relatively large	Relatively small
Transaction cost	High	Moderate and affordable
Transparency	Not transparent	Transparent and easily verifiable

and other representatives on the performance of NAIS, some modifications have been suggested in its designing to make it more effective and farmer- friendly.

Even several years after the initiation of first agriculture insurance project in 1972, the coverage and scope of agriculture insurance remains far from adequate, even-though the need for various forms of insurance for agriculture sector has been widely expressed. Some of the issues related to expansion of agriculture insurance and improving its effectiveness are discussed below.

Role of Government

As we all know, crop insurance to be successful requires public support. This could be in terms of subsidy on premium, meeting part of administrative expenditure, and reinsurance etc. Global experience shows that due to special nature of agriculture production, in several countries, premiums payable by farmers is subsidized by government. Agriculture in India is not just dependent on weather conditions, but also suffers the brunt of natural disasters. It will be quite in order for crop insurance to be regarded as a support measure in which government plays an important role, because of the benefit it provides not merely to the insured farmers, but to the entire national economy due to the forward and backward linkages with the rest of the economy. Society can significantly gain from more efficient sharing of crop and natural disaster risks. The principle behind the evaluation of crop insurance schemes all over the world is along these lines for receiving the active support and finance of the Government. Integrating the various risk mitigation methods and streamlining the funds not only injects accountability and professionalism into the system, but also increase economic efficiency. The support mechanism of major countries is given in the Table 4.5.

Government can facilitate agricultural insurance in several ways. In case farmers are asked to pay full premium themselves then chances of adoption of insurance are bleak. There is a need for some subsidization by government. It can provide information, on weather patterns, locations of farms and crops, incidence and history of perils and crop yields. It can help to meet the costs of the research to be undertaken before starting an agricultural insurance program. It can also provide reinsurance (Raju and Chand, 2010).

Conclusions

In spite of various schemes launched from time to time in the state, agriculture insurance has served very limited purpose. The coverage in terms of area and number of farmers is very small, payment of indemnity based on area approach miss affected farmers outside the compensated area, and most of the schemes are not viable. Expanding the coverage of crop insurance would therefore increase government costs considerably. Unless the programme is restructured carefully to make it viable, the prospects of its future expansion to include and impact more farmers is remote (Raju and Chand, 2010). This requires renewed efforts by Government in terms of designing appropriate mechanisms and providing financial support for agricultural insurance. Providing similar help to private sector insurers would help in increasing insurance coverage and in improving viability of the

Table 4.5: Crop Insurance Support Mechanism of Major Countries

Sl.No.	Country	Nature of Support
1.	USA(covered nearly 2 million out of total 8 million farmers and about 78 per cent of cropped area during 2003)	☆ Subsidy in premium (ranges from 38 per cent to 67 per cent; average for 2003 is 60 per cent) ☆ Reimbursement of administrative expenses of insurance companies (these were about 22 per cent of total cost of the program during 2003–04) ☆ Reinsurance support for risky crop lines ☆ Technical services in premium, policy guidelines ☆ Free insurance of catastrophic cover for resource poor farmers ☆ Non insured assistance to farmers for crops no insurance is available Over all subsidy is about 70-75 per cent
2.	Canada	☆ Subsidy in premiums (80-100 per cent for lower levels of coverage and 50-60 percent for higher levels of coverage) ☆ Significant contribution towards provincial administrative costs ☆ Provides deficit financing to provincial governments ☆ Technical services by setting premium ratesOver all subsidy is about 70 per cent
3.	Philippines	☆ Subsidy in premium (ranges from 50 per cent–60 per cent) ☆ Banks share premium of loanee farmers (15-20 per cent of total premium cost) ☆ Financial support to Philippines Crop Insurance Corporation (PCIC) in extreme adversities Over all subsidy is about 70 per cent for loanee farmers and about 50 per cent for non-loanee farmers
4.	Spain	☆ Subsidy in premium (average 58 per cent during 2003) ☆ Reinsurance support (50 per cent of reinsurance cost is paid by the government) ☆ Technical guidance Over all subsidy between 50-60 per cent

Source: Report of working group on Risk Management in Agriculture XI Five Year Plan 2007-2012.

insurance schemes over time. With the improved integration of rural countryside and communication network, the Unit area of insurance could be brought down to a village level. Insurance products for the rural areas should be simple in design and presentation so that they are easily understood. With increased commercialization of agriculture price fluctuations have become highly significant in affecting farmers' income. Accordingly, market risk is now quite important in affecting farmers' income. We feel that implementation of market insurance to cover price risk is much easier than yield insurance. There is lot of interest in private sector to invest in general insurance business. This opportunity can be used to allot some target to various general insurance companies to cover agriculture. To begin with, this target could be equal to the share of agriculture in national income.

References

Chand, Ramesh and Raju, S. S. (2008). Instability in Andhra Pradesh Agriculture – A Disaggregate Analysis. *Agricultural Economics Research Review*. 21(2): 283-288.

Chand, Ramesh and Raju, S. S. (2009). Instability in Indian agriculture during different phases of technology and policy. *Indian Journal of Agricultural Economics*. 64 (2): 187-207.

Dev, Mahendra S. (1987). Growth and instability in food gains production: An interstate analysis, *Economic and Political weekly*, 26 September:82-A 92.

Government of Madhya Pradesh (2014). Madhya Pradesh Agriculture Economic Survey, Department of Planning, Economics and Statistics.

Government of India (2011). Madhya Pradesh Development Report, Planning Commission, GoI, Published by Academic Foundation.

Hazell, Peter B.R. (1982). Instability in Indian Food grain Production, Research Report No. 30, International Food Policy Research Institute, Washington, DC, U.S.A.

Raju, S. S. and Chand, Ramesh (2007). Progress and Problems in Agricultural Insurance, *Economic and Political Weekly*. 42(21): 1905 – 1908.

Raju, S. S. and Chand, Ramesh (2008). A Study on the Performance of National Agricultural Insurance Scheme and Suggestions to make it more effective. *Agricultural Economics Research Review*. 21(1): 11-19.

Raju, S.S and Chand, Ramesh (2010). Agricultural Risk and Insurance in India: Problems and Prospects, Academic Foundation, New Delhi, 2009. p106.

Raju, S S, Chand, Ramesh and Chauhan, Sonia (2014). Instability in Indian Agriculture: An inter- state analysis, *Economic Affairs*:59 (Special Issue): 36-45.

Sharma, H.R., Singh, Kamlesh and Kumari, Shanta (2006). Extent and source of instability in food grains production in India, *Indian Journal of Agricultural Economics*, 61 (4): 648-666.

Chapter 5

Priority Setting in Indian Agriculture: Concept and Methods

Sant Kumar

ICAR-NIAP, New Delhi – 110 012

Background

Augmenting agricultural growth remains the key concern in India despite a continuous decline in the share of agricultural sector in India's gross domestic product less than 14 per cent in 2013-14 from 45 per cent in 1970-71. The significance of agriculture goes beyond its income contribution. The sector supports more than half of the country population directly, and engages millions of people indirectly in the secondary agriculture *i.e.* manufacturing and services. It is widely recognized that agricultural research has helped in increasing productivity, improving food security and reducing food prices (in real term) enabling millions of poor to have an affordable access to food (Chand *et al.*, 2012; Spielman and Pandya-Lorch, 2010; Kumar, 2001).

However, now agriculture sector is facing numerous and complex challenges of declining factor productivity, degrading soil and water resources, rising of food and energy prices, and increasing frequency of extreme climatic events. On the other hand, resources for research are scarce; India spends only about 0.6 per cent of its agricultural gross domestic product on agricultural research, much less than the average of about 2-2.5 per cent in developed countries (Beintema and Stads, 2008).

These challenges call for a careful allocation of scarce resources, so as to enhance research efficiency and improve food and nutrition security in a sustainable manner.

Priority setting exercises generate information that can aid in research resource allocation decisions whilst addressing these concerns in a more objective and transparent manner. Priority-setting is a process of making choices amongst a set of potential research activities given limited resources. Until recently, research resource allocation relied mainly on subjective assessments to manage technical constraints. However, considering the large size of the national agricultural research system (NARS) of India, emerging complex challenges and resource constraints, quantitative and formal method of assessing priorities using socio-economic data is needed to improve the allocation decisions.

Priority-setting is not a new for agricultural R&D managers. Research systems have followed either formal or informal methods of priority-setting to decide their current research agenda. Historically, the Indian agricultural research system under the aegis of the Indian Council of Agricultural Research (ICAR) and State Agricultural Universities (SAUs) have relied mainly on opinion of researchers in fixing research priorities to handle agricultural R&D issues. These decisions have formed the basis of research resource allocation choices. Analyses have demonstrated that these choices have been effective in generating high rates of returns to research investments in the past (Byerlee and Morris 1993; Alston *et al.*, 1999 and Evenson *et al.*, 1999). However, considering the size of research system and the complexities confronting, a more demand-driven, quantitative and formal method of priority-setting needed to improve the quality and transparency of complex resource allocation decisions. Quantitative method helps agricultural R&D managers in assessing research priorities objectively to achieve national goals.

Brief Overview of Priority Setting Approaches in Agriculture

Priority-setting in practice is a difficult and uncertain exercise characterized by making assumptions about futuristic trends. It is generally a multi-layer and multi-dimensional activity and sometimes involves several stakeholders. In view of emerging multiple conflicting challenges of efficiency, equity and sustainability, these exercises are an essential component of designing and managing research system. However, these require a large body of knowledge, foresightedness, stakeholders' involvement and methods to achieve the set goal. This section provides reviews on the issues and methods applied in setting research priorities in agriculture at various levels.

The early attempts in agriculture research priority-setting emphasized increasing production efficiency, thereby reducing cost of food production. However, a variety of other objectives were added over years related to equity and poverty alleviation such as farm size, per capita income, sustainability of natural resources, food security, climate change to name a few. For the past one decade or so, alleviating hunger and poverty and environmental security have been the overarching objectives/goals of priority-setting exercises across the board. The changing context of institutional and economic environment also needs to be considered in setting research priorities. For example, in view of growing importance of private investment in agricultural R&D, the role of the public sector needs to be redefined. It is argued that applied and adaptive research for commercial crops should be financed privately, either through private firms or collectively by farmers. Moreover, public sector should focus on those crops, regions, and farmers that would be by-passed by private sector, especially poorer farmers. Growing poverty and its magnitude has also drawn attention regarding resource allocation.

Therefore, in the framework of resource constraints and often multiple conflicting goals like efficiency, sustainability, equity, etc. focused research agenda becomes necessary. Using a comprehensive, transparent and robust approach is, therefore, essential. The purpose is not to overlook scientific judgment but to strengthen the decision-making process by augmenting and organizing the available information.

Priority setting is carried out explicitly or implicitly in all research programs through allocation of resources across commodities, regions, disciplines, problems, and types of technology (Anderson and Parton, 1983). In agricultural research organizations, priority setting occurs at various levels of decision making – most commonly at national, program, sub-program and project levels. Resource allocation decisions vary depending on the level at which priorities are set. Table 5.1 shows the types of decisions that are typically made at each level of priority setting.

Table 5.1: Simplified View of Decision Levels for Priority Setting in National Research Organizations

Decision	Decision Type	Common Decision-Making Bodies in Supply-Led Approach
National	By program (commodity, factor). Sometimes by regions across programs	Supreme research body such as agricultural research council or board
Program	By sub-program (disciplinary or technology type) and by region within programs	Research program coordinator or institute director
Sub-program	By project (technology type and characteristics)	Sub-program leader or departmental head
Project	By technology characteristics	Lead scientist for project

Source: Adapted from Byerlee (1999).

Priority-setting employs a set of methods that can be broadly classified into supply-driven and demand-driven, though a combination of methods are often used. In supply-driven mode, priorities are largely set in within the research system. A variety of methods could be used from informal approaches based on previous allocations (*i.e.* precedence), discussions and concerns among research managers taking into account national agricultural strategies, and formal quantitative methods, using scoring approach, congruence or economic analysis. In demand-driven framework, priorities are determined considering the perspectives of major stakeholders/donor agencies, especially outside the research system. These might employ consultative or participatory methods or users themselves be empowered to make decisions on research priorities (*i.e.* through representation in governance of research system).

There are many priority-setting methods proposed in the economic literature, *e.g.,* Shumway (1973), Norton and Davis (1981), Ruttan (1982), Anderson and Parton (1983), Parton, Anderson and Makeham (1984), Norton and Pardey (1987), Norton *et al.* (1992), Raitzer and Norton (2009), but few have been put into practice in the decision making process of the National Agricultural Research Systems. A crucial factor in the non-use of formal methods has been the lack of rigorous cost effective procedure which can incorporate a large number of commodities, research areas, multiple goals and the criteria found in most decision making situations.

The methods reported for agricultural research-priority-setting can be grouped into five categories: (i) scoring model, (ii) benefit-cost analysis, (iii) programming approach, (iv) simulation models, and (v) econometric models. A description of these methods and their merits and demerits is given below:

Scoring/Weighted Criteria Model

The scoring model is a shortcut method to incorporate multiple criteria (*i.e.* contribution of commodities or type of research) in identifying priority for the research system. Criteria may be qualitative or quantitative in nature. Information on commodities or research area may be collected on each criterion from primary and secondary sources. Finally, weights are assigned to criteria to obtain priority ranking by commodity or research area. Thus, it can be used to rank commodities or research areas according to their overall contribution to research objectives.

The credibility of a scoring model is largely determined by how rigorous ranking criteria are defined and measured. For example, carefully measured economic efficiency scores (derived from benefit/cost or economic surplus analysis) can be combined with carefully defined and measured equity criteria. Unfortunately, some scoring exercises are undertaken as substitute for systematic investment in information and analysis. The results may then be useful in building consensus within a given group of decision makers. But they may possess little external credibility.

Scoring model can be implemented in relatively short span of time and is transparent and facilitates the understanding of research administrators. Scoring model can be used to rank a long list of commodities and research areas, including a nonproduction-oriented research. These models are often criticized because of their subjective weighting of objectives. Applications of these models are found in several studies in the United States (Mahlstede, 1971) Argentia (Moscardi, 1987), The Gambia (Sompo, 1989) and TAC review of priority and strategy for CGIAR (1992).

Economic Surplus Approach

This method is simply a refinement of benefit-cost analysis method. In this method benefits to research investment are estimated (generally, an average rate of return) by estimating the benefits from research in terms of consumer and producer surpluses that result from technological change. *Ex-ante* analysis usually incorporates expert opinion to determine projected research impacts, adoption rates and probabilities of research success and provides estimates of economic efficiency and distributional implications of agricultural research resource allocation.

Economic surplus estimates are less transparent to non-economists. Sometimes an individual participating in the decision-making process intended to attribute results to the economic model and not to the data and assumptions to the technology generation and adoption underlying the model. Application of economic surplus methods, therefore, requires a well developed socioeconomic research capacity.

A major advantage of economic surplus model is its ability to incorporate concurrent changes in the commodity system in the evaluation framework (*e.g.* population growth, income changes, area expansion, research spillover, and changes in external and internal trade policies). A thorough review of economic surplus methods and possible extension for research priority-setting is provided in Science and Scarcity by Alston *et al.* (1995). This method can be difficult to apply to a large number of commodities or research areas because types of data necessary for the analysis usually do not exist for all the commodities. It is also not well suited to rank non-commodity research areas. Applications of this method are found in Peru (Norton *et al.*, 1987).

Programming Models

Programming models optimize mathematically research objective function or multiple goal function, subject to a given set of resources and other constraints of research system. They have the advantage of explicitly incorporating the budget, human resource and other constraints in the system. Like scoring method, they accommodate multiple objectives. If constructed in a multi-period format, they can guide how the research portfolio should change over time. These models are generally used in priority setting at program level by optimizing research program portfolios. Programming models can also be used in context of priority setting and research resource allocation (Alston *et al.*, 1995). However, they require a great deal of analytical ability, data and time. Use of mathematical programming model used in agricultural research resource allocation are reported by Russel (1975), De Wit (1988), Scobie and Jacobsen (1992), Multangadura and Norton (1999).

Simulation Models

In simulation models, mathematical relationships among variables are exposed to different scenarios to assess the best outcome. They can incorporate many factors that affect research priorities, such as multiple goals, research constraints, socioeconomic variables, risk and uncertainty.

These models are flexible and can be constructed as relatively simple or complex tools and can readily include probabilistic information. Their major disadvantage is that, to be useful they must be relatively complex and typically require extensive data set and time of skilled analysts. Anderson Pinstrup and Franklin (1977), Lu, Quance and Liu (1978), Berger (2001) and Yates *et al.* (2005) have use this method.

Econometric Methods

Econometric models assess the research contribution in production of commodities both in ex-ante and ex-post format. To be useful in *ex-ante* analysis, econometric methods must be applied with a high degree of disaggregation and good historical data on production, farm inputs and research expenditures.

Numerous studies have estimated models like production functions, supply functions, profit functions, etc. to evaluate impact of agricultural research. While these results have been used to justify additional research funds for particular commodity, no research system has systematically used the results of comprehensive econometric analysis for all its major commodities to determine research priorities.

Table 5.2: Comparison among Research Priority Setting Methods

Sl.No.	Features	Sc	ES	Si	MP
1.	Requires explicit elicitation of goals	Yes	No	No	Yes
2.	Determines distributional effects on consumers and producers at various income levels	No	Yes	Yes	No
3.	Considers trade-off among goals	Yes	Sometimes	Yes	Yes
4.	Evaluate benefits to "aggregate" research	No	Yes	Yes	Yes
5.	Evaluate benefits to commodity research	Yes	Yes	Yes	Yes
6.	Evaluate benefits to non-production or non-commodity oriented research	Yes	Difficult	Sometimes	Yes
7.	Provides ranking of research projects based on multiple goals	Yes	No	No	Yes
8.	Quantifies spillovers	No	Yes	Yes	No
9.	Relative ease of comprehension by decision makers	High	Medium	Low	Low

Note: Sc: Scoring; ES: Economic surplus; Si: Simulation method; MP: Mathematical programming.

Source: Jha *et al.* (1995).

There is no single method that is suitable in all the situations. Each one has merits and demerits that affect its suitability for specific evaluation purpose, and in fact, it may be appropriate to combine different methods. The scoring and economic surplus methods have been used frequently in deciding priorities. Table 5.2 presents comparison among major *ex-ante* priority-setting methods. However, the best method for specific case should include the following three characteristics: (i) efficient use of the information available, (ii) compatibility with the human resources available, and (iii) result in outputs that are clearly understood by the decision-makers and used to allocate resources between themes.

References

Alston, J.M., G.W. Norton and P.G. Pardey (1995). Science under Scarcity: Principles and Practice for Agricultural Research Evaluation and Priority Setting. Ithaca and London: Cornell University Press.

Alston, J.M., P.G. Paredey and V.H. Smith (eds.) (1999). Paying for Agricultural Productivity. John Hopkins University Press, Baltimore and London.

Anderson, J. R. and K.A. Parton (1983). Techniques for guiding the allocation of resources among rural research projects: The state of the art. Prometheus 1(1):180-201.

Anderson, Per Pinstrup and D. Franklin (1977). A Systems Approach to Agricultural Research Resources Allocation in Developing Countries. In: *Resource Allocation and Productivity in National and International Research*, C.T.M. Arndt, D.G. Dalrymple and V.W. Ruttan (eds.) Minneapolis, Minnesota.

Byerlee, Derek (1999). Targeting Poverty Alleviation in Priority Setting in National Research Organizations: Theory and Practice. Paper presented in the CIAT International Workshop, '*Assessing the Impact of Research on Poverty Alleviation*', September 14-16, San Jose, Costa Rica.

Byerlee, Derek and M. Moris (1993). Have we invested in research for marginal environments? The example of wheat breeding in developing countries. *Food Policy*. 18:381-393.

Evenson, R.E. C. Pray and M.W. Rosegrant (1999). Agricultural Research and Productivity Growth in India. Research Report 109, Washington, IFPRI.

Jha, Dayanatha, Praduman Kumar, Mruthyunjay, Suresh Pal, S. Selvarajan and Alka Singh (2005). *Research Priorities in Indian Agriculture*. Policy Paper 3, New Delhi National Centre for Agricultural Economics and Policy Research.

Lu, Y., and L. Quance and C.L. Liu (1978). Projecting Agricultural Productivity and its Economic Impact. *American Journal of Agricultural Economics*, 60 (4): 976-980.

Multangadura, Gladys and G.W. Norton (1999). Agricultural Research Priority Setting Under Multiple Objectibes: An Example from Zimbambe. *Agricultural Economics*, 20(3):277-286.

Norton, G. W., V.G. Ganoza and C. Pomareda (1987). Potential Benefits for Agricultural Research and Extension in Peru. *American Journal of Agricultural Economics*, 69: 247-257.

Norton, G.W. and J.S. Davis (1981). Evaluating Returns to Agricultural Research: A Review, *American Journal of Agricultural Economics*, 63 (4): 685-99.

Norton G.W. and P.G. Pardey (1987). Priority Setting Mechanisms for National Agricultural Research Systems: Present Experience and Future Needs, Working paper No.7, International Service for National Agricultural Research, The Hague.

Norton, G.W., P.G. Pardey and J.M. Alston (1992). Economic Issues in Agricultural Research Priority Setting. *American Journal of Agricultural Economics*, 74(5):1089-1094.

Raitzer, David A. and G.W. Norton (2009). Prioritizing Agricultural Research for Development: Experiences and Lessons (eds.) CAB international, Wallingford/Cambridge.

Russel, D.G. (1975). Resource Allocation in Agricultural Research Using Socio-economic Evaluation and Mathematical Models. *Canadian Journal of Agricultural Economics*, 23 (2): 29:52.

Ruttan, V.W. (1982). Agricultural Research Policy, University of Minnesota Press, Minneapolis, USA.

Scobie, G.M. and V. Jacobsen (1992). Allocation of R and D Funds in Australian Wool Industry. Hamilton, New Zealand: Department of Economics, University of Waikato.

Shumway, C.R. (1973). Allocation of Scarce Resources to Agricultural Research: Review of Methodology. *American Journal of Agricultural Economics*, 55(4):547-58.

Yates, David, Jack Sieber, davi Purkey and Annetee Huber Lee (2005). WEAP21— A Demand-, Priority-, and Preference-Driven Water Planning Model, Water International, 30 (4): 487:500.

Chapter 6

Simultaneous Equations: Theory and Applications in Agriculture

Smita Sirohi[1] and Bishwa Bhaskar Choudhary[2]

[1]Head and Principal Scientist, [2]Ph.D. Scholar,
Division of Dairy Economics, Statistics & Management,
ICAR-National Dairy Research Institute, Karnal – 132 001, Haryana

Introduction

Regression analysis has been extensively used in agriculture and allied sciences for modeling crop production, analyzing market behavior, yield prediction, price forecasting, *etc.* For the estimation of regression equation using the method of ordinary least squares (OLS), it is assumed that the explanatory variables are non-stochastic. In other words, it means that if we repeated the regression with a new sample, the values of the explanatory variables would remain the same, but the dependent variable would be different because the new sample would contain new values for the disturbance term. While such an assumption might sound realistic for an experiment in the physical sciences, in life sciences and social sciences most data cannot be repeated. In practice, the non-stochasticity assumption is unrealistic since the explanatory variables will themselves be determined by other relationships. This lecture note discusses in brief the key points in the technique of estimation when one or more explanatory variables instead of being exogenous are determined in simultaneity with other variables.

Simultaneous Equation Bias: Inconsistency of OLS Estimators

It is important to understand why the method of least squares may not be applied to estimate a single equation embedded in a system of simultaneous equations? When an explanatory variable is contemporaneously correlated with the disturbance term, the OLS estimator are both biased and inconsistent. One reason why contemporaneous correlation might occur in a model is because the relationship between two variables is simultaneous. Biasedness implies that the average or expected value of the estimated parameters is not equal to the true value of the population parameter. Inconsistency means that the variance of the estimated parameter does not tend to zero as sample size n tends to infinity. In simple words, biasedness and inconsistency render the estimated parameters as unreliable for any meaningful interpretation as they do not converge to their true population values no matter how large the sample size.

Identification of Equations

Before going to the estimation of the simultaneous relationships, it is important to separate endogenous from exogenous variables. For example, consider the most basic partial equilibrium supply and demand functions could be written as Q = S(P, W) and Q = D(P, Y) with W denoting the price of important factors of production and Y the income level of potential demanders. Here Q and P are endogenous while W and Y are exogenous.

For the estimation of the relationship, both the endogenous variables should be expressed in terms of exogenous variables only. The equations forming the original model are described as its *structural* equations. The equations that describe how the endogenous variables are really determined are the *reduced form* equations.

The identification problem asks whether one can obtain unique numerical estimates of the structural coefficients from the estimated reduced form coefficients. If this can be done, an equation in a system of simultaneous equations is identified. If this cannot be done, that equation is un- or under-identified. An identified equation can be just or over identified. In the former case, unique values of structural coefficients can be obtained; in the latter, there may be more than one value for one or more structural parameters. The identification problem arises because the same set of data may be compatible with different sets of structural coefficients, that is different models. Thus, in the regression of price on quantity only, it is difficult to tell whether one is estimating the supply function or the demand function, because price and quantity enter both equations.

Order Condition of Identification

A necessary (but not sufficient) of identification, known as order condition can be stated in two different equivalent ways:

1. In a model of M simultaneous equation in order for an equation to be identified, it must exclude at least M-1 variables (endogenous as well as predetermined) appearing in the model. If it excludes exactly M-1

variables, the equation is just identified. If it excludes more than M-1 variables, it is over identified.

2. In a model of M simultaneous equation in order for an equation to be identified, the number of predetermined variables excluded from the equation must not be less than the number of endogenous variables included in that equation less 1, that is, K-k e" m-1. If K-k = m-1, the equation is just identified, but if K-k > m-1, it is over identified, where K is number of predetermined variables in the model including the intercept, k is number of predetermined variables in a given equation and m is the number of endogenous variables in a given equation.

Rank Condition of Identification

A necessary and sufficient condition for identification is provided by the rank condition whereby, in a model containing M equations in M endogenous variable, an equation is identified if and only if at least one nonzero determinant of order (M-1) (M-1) can be constructed from the coefficients of the variables (both endogenous and predetermined) excluded from the particular equation but included in the other equations of the model.

Estimation Approaches

Assuming that an equation in a simultaneous equation model is identified (either exactly or over-), there are several methods to estimate it, These methods fall into two broad categories: single-equation methods also known as limited information methods, and systems method, also known as full information methods. A detailed write-up on these methods is not feasible in this short lecture note and can be referred from any standard text-book of econometrics, here only a summary of the estimation approaches has been dealt with.

Limited Information Methods

The single equation methods are by far the most popular for reasons of economy, specification errors, etc. A unique feature of these methods is that one can estimate a single-equation in a multi-equation model without worrying too much about other equations in the system, although for the identification purposes, the other equations in the system count.

The commonly used single-equation methods are, i) Ordinary Least Squares (OLS), ii) Indirect Least Squares (ILS) and iii) Two-stage least squares (2 SLS) iv) Limited Information Maximum Likelihood (LIML).

i) Although OLS is, in general, inappropriate in the context of simultaneous-equation models, it can be applied to the recursive models where there is a definite but unidirectional cause and effect relationship among the endogenous variables. For instance, consider the following equations:

$$Y_{1t} = \beta_{10} + \gamma_{11}X_{1t} + \gamma_{12}X_{2t} + u_{1t}$$

$$Y_{2t} = \beta_{20} + \beta_{21} Y_{1t} + \gamma_{21}X_{1t} + \gamma_{22}X_{2t} + u_{2t}$$

$$Y_{3t} = \beta_{30} + \beta_{31} Y_{1t} + \beta_{32} Y_{2t} + \gamma_{31}X_{1t} + \gamma_{32}X_{2t} + u_{3t}$$

where the disturbances are such that $cov(u_{1t,} u_{2t})= cov(u_{1t,} u_{3t})= cov(u_{2t,} u_{3t}) = 0$, that is, the same period disturbances in different equations are uncorrelated (zero contemporaneous correlation). The first equation satisfies all the classical assumptions and hence, its OLS estimation will produce unbiased and consistent estimates. Second equation contains the endogenous variable Y_1 as an explanatory variable so OLS estimation can be applied only if Y_{1t} is uncorrelated with u_{2t}. By assumption, u_1 which affects Y_1 is uncorrelated with u_2, hence, for all practical purposes Y_1 is predetermined variable so far Y_2 is concerned. Hence one can proceed with OLS estimation of this equation. Similarly, carrying the argument further, OLS can be applied to third equation.

ii) The method of ILS is suited for just or exactly identified equations. In this method OLS is applied to the reduced form equations, and it is from the reduced-form coefficients that one estimates the original structural coefficients.

iii) The method of 2SLS is especially designed for over identified equations, although it can also be applied to exactly identified equations. But then the results of 2SLS and ILS are identical. The basic idea behind 2SLS is to replace the stochastic explanatory variable by a linear combination of the predetermined variables in the model and use this combination as the explanatory variable in lieu of the original endogenous variable. The 2SLS method thus resembles the instrumental variable method of estimation in that the linear combination of the predetermined variables serves as an instrument, or proxy, for the endogenous regressor.

iv) Another method for obtaining the estimates of the population parameter from a random sample is maximization of the likelihood function. In this technique, the likelihood function, (which is the logarithmic form of the joint probability density function of the dependent variable Y) is estimated in such a way that the probability of observing the given Y's is as high (maximum) as possible. LIML is another method for obtaining consistent coefficient estimates of the over-identified structural equation. As in case of 2 SLS, LIML also makes use of all the predetermined variables in the entire model in order to estimate the structural parameters of a single equation. However, the computational procedure of LIML is more complicated than 2SLS as it requires constrained maximization of the maximum likelihood function that is formed for the random terms of the reduced form equations.

Full Information Methods

The full information methods, as the name suggests, are applied to all the equations of the model at the same time and give estimates of all the parameters simultaneously. The three stage least squares (3SLS) and full information maximum likelihood (FIML) two systems method for estimation of simultaneous equations.

i) 3 SLS is the combination of 2SLS and seemingly unrelated regression (SUR). The first two stages are the same as 2SLS except that we deal with all the reduced form equations of the system rather than only the over identified equation as in case of 2SLS. Hence, in the first stage, estimated values of the endogenous variables are obtained by estimating the reduce-form of all the equations of the system. In the next stage, the estimated values of the endogenous variable (obtained in the first stage) are substituted as regressors in the structural equation and least squares is applied to the transformed equations to obtain the residuals. The variance-covariance matrix of the residuals terms obtained in stage 2 are used to obtain the transformation of the original variables for the application of the Generalised Least Squares (GLS).

ii) 2SLS and 3SLS are used almost exclusively (when ordinary least squares is not used) for the estimation of simultaneous equations models because of their simplicity and asymptotic efficiency. Nonetheless, it is occasionally useful to obtain maximum likelihood estimates directly. The full-information maximum likelihood (FIML) estimator is based on the entire system of equations. With normally distributed disturbances, FIML is efficient among all estimators.

Applications in Agriculture

The estimation of demand and supply for working out elasticity and demand/supply forecasting of various agricultural commodities and inputs is perhaps the most widely used application of simultaneous equation framework in agriculture and allied sciences, as it yield more satisfactory results than ordinary least squares.

A very good practical example of the step by step estimation of simultaneous demand-supply equations has been provided by Epple and McCallum (2005), using annual U.S. time series data for 1960-1999 for broiler chickens for illustration. The paper provides the database used in the analysis and modeling of demand and supply using both, least squares and simultaneous equations to unambiguously bring out the differences in the results of these techniques. The specified basic model was as follows, with lower-case letters denoting logarithms of the underlying variables;

$$q = \beta_0 + \beta_1 p + \beta_2 y + \beta_3 pb + v \qquad \text{1 (Demand)}$$

$$q^A = \alpha_0 + \alpha_1 p + \alpha_2 pf + \alpha_3 \text{Time } \alpha_4 q^A(-1) + u \qquad \text{2 (Supply)}$$

Where, q=per capita quantity demanded, q^A =Aggregate quantity supplied i.e, q+ pop, pop= population, p= real price of chicken, pf=price of feed, Time= time trend representing technical progress, $q^A(-1)$=previous period's value of output, y = income level of potential demanders, pb= real price of beef.

In the Ordinary Least Squares (OLS) estimate of the demand equation as reproduced below as EVIEWS output, the real price of beef (pb) enters with negative sign which is contrary to the a-priori expectation for a substitute commodity and the Durbin Watson (DW) statistics is very low indicating very strong autocorrelation.

Dependent Variable: LOG(Q)

Method: Least Squares

Date: 11/09/15 Time: 23:28

Sample: 1950 2001

Included observations: 52

Variable	Coefficient	Std. Error	t-Statistic	Prob.
C	−4.679576	0.675243	−6.930214	0.0000
LOG(P)	−0.264785	0.069862	−3.790106	0.0004
LOG(Y)	0.851916	0.068589	12.42052	0.0000
LOG(PB)	−0.118367	0.083556	−1.416625	0.1631
R-squared	0.980930	Mean dependent var		3.366467
Adjusted R-squared	0.979738	S.D. dependent var		0.397546
S.E. of regression	0.056589	Akaike info criterion		−2.832214
Sum squared resid	0.153709	Schwarz criterion		−2.682118
Log likelihood	77.63755	F-statistic		823.0070
Durbin-Watson stat	0.443329	Prob(F-statistic)		0.000000

In order to resolve for autocorrelation in the model, the demand equation in the first difference form was estimated as follows:

$$\Delta q = \underset{(0.150)}{0.711\, \Delta y} - \underset{(0.058)}{0.374\, \Delta p} + \underset{(0.068)}{0.251\, \Delta pb} \qquad (3)$$

s.e.

$R^2 = 0.331$, SE = 0.0294, DW = 2.38

In the OLS estimation of the supply equation, all variables but one entered significantly and with the proper sign, the exception being the price of chicken.

$$q^A = 2.478 - 0.041\, p - 0.083\, pf + 0.0102\, time + 0.647\, qA(-1) \qquad (4)$$

(0.698) (0.052) (0.032) (0.0038) (0.108)

$R^2 = 0.997$ SE = 0.0252 DW = 1.883

As there were no signs of auto- correlated residuals and the equations' explanatory power was good, the relations (3) and (4) were adopted as a promising demand and supply specification to carry out simultaneous-equation estimation. The EVIEWS output of the 2SLS estimates of the demand and supply equation are as follows:

Demand Equation

Dependent Variable: LOG(Q)-LOG(Q(-1))

Method: Two-Stage Least Squares

Date: 11/10/15 Time: 06:23

Sample (adjusted): 1960 1999

Included observations: 40 after adjustments

Instrument list: C TIME LOG(QA(-1)) LOG(PF/CPI) LOG(Y)-LOG(Y(

-1)) LOG(PB)-LOG(PB(-1)) LOG(POP)-LOG(POP(-1)) LOG(P(

-1))

Variable	Coefficient	Std. Error	t-Statistic	Prob.
LOG(Y)-LOG(Y(-1))	0.843218	0.142954	5.898541	0.0000
LOG(P)-LOG(P(-1))	−0.404486	0.086513	−4.675441	0.0000
LOG(PB)-LOG(PB(-1))	0.279522	0.093447	2.991254	0.0049
R-squared	0.291098	Mean dependent var		0.024568
Adjusted R-squared	0.252779	S.D. dependent var		0.029251
S.E. of regression	0.025285	Sum squared resid		0.023656
Durbin-Watson stat	1.929068	Second-stage SSR		0.025944

Supply Equation

Dependent Variable: LOG(QA)

Method: Two-Stage Least Squares

Date: 11/10/15 Time: 06:28

Sample (adjusted): 1960 1999

Included observations: 40 after adjustments

Instrument list: C TIME LOG(QA(-1)) LOG(PF/CPI) LOG(Y)-LOG(Y(

-1)) LOG(PB)-LOG(PB(-1)) LOG(POP)-LOG(POP(-1)) LOG(P(

-1))

Variable	Coefficient	Std. Error	t-Statistic	Prob.
C	2.370631	0.773287	3.065655	0.0042
LOG(P)	0.105464	0.077460	1.361531	0.1820
LOG(PF/CPI)	−0.113083	0.037218	−3.038392	0.0045
TIME	0.012281	0.004307	2.851284	0.0073
LOG(QA(-1))	0.639651	0.119151	5.368395	0.0000
R-squared	0.995983	Mean dependent var		8.899071
Adjusted R-squared	0.995523	S.D. dependent var		0.416666
S.E. of regression	0.027878	Sum squared resid		0.027201
Durbin-Watson stat	1.869130	Second-stage SSR		0.021181

The results clearly indicated that all of the seven parameter estimates were of the theoretically appropriate sign and six were clearly significant. The coefficient on the price of chicken in the supply function was still the weakest link, but the sign of the estimate was positive. By and large, it is very much clear that, simultaneous estimation methods yield more plausible estimates than ordinary least squares.

Besides demand and supply estimation, simultaneous equations are used in various studies of economics, crop and animal sciences. For instance, Penn and Irwin (1971) made an initial attempt to identify and estimate the underlying relationships between the production of soybeans and other competing crops (Cotton, Rice and Corn) based on annual observations for the time period 1947-69 in the Delta Region. A four equations model was specified.

$$A_{it} = \alpha_0 + \alpha_1 A_{jt} + \alpha_2 A_{kt} + \alpha_3 A_{lt} + \alpha_4 A_{i(t-1)} + \alpha_5 SP_{it} + \alpha_6 MP_{i(t-1)} + \alpha_7 MP_{j(t-1)} + \alpha_8 MP_{k(t-1)} + \alpha_9 MP_{l(t-1)} + \varepsilon_1$$

$$A_{jt} = \beta_0 + \beta_1 A_{it} + \beta_2 A_{kt} + \beta_3 A_{lt} + \beta_4 MP_{i(t-1)} + \beta_5 MP_{j(t-1)} + \beta_6 MP_{k(t-1)} + \beta_7 MP_{l(t-1)} + \beta_8 SP_{jt} + \beta_9 A_{lj} + \beta_{10} A_{j(t-1)} + \varepsilon_2$$

$$A_{kt} = \gamma_0 + \gamma_1 A_{it} + \gamma_2 A_{jt} + \gamma_3 A_{lt} + \gamma_4 MP_{i(t-1)} + \gamma_5 MP_{j(t-1)} + \gamma_6 MP_{k(t-1)} + \gamma_7 MP_{l(t-1)} + \gamma_8 SP_{it} + \gamma_9 Al_i + \gamma_{10} A_{k(t-1)} + \varepsilon_3$$

$$A_{lt} = \delta_0 + \delta_1 A_{it} + \delta_2 A_{jt} + \delta_3 A_{kt} + \delta_4 MP_{i(t-1)} + \delta_5 MP_{j(t-1)} + \delta_6 MP_{k(t-1)} + \delta_7 MP_{l(t-1)} + \delta_8 SP_{lt} + \delta_9 A_{l(t-1)} + \varepsilon_4$$

where, i=Soybean, j=Cotton, k=Rice, l= Corn A= Acreage, SP = Support Price, MP= Market Price, Al= Acreage allotment

The pre-estimation identification properties of the model were examined and the system was found to be overidentified, therefore it was estimated by two stage least squares (2SLS). The estimation results were quite interesting. The soybean price variable found to exert substantial effect on the acreages of all crops-more so than the other price variables. Thus, it was concluded that the world market expectations for soybeans were crucially interdependent in setting necessary program variables for the other crops. The magnitudes of the coefficients for yield index variable in the four equations suggested that effects of changes in yields had most affected cotton acreage, followed by rice, soybeans, and corn, in that order. Also, the coefficients for soybeans and cotton support price were of the expected sign and both appeared to be somewhat stronger than the market price variable indicating that program dependence was high for cotton, and that soybean acreage expansion was key to removal of price uncertainty.

The simultaneous equation model was applied by Chakir and Hardelin (2010) to investigate the crop insurance and pesticide use decisions for risk management in French agriculture. Economic theory suggests that insurance and prevention decisions are not independent due to risk reduction and/or moral hazard effects. Statistical tests confirmed that chemical and insurance demands are endogenous to each other and simultaneously determined. An econometric model involving two simultaneous equations with mixed censored/continuous dependent variables was thus estimated for rapeseed. Estimation results showed that rapeseed insurance demand has a positive and significant effect on pesticide use and vice versa.

Another example of an interesting application of simultaneous equations is exploration of the three way linkage between weather variability, agricultural performance and internal migration in India at state and district level using

Indian Census data for years 1981, 1991 and 2001 (Vishwanathan and Kavi Kumar, 2013). The analyses were based on a simultaneous equation model for panel data employing 2SLS/LIML estimation techniques. A two equation model was specified

$$M_{it} = \alpha + \beta Y_{it} + d_i + r_t + \varepsilon_{it} \tag{1}$$

$$Y_{it} = \gamma + \delta T_{it} + p_i + c_t + v_{it} \tag{2}$$

where M_{it} was the out-migration (in-migration) rate from (to) region 'i' at period 't', Y_{it} was one of the agriculture variables (wheat yield or rice yield or per capita net state domestic product from agriculture for region 'i' at period 't'), T_{it} represented the set of weather variables of region 'i' at period 't'. The d_i and p_i were the coefficients for the regional (fixed) effects; r_t and c_t were coefficients to capture time (fixed) effect.

The first equation captured the migration-agriculture linkage while the second equation assumed yield to be endogenous in the first equation, thus using weather variables as instruments to correct for the simultaneity bias of the coefficient of yield in equation (1).

The study on determinants of capital formation and their impact on growth of Indian agriculture conducted by Chand and Kumar (2004) estimated simultaneous equation model for the period 1974-75 to 2001-02. The model comprised of three equation framework:

$$gdpaa = \alpha_1 + \alpha_2 nsa + \alpha_3 rain + \alpha_4 totmf(-1) + \alpha_5 wrkr + \alpha_6 nfcsto(-1) + \alpha_7 subsd \tag{1}$$

$$gfcfpv = \beta_1 + \beta_2 gfcfpb(-1) + \beta_3 rorpv(-1) + \beta_4 crdtt + \beta_5 subsd + \beta_6 addhold \tag{2}$$

$$gfcfpb = \gamma 1 + \gamma\, 2subsd/gdpaa + \gamma\, 3revrec(1)\, gdpaa(-1) + \gamma\, 4gfcfpb\, (-1)$$
$$+ \gamma\, 5gfcfpb\, (-2) \tag{3}$$

where:

gdpaa = Gross domestic product from agriculture and allied activities, at 1993-94 prices (Rs crore).

gfcpv = Gross fixed capital formation in agriculture in private sector, at 1993-94 prices (Rs crore).

gfcpb = Gross fixed capital formation in agriculture in public sector, at 1993-94 prices (Rs crore).

nsa = Net sown area in crore hectare.

totmf = Terms of trade for agriculture relative to manufacturing sector.

wrkr = Number of agriculture workers, crore persons.

rain = Index of June to September (monsoon) rainfall in relation to long-term average of rainfall.

nfcsto = Net fixed capital stock in agriculture at 1993-94 prices (Rs crore).

subsd = Subsidies in agriculture sector as estimated by CSO in (Rs crore).

revrc = Revenue receipts from agriculture in all states, as reported by RBI.

addhold= Number of operational holdings added during the year.

crdtt = Amount of institutional credit supplied to agriculture sector during a year by cooperatives, regional rural banks and commercial banks.

rorpv = Rate of return to private investments.

The estimated results provides some new insights to understand the behavior of private investments, and quantified the trade-offs between public investments and subsidies. The most important determinant of private capital formation was found to be rate of return on private investments, which in turn depends on the terms of trade and technology. The effect of rising and falling public investments on private investments was asymmetric, that is, an increase in public investment induced a rise in private investments, while a decline forced farmers to cope with its adverse impact, again by increasing private investment. Another interesting result was that the increase in farm subsidies and decrease in revenue receipts from agriculture was causing an adverse impact on public sector capital formation. The authors opined that long-term returns from capital formation were more than double the returns from subsidies; therefore diverting resources from subsidies to public sector capital formation was highly desirable to ensure growth in Indian agriculture.

The examples referred in this Chapter are by no means exhaustive. To get a bird's eye view of the applications of simultaneous equations in agriculture, the references in the bibliography section may provide a useful reading.

References

Acharya, S S. An analysis of farm income and demand for inputs. *Rajasthan Economic Journal*. 1978; 2(1): 15-29.

Bhati, U N. An analysis of aggregate labour demand and supply relationships for Australian agriculture. *Quarterly Review of Agricultural Economics*. 1978; 31(2/3): 106-123.

Chakir, R. and Hardelin, J. Crop insurance and pesticides in French agriculture:An empirical analysis of multiple risks management. 2010; Working paper 2010/04. Joint Research Unit in Public Economics, Paris, France.

C Gundersen. The food stamp program and food insufficiency. *American Journal of Agricultural Economics*. 2001 83(4).

Dijk, G van; Smit, L. Land prices and technological development. *European Review of Agricultural Economics*. 1986; 13(4): 495-515.

El Bably, A Z. Estimation of evapotranspiration using statistical model. Options Mediterraneennes Serie A, Seminaires Mediterraneens. 2003; (57): 441-449 http://www.ciheam.org.

Epple, D. and McCallum, B.T. Simultaneous Equation Econometrics: The Missing Example. *Economic Inquiry*.2005; 44, 374-384.

Fuglie, K O; Bosch, D J. Economic and environmental implications of soil nitrogen testing: a switching regression analysis. *American Journal of Agricultural Economics*. 1995; 77(4): 891-900.

Negatu, W; Parikh, A. The impact of perception and other factors on the adoption of agricultural technology in the Moret and Jiru woreda (district) of Ethiopia. *Agricultural Economics*. 1999; 21(2): 205-216.

Nelsen, T C; Short, R E; Urick, J J; Reynolds, W L. Genetic variance components of birth weight in a herd of unselected cattle. *Journal of Animal Science*. 1984; 59(6): 1459-1466.

Nieuwoudt, W L; Bullock, J B. The demand for crop insurance. Agriculture in a turbulent world economy Proceedings, *Nineteenth International Conference of Agricultural Economists*, held at Malaga, Spain, 26 August 4 September 1985. 1986; 655-661.

Ortiz, J .Welfare implications on Chilean agriculture as a result of collective action. *Food Policy*. 2000; 25(2): 169-188.

Penn, J. B. and Irwin, G. D. A Simultaneous Equation Approach to Production Response: Delta Region. *Southern Journal of Agricultural Economics*, December 1971.

Chand, R. and Kumar, P. Determinants of Capital Formation and Agriculture Growth: Some New Explorations. *Economic and Political Weekly*. December 25, 2004.

Sharma Pradeep, K. Foodgrain economy of India: government intervention in rice and wheat markets. Foodgrain economy of India: government intervention in rice and wheat markets. 1997; viii+160 pp. New Delhi, India: Shipra Publications.

Smit,B.E. Employment of family and non family labour in agriculture. *Canadian Journal of Agricultural Economics*. 1977; 26(1): 35-42.

Uri, N D. Industry structure and economic performance in the food manufacturing industries. *Journal of International Food and Agribusiness Marketing*. 1992; 4(1): 95-123.

Viswanathan, B. and Kavi Kumar, K.S. Rural Migration, Weather and Agriculture: Evidence from Indian Census Data. 2013, Working Paper 80/2013, Madras School of Economics, Chennai.

Wahl, T I; Williams, G W; Hayes, D J. 1988. Japanese beef market access agreement: forecast simulation analysis. *IAAE Occasional Paper*. 1989; (5): 158-167.

Wakatsuki, T; Rasyidin, A. Rates of weathering and soil formation. *Geoderma*. 1992; 52(3/4): 251-263.

Yaqoob, M M; Netke, S P. Studies on the incorporation of triticale in diets for growing chicks. *British Poultry Science*. 1975; 16(1): 45-54.

Zhang, S H; Terao, H; Ueno, M; Fujita, K. Dynamic performances of tractor trailer combinations for farm use. (IV). Introduction of state equations and dynamic characteristic. *Journal of the Japanese Society of Agricultural Machinery*. 1991; 53(3): 15-23.

Chapter 7

Short Run Forecast of Food Inflation using ARIMA: A Combination Approach

S.K. Srivastava

ICAR-NIAP, New Delhi – 110 012

Introduction

The rising food inflation in India has been a major challenge for the policy makers during the recent year. Over the past few years, food prices in India have increases at faster rate than the non-food inflation. This has a strong implication especially for poor households who spend more than half of their expenditure on food products. Many studies have explored the causes of recent rise in food inflation and provided plausible explanations. Chand (2010) and World Bank (2010), argue that food inflation is a result of supply shocks due to droughts and floods. On the other hand, Landes (2007) and Gokarn (2010) attribute food inflation to demand shocks. Mitra and Josling (2009) and Sharma, Gummagolmath and Sharma (2011), believe that India's food inflation is a product of maladministration in national food institutions, especially the public distribution system (PDS). However, little has been done to provide a reliable forecast of food inflation, probably because of complexity of the subject. The present study attempts to fill this void and tests the accuracy of alternative models to arrive at better forecast of the food inflation. The specific objectives of the study are to study the long run trends and provide short run forecast of the food inflation in India.

Data and Methodology

The long run trend in food inflation was studied using the official data on monthly wholesale price index (WPI) at disaggregated level. The monthly WPI was converted into a common base year (2004-05) using ratio method. Thereafter, year-on-year (y-o-y) inflation was calculated using the WPI (constant prices). Trend in food inflation was estimated using Hodrick-Prescot filter (HP filter). The details of HP filter method is given below;

Hodrick-Prescot Filter (HP Filter)

The HP filter is a model-free based approach to decomposing a time series into its trend and cyclical components. The HP filter is an algorithm that "smooths" the original time series y_t to estimate its trend component, τ_t. The cyclical component is, as usual, the difference between the original series and its trend, *i.e.*,

$$y_t = \tau_t + c_t \tag{1}$$

where τ_t is constructed to minimize:

$$\sum_{1}^{T}(y_t - \tau_t)^2 + \lambda \sum_{2}^{T-1}[(\tau_{t+1} - \tau_t) - (\tau_t - \tau_{t-1})]^2 \tag{2}$$

$$\sum_{1}^{T}(y_t - \tau_t)^2 + \lambda \sum_{2}^{T-1}[(\tau_{t+1} - \tau_t) - (\tau_t - \tau_{t-1})]^2 \tag{3}$$

The first term is the sum of the squared deviations of y_t from the trend and the second term, which is the sum of squared second differences in the trend, is a penalty for changes in the trend's growth rate. The larger the value of the positive parameter λ, the greater the penalty and the smoother the resulting trend will be.

If, *e.g.*, $\lambda = 0$, then $\tau_t = y_t$, t = 1,...,t.

If $\lambda \to \infty$, then τ_t is the linear trend obtained by fitting y_t to a linear trend model by OLS.

Hodrick and Prescott suggest that $\lambda = 1600$ is a reasonable choice for quarterly data and that suggestion is usually followed in applied work. For monthly data a value in the range of 100,000-150,000 has been suggested and for annual data a value in the range of 5-15 has been suggested. For the present analysis, Eviews software was used which uses 14400 value to estimate trend.

Short Run Forecast of Food Inflation: ARIMA Model

The short run forecast of food inflation was made using ARIMA (Autoregressive Integrated Moving Average) model on the basis of Box-Jenkins approach to model time series. The Box-Jenkins approach to modelling time series is summarize in Figure 7.1. This approach consists of three phases: identification, estimation and testing, and application. The identification phases starts with data preparation. For time series analysis, data should be stationary *i.e.* data fluctuate around a constant

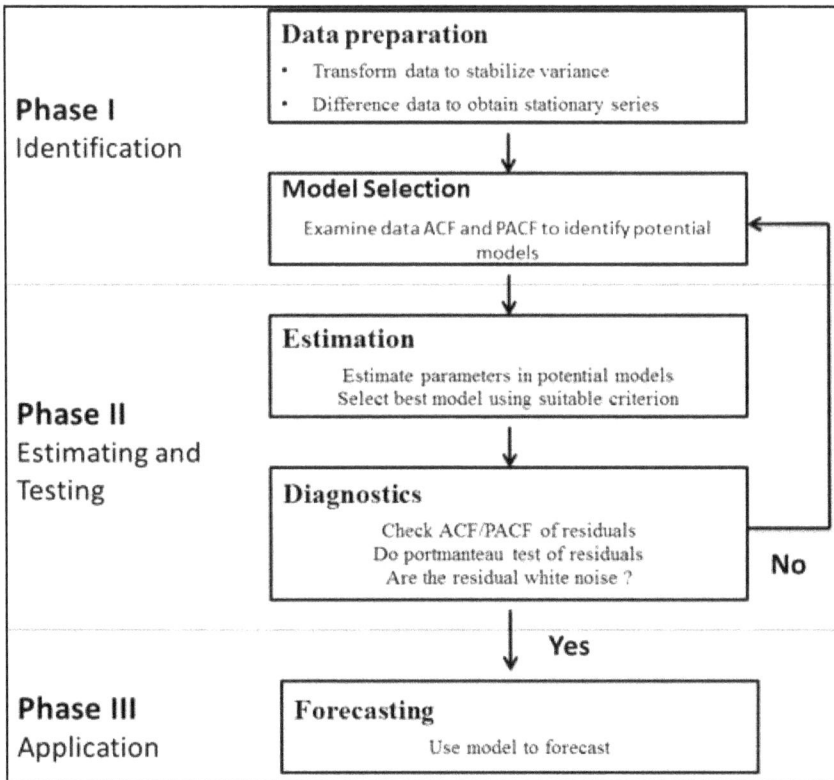

Figure 7.1: Schematic Representation of the Box-Jenkins Methodology for time Series Modeling (*Source*: Makrtidakis *et al.*, 1998).

means, independent of time, and the variance of the fluctuation remains essentially constant over time. Stationarity condition of each time series was checked using **Augmented Dickey Fuller (ADF) test** and **Kwiatkowski, Phillips, Schmidt, and Shin (KPSS) test.** If the data is not found stationary through these tests, suitable data transformation and differencing is done to make it stationary. The original WPI series were not found to be stationary based on above tests. Therefore following transformation was applied to make the series stationary.

$$Z_t = (\ln X_t - \ln X_{t-1})_y - (\ln X_t - \ln X_{t-1})_{y-1} \qquad (4)$$

where X_t is wholesale price index of the respective food commodity. This transformation leads to seasonally adjusted monthly changes in wholesale price index, which captures inter-month fluctuations in prices of food commodities.

The second step in identification is to short list potential ARIMA models based on autocorrelation functions (ACF) and partial autocorrelation functions (PACF). The examination of ACF and PACF helps in identification of AR (p), I (d) and MA (q) components of ARIMA. ACF is a valuable tool for investigating properties of an empirical time series. The autocorrelation coefficient is estimated as follows;

$$r_k = \frac{\sum_{t=k+1}^{n} \left([(Y)]t + \overline{Y}\right)\left(Y_{t-k} - \overline{Y}\right)}{\sum_{t=1}^{n} \left([(Y_t)] + \overline{Y}\right)^2}$$

(5)

where r_k is the correlation of the time series with itself lagged by 1,2,.k period. For example, r_1 indicates how successive a values of Y relate to each other, r_2 indicates how Y values two period apart relate to each other, and so on. Together, autocorrelation at lags 1,2,., make up the autocorrelation function or ACF. Partial autocorrelation (PACF) are used to measure degree of association between Y_t and Y_{t-k}, when the effect of of other tome lags - 1,2,3,.k-1 - are removed. The plots of estimated ACF and PACF is compared with theoratical values of ACF and PACF to identify potential value of p,d, and q in the model.

Potential ARIMA models are then estimated and the best model is selected based on suitable criteria *i.e.* Akaike's Information Criteria (AIC). Lower AIC value from a model indicates better fit and out of several fitted models, model with lest AIC value is retained. Estimation of the model is followed by residual diagnostic check. The residual obtained from the model are subject to ACF, PACF and unit root tests. A good fitted should have the residual with "white noise" property. If the model is white noise then it is used for forecasting purpose. The forecasted value are subsequently subjected to forecast evaluation procedures which comprises of estimating following statistics;

Mean absolute deviation,
$$MAD = \sum_{i=1}^{n} \frac{|Y_i - Y_i|}{n}$$

(6)

Mean Absolute percentage error,
$$MAPE = \frac{100}{n} \sum_{i=1}^{n} \frac{|Y_i - Y_i|}{Y_i}$$

(7)

Root mean square error,
$$RMSE = \sum_{i=1}^{n} \frac{(Y_i - Y_i)^2}{n}$$

(8)

Root mean square per cent error,
$$RMSPE = \frac{100}{n} \sum_{i=1}^{n} \frac{(Y_i - Y_i)^2}{Y_i}$$

(9)

U theil statistics,
$$U = \sqrt{\sum_{i-1}^{n-1} \frac{\left(\frac{Y_{i+1} - Y_{i-1}}{Y_i}\right)^2}{\sum_{i=1}^{n-1}\left(\frac{Y_{i+1} - Y_i}{Y_i}\right)^2}}$$

(10)

The lower the values of above statistics, better is the forecasted ability is of the model. For U-theil statistics, value less than 1 indicates better model.

Model Formulation

ARIMA was fitted for 3 alternative models *i.e.* Aggregate food model, GROUP2 model and GROUP 7 model. Aggregate model consists of fitting ARIMA for aggregate food WPI series. In GROUP2 model, overall food WPI was disaggregated into two components *i.e.* primary food articles WPI and manufactured food products WPI. Thereafter, ARIMA was fitted separately for each component and forecasted values were aggregated using simple weighted average. Similarly, in GROUP7 model, overall food WPI was disaggregated into seven food groups *i.e.* Cereals, Pulses, Fruits and vegetables, Milk, Eggs, meat and fish, Manufactures food products and other food products. ARIMA was fitted for each food groups and forecasted values were aggregated using weights of respective food products.

The forecast obtained from each model (aggregate, GROUP2 and GROUP7) was evaluated and best model was retained based on selected evaluation criteria. Further, forecasts obtained from each models were combined using simple average method and resultant forecast was evaluated.

Results and Discussion

Long Run Changes/Trend in Food Inflation

In India, officially food inflation is estimated using wholesale price index (WPI) which comprises of 674 commodities having different weights. The WPI for food as well as non-food commodities at (at 2004-05) witnessed a rising trend (Figure 7.2) in the last three decade. In the recent years after 2008, food prices have increased at much higher rate than non-food prices. The estimated year-on-year inflation based on WPI showed that food inflation has higher volatility than non-food inflation (Figure 7.3). Both food and non-food inflation witnessed cyclical trend in long run. The increasing trend in inflation before 1990 was followed by a almost a decade of declining inflation particularly by food commodities. The food inflation reached at its lowest level of less than 2 per cent in 2000. But, afterwards food prices started soaring till July 2010 and the food inflation reached to a double digit mark.

The overall trend in food inflation was not uniform across different food commodities. Primary food articles witnessed higher fluctuation than the manufactured food products. The difference between primary food articles and manufactured food products increased upto 17 percentage points in December 2009. This indicates the primary food article, a major contributor of recent rise in food inflation in the country. Further, different food products witnessed differential cyclical trend in food inflation as indicated by HP filter plotted in Figure 7.3.

Short Run Forecast of Food Inflation

Three model formulation were constructed to provide a reliable estimate of short run inflation forecast. These formulations were aggregate model, GROUP2 (Primary food articles and Manufactured food products components) and GROUP7 model (Cereals, Pulses, Fruits and Vegetables, Milk, Non-veg, Manufactured and Other food products). Box-Jenkins approach (ARIMA) was used for model fitting and forecast. The time series WPI for each food products was divided into two

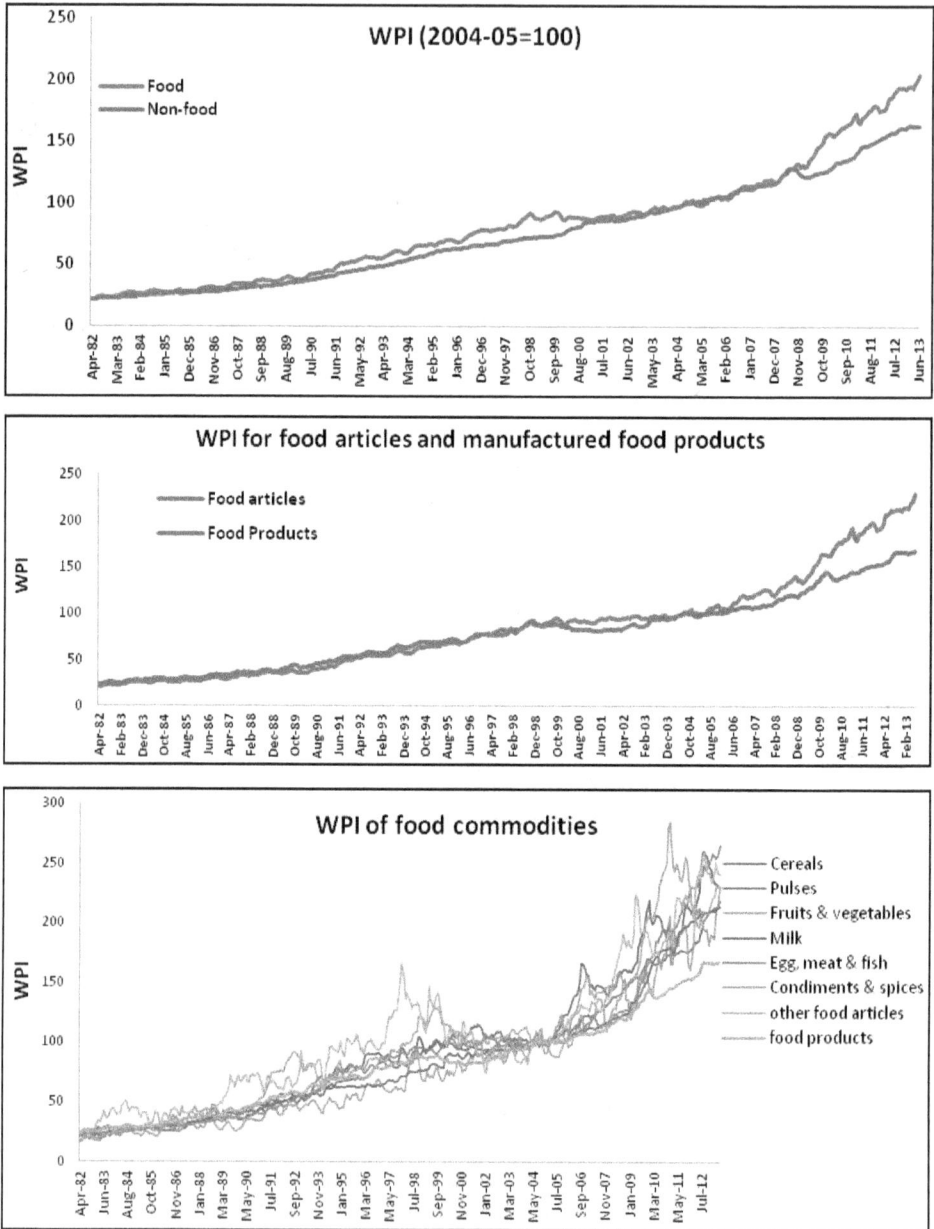

Figure 7.2: Long Run Trend in WPI (2004-05 =100) of Food Products.

part *i.e.* estimation period (April 1982 to May 2010) and forecast evaluation period (June 2010 to June 2013). To test stationarity of WPIs, KPSS and ADF tests were conducted which confirmed that original series (WPI) were non-stationary (Table 7.1). Therefore, original series were transformed using $Z_t = (\ln X_t - \ln X_{t-1})_y - (\ln X_t -$

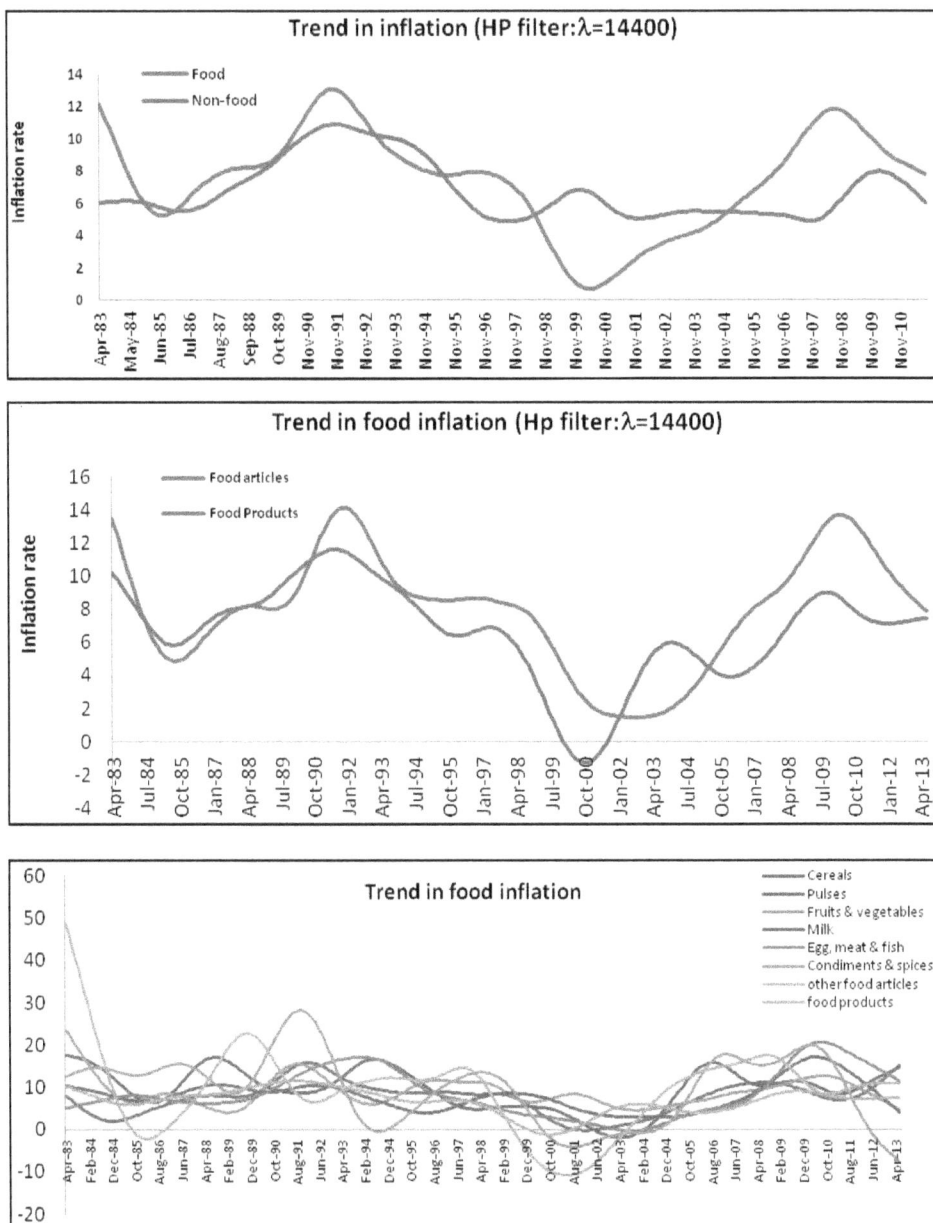

Figure 7.3: Long Run Trend in Inflation of Food Products (HP filter).

ln $X_{t-1})_{y-1}$. This transformation stabilizes the short run and seasonal fluctuation in prices and gives the month-over-month (m-o-m) estimate of inflation. The KPSS and ADF tests confirmed that transformed series was stationary and can be used ARIMA estimation.

Table 7.1: Unit Root Tests for Stationarity

Model	KPSS[a] Test Statistics $\{H_0 = I(0)\}$		ADF[b] Test Statistics $\{H_0 = I(1)\}$	
	Original Series	Transformed Series	Original Series	Transformed Series
Aggregate food	2.27**	0.03	4.31	−7.81**
GROUP2 model				
Primary Food Article	2.22**	0.05	2.25	−7.88**
Manufactured Food	2.20**	0.02	2.13	−8.53**
GROUP7 model				
Cereals	2.29**	0.03	4.04	−9.51**
Pulses	2.24**	0.02	0.22	−7.57**
Fruits and vegetables	2.25**	0.07	3.14	−9.37**
Milk	2.08**	0.02	3.95	−8.33**
Eggs, meat and fish	2.01**	0.05	5.04	−8.42**
Manufactured	2.20**	0.02	2.13	−8.53**
Others	2.06**	0.02	0.66	−8.17**

a: Kwiatkowski, Phillips, Schmidt and Shin (1992) test for stationarity I(0).

b: Augmented Dickey-Fuller test for stationarity I(1).

** Significant at 1 per cent level of significance.

Table 7.2: Optimum ARIMA Models for different Food Commodities

Model	ARIMA (p,d,q) (P,D,Q)	AIC	Observations
Aggregate food	(2,0, 3) (12,0,12)	−6.32	311
GROUP2 model			
Primary Food Article	(1,0,1) (0,0,12)	−5.71	324
Manufactured Food	(2,0, 3) (0,0,12)	−6.13	323
GROUP7 model			
Cereals	(2,0,1) (6,0,12)	−5.65	317
Pulses	(2,0, 3) (12,0,12)	−4.43	311
Fruits and vegetables	(1,0,2) (0,0,12)	−3.49	324
Milk	(2,0,2) (0,0,12)	−5.48	323
Eggs, meat and fish	(0,0,1) (0,0,12)	−4.75	325
Manufactured	(2,0, 3) (0,0,12)	−6.13	323
Others	(2,0, 3) (12,0,12)	−3.89	311

Based on estimated ACF and PACF, tentative parameters of ARIMA (p,d,q) (P,D,Q) were identified and potential models were fitted for each of the transformed series. Out of the several fitted ARIMA model, best model for each series was identified based on AIC value. The best fitted models are given in Table 7.2 and

Table 7.3: Estimated Model Equations for different Food Products

Model	Estimated Model Equation
Aggregate food	$Y_t^{Food} = -1.01\,E - 05 - 0.28\,Y_{t-1}^{Food} - 0.93\,Y_{t-2}^{Food} + 0.03\,Y_{t-12}^{Food} + 0.61\epsilon_{t-1}^{food} + 1.06\,\epsilon_{t-2}^{food} + 0.42\,\epsilon_{t-3}^{food} - 0.90\,\epsilon_{t-12}^{food}$
Primary Food Article	$Y_t^{PFA} = 2.97E - 05 - 0.37\,Y_{t-1}^{PFA} + 0.63\,\epsilon_{t-1}^{PFA} - 0.92\,\epsilon_{t-12}^{PFA}$
Manufactured Food	$Y_t^{mfp} = -0.0001 - 0.16\,Y_{t-1}^{mfp} - 0.87\,Y_{t-2}^{mfp} + 0.44\,\epsilon_{t-1}^{mfp} + 1.00\,\epsilon_{t-2}^{mfp} + 0.37\,\epsilon_{t-3}^{mfp} - 0.89\,\epsilon_{t-12}^{mfp}$
Cereals	$Y_t^{Cereals} = -3.5E - 05 - 0.47\,Y_{t-1}^{Cereals} + 0.17\,Y_{t-2}^{Cereals} + 0.12\,Y_{t-6}^{Cereals} + 0.80\,\epsilon_{t-1}^{Cereals} - 0.95\,\epsilon_{t-12}^{Cereals}$
Pulses	$Y_t^{Pulses} = -4.5E - 05 - 0.48\,Y_{t-1}^{Pulses} - 0.98\,Y_{t-2}^{Pulses} - 0.11\,Y_{t-12}^{Pulses} + 0.82\,\epsilon_{t-1}^{Pulses} + 1.16\,\epsilon_{t-1}^{Pulses} + 0.32\,\epsilon_{t-1}^{Pulses} - 0.93\,\epsilon_{t-12}^{Pulses}$
Fruits and vegetables	$Y_t^{F\&V} = -4.15E - 05 + 0.81\,Y_{t-1}^{F\&V} - 0.78\,\epsilon_{t-1}^{F\&V} - 0.20\,\epsilon_{t-2}^{F\&V} - 0.88\,\epsilon_{t-12}^{F\&V}$
Milk	$Y_t^{milk} = 1.61E - 05 - 0.95\,Y_{t-1}^{milk} - 0.94\,Y_{t-1}^{milk} + 1.05\,\epsilon_{t-1}^{milk} + 0.98\,\epsilon_{t-1}^{milk} - 0.90\,\epsilon_{t-12}^{milk}$
Eggs, meat and fish	$Y_t^{non-veg} = 2.53E - 05 + 0.11\,\epsilon_{t-1}^{non-veg} - 0.93\,\epsilon_{t-12}^{non-veg}$
Others	$Y_t^{ofp} = 4.58E - 05 + 0.94\,Y_{t-1}^{ofp} - 0.93\,Y_{t-1}^{ofp} - 0.15\,Y_{t-12}^{ofp} - 0.78\,\epsilon_{t-1}^{ofp} + 0.70\,\epsilon_{t-2}^{ofp} + 0.20\,\epsilon_{t-2}^{ofp} - 0.93\,\epsilon_{t-12}^{ofp}$

Table 7.3. The examination of residuals using unit root tests indicated that residuals obtained from model were stationary and follow white noise process (Table 7.4). These univariate models can be used for short run inflation forecast.

Table 7.4: Unit Root Tests for Residuals of Estimated Models

Model	KPSS[a] Test Statistics $\{H_0 = I(0)\}$	ADF[b] Test Statistics $\{H_0 = I(1)\}$
Aggregate food	0.17	−17.70**
GROUP2 model		
Primary Food Article	0.18	−18.07**
Manufactured Food	0.09	−18.08**
GROUP7 model		
Cereals	0.08	−17.73**
Pulses	0.11	−17.46**
Fruits and vegetables	0.05	−18.11**
Milk	0.21	−18.65**
Eggs, meat and fish	0.17	−18.07**
Manufactured	0.09	−18.08**
Others	0.14	−17.66**

**Significant at 1 percent level of significance.

The out of sample forecast for the 36 months (June 2010 to June 2013) were made using the best fitted model for each disaggregated food commodity. Subsequently, these forecasts were combined to produce overall food inflation forecast from three alternative models *i.e.* aggregate model, GROUP2 model and GROUP7 model. The forecasting ability of these models was tested by estimating measures such as RMSE, RMSSE, MAE, MAPE, U-Theil (Table 7.5). Additionally, the forecast obtained from each of three models were combined using simple average to produce a combined forecast and forecast evaluation was made. The results showed that GROUP7 model was the best model followed by Combined forecast. The aggregate model possesses highest value of evaluation criteria. This indicate that obtaining forecast of disaggregated food commodities and combining them is better than forecasting using aggregate time series.

Table 7.5: Forecast Evaluation Criteria of Alternative Models as well as its Combination

Model	RMSE	RMSPE	MAE	MAPE	U- Theil	Rank
Aggregate	1.90	1.08	1.39	0.78	0.84	4
GROUP2	1.72	0.99	1.17	0.66	0.80	3
GROUP7	1.57	0.90	1.15	0.65	0.78	1
Combination (Simple average)	1.68	0.96	1.19	0.67	0.79	2

Food Inflation Forecast for June, 2014

The estimated models were used to forecast monthly WPI for the next twelve months *i.e.* July 2013 to June 2014. Based on these values year-on-year forecast of food inflation was calculated for June 2014 (Table 7.6). The food inflation using the best model (GROUP7) will be about 7 per cent in June 2014 (over June 2013). The forecasted value of food inflation using Aggregate model, GROUP2 model and combined forecast in June 2014 will be 6.8 per cent, 5.8 per cent and 6.57 per cent, respectively. Among the disaggregated food products, non-vegetarian products will have highest inflation followed by pulses and milk. The expected value of inflation in near future will help policy makers to take corrective measures to augment food supply or manage demand to control the prices.

Table 7.6: Inflation Forecast for Food Commodities Using Alternative Models for June 2014

Commodity	Inflation Forecast
Primary food articles	8.70
Manufactured food	4.77
Cereals	6.96
Pulses	8.41
Fruits and Vegetables	2.14
Milk	8.40
Eggs, meat and fish	9.79
Others	7.61
Total food	
Aggregate model	6.81
GROUP2 Model	5.84
GROUP7 Model	7.08
Combined forecast	6.57

Conclusions

The study revealed that the WPI for food as well as non-food commodities at (at 2004-05) witnessed a rising trend in the last three decade. The food inflation was found to be more volatile as compared to non-food inflation and followed a cyclical trend. Further, trend in food inflation was not uniform across different food commodities. Primary food articles were the found to be the driving force for the overall food inflation. The improvement in marketing and processing infrastructure will help in reducing the food inflation. Forecast of food inflation by alternative model formulations suggested that forecasting inflation of disaggregated food commodities and combining individual forecast improves the forecast accuracy.

References

Chand R. (2010). Understanding the nature and courses of inflation. *Economic and Political Weekly*, XLV(9), 10–13.

Gokarn, S. (2010). The price of protein. Monthly Bulletin, Reserve Bank of India, November.

Landes (2007), Landes, M. (2007). Indian agriculture and policy in transition. USDA Economic Research Service, Economic Research service, US Department of Agriculture.

Mitra and Josling (2009) Mitra, S. and Josling, T. (2009). Agricultural export restrictions: Welfare implications and trade disciplines (IPC Position Paper, Agricultural and Rural Development Policy Series). Washington, DC: International Food and Agricultural Trade Policy Council.

Sharma, P.,Gummagolmath, K. and Sharma, R. (2011). Prices of onions: An analysis. *Economic and Political Weekly*, XLVI(2), 22–25.

World Bank (2010). World Bank South Asia economic updates 2010: Moving up, looking East.Washington, DC: The World Bank.

Chapter 8

Impact Assessment of Natural Resource Conservation Programmes: A Case Study of Watersheds

Subhash Chand

Principal Scientist (Agricultural Economics),
ICAR-NIAP, New Delhi-110012

Introduction

Economic development projects brought innumerable benefits but also had unintended detrimental effects on people and natural resources. Human activities have resulted in the disruption of social and communal harmony, the loss of human livelihood and life, the introduction of new diseases, and the destruction of renewable resources. These and other consequences can negate the positive benefits of economic development. A balanced development planning takes into account the environmental, social and biodiversity impacts of economic development. Environmental Impact Assessment (EIA), Social Impact Assessment (SIA) and biodiversity impact assessments are some of the methods that aid in the planning and decision making process. These impact assessments help in identifying the likely positive and negative impacts of proposed policy actions, likely trade-offs and synergies, and thus facilitate informed decision-making. The Inter-organisational Committee on Guidelines and Principles for Social Assessment (1994) (cited in Glasson 2000) defined social impacts as 'the consequences to human populations of any public or private actions that alter the ways in which people live, work, play, relate to one another, organize to meet their needs, and generally cope as members of society'. Social impacts include changes in people's way of life, their culture, community, political systems, environment, health and wellbeing, their personal and property rights and their fears and aspirations.

Dimensions of Impact Assessment

Social impact assessment can be performed some times to get an overview of the social issues associated with the project in terms of some of the parameters:

(a) *Demographic factors:* number of people, location, population density, age etc.

(b) *Socio-economic determinants:* factors affecting income and productivity, such as risk aversion of the poorest groups, land tenure, access to productive inputs and markets, family composition, kinship reciprocity, and access to labour opportunities and migration.

(c) *Social organization:* organization and capacity at the household and community levels affecting participation in local level institutions as well as access to services and information.

(d) *Socio-political context:* implementing agencies' development goals, priorities, commitment to project objectives, control over resources, experience, and relationship with other stakeholder groups.

(e) *Needs and values:* stakeholder attitudes and values determining whether development interventions are needed and wanted, appropriate incentives for change and capacity of stakeholders to manage the process of change.

Impact Assessment of Watershed

Watershed management programmes are receiving widespread attention for development and management of dryland/rainfed areas, wastelands and degraded lands for sustained production and enhanced biomass. This holistic approach to resource management is ultimately aimed at understanding the interactive and cumulative effects of a variety of impacts on the watersheds and manages them to protect valued ecosystem and improve overall condition of a watershed. Watershed impact assessment is essentially a part of the comprehensive process of watershed management.

A major area of concern in the realm of watershed management is the inadequate monitoring and impact assessment of various watershed programme. Watershed development projects affect social, economic and environmental activities. Therefore, apart from using the traditional economic measures such as benefit cost ratio, internal rate of return (IRR) alone, it is essential to use suitable measures for social and environmental benefits. Such projects may generate productive (or direct), protective/reclamative, ecological and employment generation benefits. The monitoring and evaluation in a watershed will not only help in analysing impacts of current and future activities but also plan corrective measures after mid-term evaluation. This will also help in monitoring and evaluating the performance of various agencies involved at different levels of watershed project.

There are no single definitive indicators or measures or indices for overall impact assessment in view of its complexities and diverse/multiple objectives. The paper presents some simple surrogate measures or a set of indicators and indices that could be used to assess changes in watershed condition for impact assessment.

Main Issues of Monitoring and Evaluation

a) What indicators to be monitored?
b) What frequency?
c) What measures or indices or tools are used?
d) How and who to do what?

Characteristics of Good Indicators

a) Simple and easy to measure,
b) Reliable and replicable,
c) Sensitive to changes,
d) Simple to compute,
e) Easy to understand and interpret.

Methods of Data Collection for Impact Evaluation

Sample surveys, field observations, discussion with community members, community organizers and line department staff are used for data/information collection. Some of the methods that can be used for information collection are as follows:

☆ Transect
☆ Direct Observation
☆ Semi-structured interview technique
☆ Resource mapping
☆ Scoring, ranking and matrices
☆ Focus group discussion
☆ Self assessment through scoring technique
☆ Sustainability analysis
☆ Garrett ranking
☆ SWOT analysis
☆ Perusal of Records/Registers/Account books maintained by farmer and other agencies.

The selection of indicators is of crucial importance and is a highly skilled task. It depends on the nature of the objectives and intended effects and impacts of the project. Therefore, the first and foremost step is to have a clear and unambiguous statement of short-term, intermediate long-term objectives of the projects *e.g.* water resource development (short-term), runoff and soil loss reduction (intermediate term) and increased production on sustainable basis (long-term). Therefore, the choice of selection of an indicator will depend on users, reporting period and data collection. Generally, the choice of indicators is also guided by common sense, experience, knowledge, statistical data sources, and choice of the project staff, farmers and stakeholders. Before identifying and selecting indicators, project plans should be carefully examined.

Since most of the time bench mark data is not available or inadequate, participatory impact evaluation may be adopted. The evaluation team may largely use PRA techniques for information/data collection during field visits. Sample surveys, field observations, discussion with community members and community organizers and line department staff are used for data/information collection.

Some Impact Evaluation Indices

The following are the some indices use for detail study of impact of the watershed programme.

A. Hydrological Indices

 (a) Changes in runoff depth or water yield.
 (b) Ratio of peak runoff before and after.
 (c) Changes in duration of flow in the stream (*i.e.*, enhanced perennniality of flow).

B. Water Resource Generation Indices

 (a). Changes in surface water storage *e.g.*, ponds, tanks capacities, etc. (b). Change in ground water table (*i.e.*, water table rise) (Table 8.1). Ground water levels as observed from open wells can be used for determining changes by comparing water table with that of outside the watershed or before implementation of works Figure 8.1, (c). Increase in well yield/recuperation, (d). Change in perenniality (*i.e.*, duration of water availability over the year) of water in wells, (e). Some indirect measures include increase in number of wells; increase in irrigated area, duration of pumping before well goes dry and time it takes to recuperate crop diversification (*i.e.*, switching over to cash crops like vegetables, etc.).

C. Soil Erosion and Sedimentation Indices

 (a) Changes in soil loss due to watershed interventions,
 (b) Changes in sediment yield to pond/tank
 (c) Silt deposition in channel bed behind structures and in ponds/tanks.

D. Land Development/Improvement Indices

 (a) Land Improvement Index (LII) (ratio of recommended safe limit of slope to the existing field slope) evolved and demonstrated by Sikka *et al.* (1998) can be used for evaluating impact on land levelling. This was found to

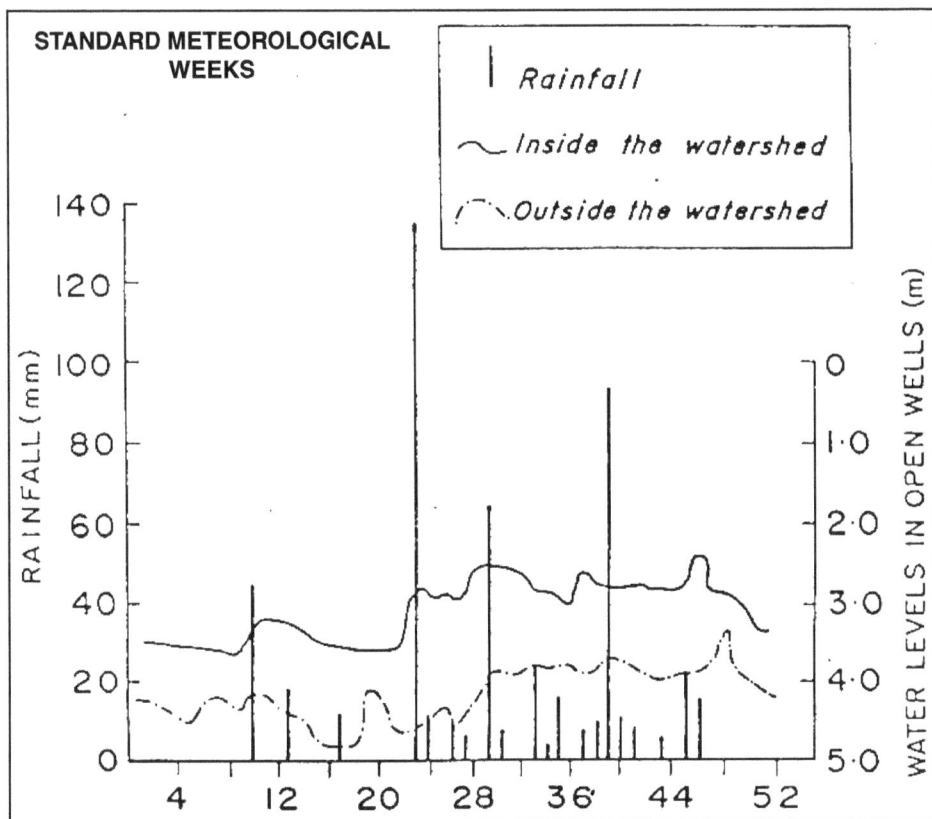

Figure 8.1: Effect of Watershed Management Programme on Groundwater under Recharge in Watershed of Andhra Pradesh (1120 ha).

have increased from a low of 0.22 to 0.61 in just two years after project implementation at Relmajra in Shiwalik foothills of Punjab.

(b) Similarly, an index of area covered under bunding and its condition can be used for evaluating impact of bunding, etc.

Table 8.1: Groundwater Recharge through Percolation Tanks, Water Harvesting Structures and Soil Conservation Measures

Region	Type of Measures	Rise in Water Table (m)
Basaltic formations of Central Maharashtra	Percolation Tank	2.5
Coimbatore district of Tamil Nadu	– Do –	1.0 to 2.5
Chinnatekur, Kurnool, A.P.	Check Dams, bunds and weirs	0.5 to 1.0
Anantapur, A.P.	Water Harvesting Structures	2.0 to 3.0
G.R. Halli, Karnataka	– Do –	1.5
Parbhani, M.S.	Nala bund, gully plugs	0.3 to 2.5

E. Land Use and Productivity Indices

(a) Crop Yield Index

A measure of comparison of the yield of all the crops in a given farm/watershed with the average yield of these crops in the locality/taluk/district/state/country. The relationship is expressed in per cent.

$$\text{Crop Yield Index} = \frac{\text{Average yield in the watershed (q/ha)}}{\text{Average yield in the area (q/ha)}} \times 100$$

Apart from annual crops, yield of fruit, fodder and fuel wood may also be measured similarly.

(b) Crop Diversification Index (DI)

A measure of diversification of crops from less economical to cash crops after implementation.

$$DI = \sum_{i=1}^{n} Pi \log \frac{i}{Pi}$$

Where, Pi is proportion of area sown under crop i.

It can be worked out for both the growing seasons separately.

(c) Cropping Intensity

$$\text{Cropping intensity (CI)} = \frac{\text{Gross cropped area of watershed}}{\text{Total watershed area}} \times 100$$

(d) Crop Fertilization Index

This indicates extent of crop mixtures (NPK) applied to the crop in comparison to the recommended level of nutrients to that crop.

(e) Cultivated Land Utilization Index (CLUI)

The cultivated land utilization index is calculated by summing the products of land planted to each crop, multiplied by actual duration in days of that crop, divided by the total cultivated land area times 365 days.

$$CLUI = \frac{\sum_{i=1}^{n} a_i \, d_i}{A \times 365}$$

where,

$$i = 1,2,3 - n$$

$$n = \text{Total number of crops}$$

ai = Area occupied by the ith crop

di = Days that the ith crop occupied

A = Total cultivated land area available during the 365 days period.

This indicates the duration for which land is being utilized. Prior to the implementation of watershed programme, most of the wastelands in the project area are either fallows or farmers raising only a low value crop for a short period in a year. After the implementation of Project, the wastelands of project area are planted with tree species and the land area in the project site is better utilized by covering the land with permanent vegetation and this quantification is reflected by the CLUI.

(f) Biometric Measures of Trees

This may include important growth parameters of trees such as plant height, girth, and biomass and survival percentage.

(g) Watershed Eco-index

It is the ratio or percentage of watershed area that has been made green through annuals and/or perennials. Induced WEI therefore is used to represent additional area made green through watershed treatment.

Tables 8.2–8.6 illustrate the impact assessment of few case studies using these indices.

Table 8.2: Production and Protection Impact of Watershed Programme (Fakot, UP hills, 327 ha)

Product	Pre-project (1974-75)	During Interventions (1975-86)	After Withdrawal (1987-95)
Food crops (q)	882	4015	5843
Fruit (q)	Neg.	62	1962
Milk ('000 lit.)	56.6	184.8	237.6
Floriculture* ('000 Rs.)	Nil	Nil	120.0* (1994-95)
Cash Crops ('000 Rs.)	6.5	24.8	202.5
Animal rearing method	Heavily grazing	Partially grazing	Stall feeding
Dependency on forest Fodder (per cent)	60	46	18
Runoff (per cent)	42	18.3	13.7
Soil loss (t/ha/annum)	11	4.5	2.0

Source: CSWCRTI, Annual Report 2000.

Table 8.3: Socio-Economic Indicators of Watersheds Implemented by different Agencies

Particulars	Name of the Watershed		
	DPAP	Kattery	CWDP
Literacy (per cent)	49	68	73
Credit Repayment (per cent)	39.16	59	27
Benefit Cost Ratio (BCR at 15 per cent)	1.15:1	–	–
Internal Rate of Return (per cent)	22	–	–
Per Capita Income Before (Rs)	5539	–	5957
After (Rs)	6804		9018
Land value appreciation	–	–	Dry and wastelands (10 to 18 fold)
Employment generation	–	–	man days 66200
Infrastructure Development Index (per cent)	36		

Table 8.4: Participatory Indicators of Watersheds Implemented by different Agencies

Particulars		Name of the Watershed		
		DPAP	Kattery	CWDP
People's Participation	Planning	0.55	0.71	0.52
Index (PPI)	Implementation	0.44	0.56	0.66
Maintenance		0.27	0. 46	0.57
Peoples Participation in different Trainings (No.)		722	277	9081
Community contribution to project activities (per cent)		–	14.71	40
No of SHG's		–	60	173
Women's representation in SHG's (per cent)		22	80	33
Awareness (per cent)		62	82	70

Table 8.35: Productivity Indicators of Watersheds Implemented by different Agencies

Particulars	Before		After	
	DPAP	CWDP	DPAP	CWDP
Cropping Intensity (per cent)	57	–	75	–
Crop Fertilization Index (CFI)	0.67	0.49	0.86	0.63
Index of Crop Productivity (ICP)	0.62	–	0.70	–
Crop Diversification Index CDI_1	0.83	–	0.98	–
CDI_2	0.50	–	0.64	–
Cultivated Land Utilization Index (CLUI)		0.27		1.00
Horticulture plantation (Private land) (per cent)	–	50-68		55-77
Afforestation (Common land) (per cent)	–	6-7		–
Watershed Eco-Index (IWEI)	–	0.20		0.17

Table 8.6: Water Resource Indicators (DPAP Watersheds)

Particulars	Extent	
Additional Capacity created (ha-cm)	1381.54	
Rise in water table (m)	1 – 2.5	
Perenniality of water in wells (per cent)	**Before**	**After**
12 months	14.8	33.3
9 months	51.9	63.0
6 months	33.3	03.7
Increased irrigated area (per cent)	**7**	**21**

**Table 8.7: Impact of Watershed Development Programme
using Remote Sensing Techniques**

Name of the District	Name of the Watershed	Area (hectares)	Period of Study	Increase in NDVI (Percentage)
Ananthapur	Chiyyedu	1000	1992-1997	40
	a. Somagatta	4290	1992-1997	35
	b. Cheegicherla	1500	1992-1997	32
	c. Vanjuvanka	13450	1992-1997	40
	d. Salkamcheruvu	5840	1992-1997	35
	e. Itodu	2200	1992-1997	30
Prakasam	a. Tadivaripalli	1325	1994-1998	30
	b. Vemulakota	2050	1994-1998	42
Kurnool	a. S. Rangapuram	910	1995-1998	240

(h) Application of Remote Sensing to Watershed Monitoring and Evaluation

The repetitive nature of satellite derived data provides near real time information and helps improve the prospects of monitoring changes in land use, vegetation, erosion pattern, etc., in a watershed. Remotely sensed satellite data integrated with the ancillary data using an appropriate GIS can provide a cost-effective tool for monitoring and evaluation of watershed changes. Monitoring of changes in bio-mass, water bodies, etc., is one of the common tool for monitoring watershed impacts. Changes in crop conditions and vegetation detected from remotely sensed data can be used in evaluating the effect of conservation measures on vigour and extent of crops/bio-mass for impact assessment. Vegetation index computed as the ratio of reflectance in near infra-red (NIR) to red ® reflectance or its normalized form (Normalized Difference Vegetation Index NDVI = NIR - R/ NIR + R) computed from reflectance values, is a surrogate measure of the crop or vegetation condition. NDVI of different periods (pre-treatment and post-treatment) can be used to monitor the changes in the condition/vigor of the vegetation and to assess the impact or change in bio-mass production. This has been used for monitoring impact of watershed programmes in a number of districts in Andhra Pradesh. The comparison of vegetation index images of two periods and the charges derived clearly indicated an increase in the crop land and bio-mass in the recent image and this could be attributed to various development activities taken up in the watersheds (Table 8.7).

Socio-Economic Indices/Measures Used in Watershed Impact Assessment

There are a number of direct and also indirect outcome of the project that can be associated with the impact of WSM. As a result of this, level of awareness, education, buying capacity for household assets, infrastructural development is likely to improve. Some of the important socio-economic measures (possession of assets, consumer durables, per capita availability of watershed produce, attendance in school, improvement in housing pattern, literacy) are being used in WSM projects for impact assessment. Per capita availability of agricultural and horticultural produce, milk, etc. can also be taken as a surrogate index. Growth of infrastructures and developmental institutions is also taken as an indirect measure of the watershed impact.

Apart from above socio-economic measures, the following indices can be used to measure the level of community participation, rate of adoption of technology, employment generation, change in borrowing pattern, performance of SHGs, etc. These indices can also be used to monitor and evaluate the performance and community organization activities in the watershed.

(i) People's Participation Index (PPI)

PPI may range from 0 (no participation) to 100 per cent (full participation). This can be used to assess participation at various levels such as planning, implementation and maintenance. A set of questions are framed and answer to each could be assigned scores based on extent of reply. Based on this, scores for each respondent are computed. The same are averaged over the chosen number of respondents to find out the mean participation rate.

$$P = \sum_{i=1}^{N} Pi/N$$

where, Pi is the score of ith respondent and N the number of respondents.

Overall PPI is determined by dividing mean participation by maximum participation score. Based on the mean and standard deviation, this can be grouped into low, medium and high level of participation.

Economic Indices

Economic indices/measures evaluate the project worth by comparing the values of goods and services produced or conserved with the cost for assessing its effect on social welfare needs and viability. The following discounting techniques can be used for this purpose.

(i) Net Present Worth (NPW) Method

This is the most widely used measure. This is the difference between the discounted value of gross benefits and the discounted value of gross costs of the project over its life.

The general formula for NPW is,

$$NPW = \sum_{t=1}^{N} \frac{B_t - C_t}{(1+r)^t}$$

where,

B_t = Gross benefits from the a project in year t

C_t = Gross costs from the project in year t

r = Discount rate

t = time, year 1 to n (life of the project)

The decision rule is to select the projects when NPW is greater than zero, otherwise reject. Higher the NPW, better is the project. Select that project which has highest NPW.

The demerit of this criterion is that it does not reflect the return per rupee invested on the project. The project 'A' may lead to more net present worth than project 'B'. But 'A' also may have more cost than 'B' and the return to per rupee invested (cost) on project 'A' may be less than project 'B'. An example for calculating NPW is given in Example.

(ii) Internal Rate of Return (IRR)

Internal rate of return is frequently used in the evaluation of projects by banks and other organizations. It is the rate of discount, which makes the present value (value today), of benefits equal to present value of costs, thus, IRR does not use a pre- determined discount rate.

The IRR is the discount rate, r such that,

$$IRR = \sum_{t=1}^{n} \frac{B_t}{(1+r)_t} = \sum_{t=1}^{n} \frac{C_t}{(1+r)_t} \text{ or } \sum_{t=1}^{n} \frac{B_t - C_t}{(1+r)_t} = 0$$

In an analysis using IRR measure, the calculated IRR is compared to some prescribed discount rate (generally the interest rate chargeable on money to be invested or the value that invest-ed resources would earn in other opportunities (the opportunity cost of capital) to decide whether the project is worth to take or not? The decision rule applied is to select the project if calculated discount rate IRR is greater than predetermined dis-count rate, otherwise reject it.

The advantages of this measure are: IRR is well known; oftenly used and easily understood; and ranking of projects can be done easily on this basis. However, IRR has some disadvantag-es too. It may be misleading in a situation where selection has to be made among mutually exclusive projects. The reason is that IRR may be higher for project 'A' that in fact produces less benefit than project 'B' having lower IRR but produces more benefits. Calculation of IRR is shown in Example.

(iii) Benefit-Cost Ratio (BCR)

This ratio simply compares the present value of benefits to present value of costs, obtained by dividing the present value of all benefits (sum of discounted benefits) by the present value of all costs (sum of discounted costs).

$$BCR = \sum_{t=1}^{n} \frac{B_t/(1+r)^t}{C_t/(1+r)^t}$$

The decision rule applied is, if the B:C ratio is greater than unity (1), select the project otherwise reject it. The advantages of this measure are: easily understood; easy to convince the planner or decision maker; easy to compute; and it can easily see how much cost is to be allowed to increase before a project is to be rejected.

The use of B:C ratio has two disadvantages. The first one is just as with IRR that BCR favours low cost projects. The second disadvantage is related to computational procedure and interpretation of BCRs.

If we are to simply evaluate one project, the decision criterion is to accept the project as economically feasible if its net present worth (NPW) is greater than zero. Equivalently, the project is accepted if its benefit-cost ratio (B:C) is great-er than one or its internal rate of return (IRR) exceeds the appropriate (pre-determined) rate of discount.

References

A.K. Sikka, M. Madhu, Subhash Chand, D.V. Singh, V. Selvi, P. Sundarambal,K. Jeevarathnam and M Murgaiah (2014). Impact analysis of participatory integrated watershed management progaramme in semi- arid region of Tamil Nadu. *Indian Journal of Soil Conservation,* vol. 42(2):pp. 98-106.

Arya, Swarn Lata and Samra, J.S. (1995). Socio-economic Implications and Participatory Appraisal of Integrated Watershed Management project at Bunga. Bulletin No.T-27/C-6, CSWCRTI, Research Centre, Chandigarh.

Dhruvanarayan, V.V., Bhardwaj, S.P., Sikka, A.K., Singh, R.P., sharma, S.N., Vittal, K.P.R and Das, S.K. (1987). Watershed Management for Drought Mitigation. Bulletin, ICAR, New Delhi.

Glasson, J. (2000). Socio-economic impacts 1: overview and economic impacts, in: Morris, P. and Therivel, R. (2000) (ed), Methods of Environmental Impact Assessment, Spon Press, London and New York.

Grewal, S.S., Samra, J.S., Mittal, S.P and Agnitotri, Y. (1995). Sukhomajri Concept of Integrated Watershed Management. Bulletin No.T-26/C-5, CSWCRTI, Research Centre, Chandigarh.

P. Sundrambal, Subhash Chand and A.K. Sikka (2004). Constraints experienced in attending various trainings by women in Nilgiris, *Indian J. Soil Cons.,* 32(2) pp. 81-90.

Samra, J.S., Bansal, R.C., Sikka, A.K., Mittal, S.P and Agnihotri, Y. (1995). Resource Conservation Through Watershed Management in Shiwalik Foothills – Relmajra. Bulletin No.T-28/C-7, CSSWCRTI, Research Centre, Chandigarh.

Singh, Katar, (1994). People's participation in micro watershed management – case study of an NGO Gujarat. *Indian Jour. Soil Conservation*, 22(1-2), pp. 271-278.

Subhash Chand, A. K. Sikka, R. C. Srivastava and Sundarambal (2009). Constraints Faced by Functionaries in Watershed Management: A Case Study. *Indian Research Journal of Extension Education*, Vol.9 (2): 68-71.

Subhash Chand, A.K. Sikka, R. Raghupathy, P. Samraj and C. Henry (2002). Economic evaluation of Agro-forestry Systems on Sloping lands of Nilgiris",. Published in *Indian J. Agricultural Economics*, vol. 57(4):pp. 736-740.

Subhash Chand, Alok K. Sikka and V.N. Sharda (2009). Environmental Implications of Converting Natural Grass Land into Eucalyptus Plantations in Hydro Power Catchments in Nilgiris, Tamil Nadu: An Economic Analysis, *Indian J. of Agricultural Economics*, vol. 64(4):618-627.

Subhash Chand, Sikka. A.K. Sikka, Madhu. M., Singh. D.V and Sundarambal, P. (2003). Impact Assessment on Socio-Economic aspects of Watershed Programmes: A case study. *Journal of Rural Development*, Vol. 22(4), pp. 487-500.

Subhash Chand, Sikka. A.K. Sikka, Rajkumar, S., Sundarambal, P., M.J. Sam and Madhu. M. (2002). Capacity building of informal institutions through watershed management Programmes in hilly areas: An experience in Nilgiris. *Journal of Rural Development*, NIRD, Hyderabad 29(4): 757-768.

Chapter 9

Technologies for Conservation Agriculture

Usha Ahuja

ICAR- NIAP, New Delhi – 110 012

Introduction

Presently agricultural sustainability, resource conservation and food problem are the important issues debated at national and international levels. Therefore, agricultural technology that can save resources, reduce production costs and improve production while sustaining environmental quality is becoming increasingly important. Conservation agriculture offers a powerful option for meeting future food demands while also contributing to sustainable agriculture and rural development. CA methods can improve the efficiency of input, increase farm income, improve or sustain crop yields, and protect and revitalize soil, biodiversity and the natural resource base. Conservation agriculture (CA) aims to conserve, improve and make more efficient use of natural resources through integrated management of available soil, water and biological resources combined with external inputs. It contributes to environmental conservation as well as to enhanced and sustained agricultural production. It can also be referred to as resource efficient or resource effective agriculture (FAO). Conservation agriculture permits management of soils for sustainable agricultural production without excessively disturbing the soils, while protecting it from the processes of soil degradation like erosion, compaction, aggregate breakdown, loss of organic matter, leaching of nutrients, and processes that are accentuating by anthropogenic interactions in the presence of extremes of weather and management practices. Conservation agriculture is used in most of the world's high-performing food production systems to strengthen soil structure and fertility, improve water retention and bring farmers savings in cost and labor for comparable yields. But conservation practices have yet to be taken-up in many low-income countries with fragile ecosystems as this technology is suitable for both irrigated and rain fed systems, but particularly for subsistence farmers in dry areas with poor soils.

Meaning of CA

Conservation agriculture combines minimum tillage, retention of crop stubble, and use of crop rotations. It significantly reduces production costs, while improving crop yields, soil health and nutrient recycling.

The FAO has characterized CA as follows:

Conservation Agriculture maintains a permanent or semi-permanent organic soil cover. This can be a growing crop or dead mulch. Its function is to protect the soil physically from sun, rain and wind and to feed soil biota. The soil micro-organisms and soil fauna take over the tillage function and soil nutrient balancing. Mechanical tillage disturbs this process. Therefore, zero or minimum tillage and direct seeding are important elements of CA. A varied crop rotation is also important to avoid disease and pest problems.(see FAO web site)

The three "pillars" of conservation agriculture are:

1. Minimum soil disturbance
2. Maintaining soil cover, and
3. Diverse crop rotations.

So Appropriate CA technologies encompass innovative crop production systems that combine the following basic tenets

Zero Tillage

Studies conducted for agricultural conservation, resulted in different mechanized technologies, out of those zero tillage is one of the successful technologies for conservation agriculture. To date, the most successful resource conserving technology in the rice–wheat systems has been zero-tillage and now it is being adopted in other cropping systems also.Tillage systems influence physical, chemical, and biological properties of soil and have a major impact on soil productivity and sustainability. Conventional tillage (CT) practices may adversely affect long-term soil productivity due to erosion and loss of organic matter in soils. Sustainable soil management can be practiced through conservation tillage (including no-tillage). Studies conducted under a wide range of climatic conditions, soil types, and crop rotation systems showed that soils under no-tillage and reduced tillage have significantly higher soil organic matter contents compared with conventionally tilled soils

Zero tillage generally reported to save irrigation water in the range of 20–35 per cent in the wheat crop compared to CT, reducing water usage by about 10 cm ha–1, According to various studies, excessive tillage leads to degradation of land and environment pollution. Zero tillage has changed the proverb of *Dab keVaho,*

Raazhkekhao. Zero tillage specialized machine can directly sow a crop in standing stubbles without the land preparation. Results of number of studies which are related to zero tillage, showed reduction in the cost of cultivation, saving in fuel, at the same time escape from excessive use of fertilizers, seeds, pesticides and water. It is noticed that most of the time the farmers burn the stubbles as a result create the pollution as well destroy the beneficial pest those are helpful to increase the productivity of crops.

Retention of Adequate Levels of Crop Residues on the Soil Surface

Surface retention of sufficient crop residues to protect the soil from water run-off and erosion; improve water infiltration and reduce evaporation to improve water productivity; increase soil organic matter and biological activity; and enhance long-term sustainability. Soil microbial biomass (SMB) has commonly been used to assess below-ground microbial activity and is a sink and source for plant nutrients. Amendments such as residues and manures promote while burning and removal of residues decrease SMB.Cover crops help promote biological soil tillage through their rooting; the surface mulch provides food, nutrients and energy for earthworms, arthropods and micro-organisms below ground that also biologically till soils. Burring stubbles, destroys the organic productive pest which leads to use of more fertilizers by the farmers for increasing the productivity resultantly land has become habitual of more fertilizers but the productivity is stagnant. Moreover excessive use of fertilizers is harmful for future agriculture. Ground cover promotes an increase in biological diversity not only below ground but also above ground.

Use of Sensible Crop Rotations

Crop rotation is an agricultural management tool with ancient origins. Employ economically viable, diversified crop rotations to help moderate possible weed, disease, and pest problems; enhance soil biodiversity; take advantage of biological nitrogen fixation and soil enhancing properties of different crops; reduce labor peaks; and provide farmers with new risk management opportunities

The rotation of different crops with different rooting patterns combined with minimal soil disturbance in zero-till systems promotes a more extensive network of root channels and macro pores in the soil. This helps in water infiltration to deeper depths. Because rotations increase microbial diversity, the risk of pests and disease outbreaks from pathogenic organisms is reduced, since the biological diversity helps keep pathogenic organisms in check.

Other interventions being tested and promoted include raised-bed planting, laser-aided land-leveling, residue management alternatives, and alternatives to rice–wheat cropping system in relation to CA technologies. Adopting CA systems further offers opportunities for achieving greater crop diversification. Direct seeded rice has been evaluated as an alternative to transplanted rice in view of increasing water and labour crisis and the adverse effect of greenhouse gas emissions like methane and nitrous oxide. The work on system rice intensification in rice based production systems is also being worked out for saving water, chemical fertilizers and plant protection chemicals, and reducing greenhouse gas emissions and also improving soil health. Information on efficient alternatives to rice-wheat cropping system

Crop Management with Conservation Agriculture

International Centre for Agricultural research in the Dry Areas (ICARDA) has given following recommendations for sound crop management with Conservation Agriculture.

☆ Do not till fields. Ploughing is unnecessary, takes time and money, and robs soil of moisture, organic matter, and structure.

☆ If required, kill off weeds with a non-selective herbicide before planting. This may not be necessary where there is little weed growth after harvest, *e.g.* where summers are hot and dry.

☆ Sow as early as possible. This is usually immediately after the first effective rains when soil moisture is favourable. If the rains are late, consider sowing into dry soil—the seeds will remain viable for many weeks and when the rains come establishment should be satisfactory.

☆ Sow seed and apply fertilizer using a zero-tillage or minimum-tillage seeder. Ensure seed depth and distribution are uniform.

☆ Use reduced seed rates. Seed establishment rates with zero-tillage seeders should be high, so high seed rates are not required; 50–100 kg/ha for cereals and 100–150 kg/ha for pulses are recommended, depending upon expected rainfall.

☆ Manage crop nutrition and control pests, diseases and weeds according to the best local practices. These may need to be modified to suit CA systems. In medium- and high-rainfall regions pay special attention to weed management with the use of selective herbicides.

☆ If possible, leave crop residues on the soil surface after harvest. This protects the soil from wind and water erosion and returns nutrients to the soil.

☆ If needed, allow livestock to graze on stubble and crop residues. While this is not ideal, livestock production is important for many farmers in the region.

☆ Do not burn crop residues.

☆ Wherever possible, rotate crops between cereals, legumes and other crops. this will help avoid build-up of cereal weeds, pests, and diseases.

Constraints in Adoption of CA Practices

In India, efforts to adopt and promote CA practices are in increasing demand among stakeholders in intensively copped areas as in IGP. There is also limited use in other parts of India due to inappropriate knowledge about CA technologies, unavailability of machinery and shortage of fodder and fuel in rural areas. The Northern and Eastern IGP, black soil belts of central plateau, Odisha-upland systems,

Coastal high rainfall regions and rainfed regions are the areas where there is a potential to improve crop productivity through CA technologies. In IGP, some of the CA components have gone to field implementation whereas in other parts of India efforts are made to popularize such technologies. Developing location specific CA practices in these regions are urgently required.

Steps to Encourage Adoption

Given the chance, the financial and environmental benefits of conservation agriculture (CA) can sell themselves. The task for policy-makers and development partners is to give this innovative approach to agriculture a chance with farmers who are skeptical that crops can grow on land that has not been prepared with heavy plowing.

ICARDA's experience has shown that three key steps can lead to widespread adoption of conservation tillage:

1. Raise Awareness

Farmers and the national agricultural research and extension systems they depend on must be made aware of the principles and benefits of CA. This can be done by showing them how CA has worked in similar circumstances, preferably in neighboring countries. Field experiments on research stations can help convince them that the system works, and help fine-tune the system for local conditions and practices. Field days and training courses are the main avenues for raising initial awareness.

2. Provide Appropriate and Affordable Seeders

Farmers must have access to seeders that they can afford, operate, and maintain with their own resources. As farmers become interested in continuing to use CA they will create local demand for affordable seeders. Policy-makers and development partners can help local entrepreneurs acquire the capacity to manufacture seeders and kits for converting conventional seeders that are already being used to zero-tillage seeders. Manufacturers may require specialized training to improve their knowledge and skills, and access to quality parts and materials. Custom hiring of zero-tillage seeders can also be a feasible alternative

3. Establish Participatory Extension Groups

Once researchers, extensionists, and farmers understand CA principles, they need to see it in practice. ICARDA's experience shows that the best way to do this is using a participatory extension approach, enlisting the collaboration of scientists, extension officers, socio-economists, policy-makers, machinery manufacturers, and farmers. To begin with, farmers should be able to test seeders free of charge. Above all, this phase must take a flexible approach to testing CA under local conditions and adapting it to meet farmers' circumstances and resources. Farmers may require concessions that allow them to participate without fear of the consequences of crop failure.

References

FAO, (2008). Investing in Sustainable Agricultural Intensification. The Role of ConservationAgriculture. A Framework for Action. Food and Agriculture Organization of the United Nations, Rome.

FAO, 2008. Conservation Agriculture. 2008-07-08 http://www.fao.org/ag/ca/index.html.

Ito, M., Matsumoto, T., Quinones, M.A., 2007. Conservation tillage practice in sub-Saharan Africa: the experience of Sasakawa Global 2000. *Crop Prot.* 26, 417–423.

Case Study 1

Socio-Economic Impact of Zero Tillage in Mewat District of Haryana State

Zero tillage is one of the successful technologies for conservation agriculture. The study was conducted in the ten villages of the district with a sample of 100 farmers who adopted zero tillage for the cultivation of wheat.Qualitative and quantitative data were collected through focus group discussions and a well-structured schedule regarding cost and benefits of zero tillage as compared to conventional tillage. Data were analyzed to see the efficiency, equity, and sustainability of zero tillage compared to conventional method of tillage by adopting before and after technique of impact assessment.

Results regarding socio economic impact of Zero tillage (Table 9.1) revealed that this intervention reduced the cost of cultivation by 15 percent; increased crop yield by 7 percent and net income is enhanced by 45 percent. Moreover, energy requirement is reduced to an enormous extent (85 per cent), labor and irrigation also got reduced by this intervention. Moreover, there are other intangible benefits which need to be seen further. Economically zero tillage is superior over conventional method of sowing because more net returns were recorded on zero tillage farms than that of conventional wheat farms in addition to its edge of eco-friendly practice (Nagarajan *et al.*, 2002). For a technology to be adopted, it is pre-requisite that it has been evaluated with respect to its economic feasibility and viability which is a major determinant of its adoption. Regarding adoption and up scaling of this intervention it has been observed that in the study area, the interest of the farmers in the purchase of zero tillage seed drill is so intense that the applicants for subsidized Zero Tillage machines are more than the target with the state Department of Agriculture in district Mewat. So it can be concluded that by addressing the existing knowledge gaps regarding zero tillage and assessing socio economic, livelihood, and environmental impacts would enhance the ability to out scale it in a cost-effective, equitable, and sustainable manner.

Table 9.1: Effect of Zero Tillage on Yield, Cost of Cultivation, Fuel Saving, Labor Saving and Net Income

Indicator	Particulars	Before	After	Change	
				Absolute	*(Per cent)*
Efficiency	Reduction in Cultivation Cost (Rs/acre)	10192	8716	1476	14.5
	Reduction in tractor fuel (litre/acre)	18.5	2.5	16	85
	Increase in Net Income (Rs/acre)	11025	15992	4966	45
Equity	Labour saving M/days	16	11	5	
Sustainability (Water saving)	Pumping hours/acre	11.6	9	2.6	24

Chapter 10

Agricultural Prices and Market Intelligence in India*

Raka Saxena and S. Pavithra

Senior Scientist and Scientist,
ICAR-NIAP, New Delhi-110012

Backdrop

It is evident that India has marched through a long way in achieving a significant increase in the overall production of agricultural commodities particularly the food grains. The total food grain production in the country has increased from 50 million tonnes during the period 1950-51 to 264 million tonnes in 2013-14. Though there was a notable expansion in the area under food grains prior to 1960's, during the last two decades the total area under food grains has been pegged at around 121-125 million hectares indicating that the area expansion has played a limited role in the increase in agricultural output as compared to the productivity of crops. These noticeable achievements on the production front have transformed Indian agriculture towards higher commercialization from the status of a mere subsistence level activity. Over the years, increase in area and production of major agricultural commodities has not only resulted in attaining self-sufficiency in food production in India, but has also helped in increased participation in agricultural trade through the promotion of agricultural exports thus, building the foreign exchange reserves.

---

* This chapter is an output of the SSN Project on Market Intelligence awarded to NIAP by the Indian Council of Agricultural Research and is largely drawn from Chapters 1 and 2 of the Manual on Price Forecasting Techniques, ICAR-National Institute of Agricultural Economics and Policy Research, New Delhi.

In the year 2013-14, agricultural exports accounted for about 14 per cent of the value of the total national exports of the country (GOI, 2014)

Marketed Surplus Ratio (MSR), expressed as the ratio of output marketed to the total output produced, serves as an indicator for the extent of output traded in the commodity markets in relation to the crop output consumed at farm household level for meeting the requirement of home consumption, seed, feed and wastages in handling. The change in MSR for the major agricultural commodities of the country is presented in Table 10.1. The marketed surplus ratio for most of the crops has increased appreciably during last 13 years from 1999-2000 to 2011-12. The increase was more prominent during 1999-2000 to 2004-05. As far as the food grains are concerned, maize was the highest marketed crop in India. The marketed surplus ratio was highest for cotton and some of the oilseeds due to obvious reasons. Thus, the higher MSR clearly indicates the increasing commercialization of Indian agriculture in terms of commodity marketing and trade. Efficient marketing and trade of agricultural commodities require modern market infrastructure, processing facilities, efficient distribution channels, enabling institutions and policies as well as better marketing networks in place to ensure remunerative returns to the farmers.

Table 10.1: Marketed Surplus Ratio of Important Agricultural Commodities in India

Crops	1999-00	2004-05	2011-12
Rice	60.32	71.37	77.20
Wheat	54.48	63.33	70.00
Maize	62.79	76.22	83.32
Jowar	46.83	53.44	53.46
Arhar	62.93	79.52	81.45
Gram	65.63	93.76	85.25
Urad	80.91	85.76	70.04
Moong	70.13	76.79	87.32
Lentil	59.87	85.86	88.14
Groundnut	63.34	88.75	90.78
Rapeseed and Mustard	71.57	89.66	82.08
Soybean	94.95	94.99	94.41
Sunflower	99.30	98.32	65.62
Sugarcane	82.50	98.23	78.02
Cotton	94.58	94.94	98.36
Jute	97.50	90.72	83.50
Onion	–	82.91	75.36
Potato	45.90	85.00	77.40

Source: Agricultural Statistics at a Glance, various years.

The achievement on the production front in terms of a significant increase in production would translate into higher farm incomes, consumer welfare and poverty reduction only when it is supported by an efficient and competitive marketing system. Agricultural marketing system plays a pivotal role in fostering and sustaining the tempo of rural development and it also triggers the process of agricultural development. An efficient and competitive agricultural marketing system is crucial not only to ensure an effective transfer of agricultural commodities from farmer to the consumers but also in achieving its broader objectives of providing market signals and production incentive to farmers, balancing the demand and supply of agricultural commodities and in ensuring efficient utilization of production resources (Acharya, 2003; Chand, 2012).

Challenges in Agricultural Marketing

Agricultural marketing in India is facilitated through a network of regulated markets established under the APMC Act. The objective of such intervention was to ensure regulation of marketing practices and protect the farmers from the exploitation of intermediaries. However, there is an argument that over a period, market regulation has taken the form of restrictive and monopolistic trade and the balance of power in transactions has moved in the favour of middle men and traders (Chand, 2012). In fact, Acharya (2006) attributes the failure of agricultural marketing system in India to an excessive state intervention. As a result, the prices realized by the farmers still remain low.

Adequate marketing infrastructure helps in maintaining the quality of agricultural produce as well as in reducing the losses in handling. There is still a lack of conducive market infrastructure facilities for the sale of agricultural produce. Several markets are still found to be poorly equipped to handle the agricultural produce. It is unfortunate that the existing number of regulated markets are not sufficient enough to cater to the expanding agricultural production of the country. The total number of regulated markets in India as on 31.3.2014 was 7114, and the number of rural periodical markets was 22759. Area covered by each regulated market was as low as 118 per sq km in Punjab to 1031 per sq km in Himachal Pradesh considering only the major states (AGMARKNET). This leads to congestion in the regulated markets during the peak arrival seasons ultimately leading to delay in the disposal of the farm produce. There is also a dearth for well linked cold storage system in the country.

Studies have indicated that only two third of the regulated markets are equipped with covered and open auction platforms; only one fourth of the markets have common drying yards; whereas, grading facilities are found in one third of the regulated markets. Only few markets are found to have electric weigh bridges. Even the Azadpur mandi, which is the biggest mandi of Asia, handling bulk of the produce through all India feeding markets, is not able to efficiently handle the produce and not able to provide the congenial atmosphere for trading. A common auction platform is not available in one-third of the markets, necessitating the use of private platforms or the conduct of auctions without the proper display of produce (Chand, 2012).

Inadequate cold storage facility is the major constraint in the case of horticultural commodities because of high perishability of the products and less retention capacity of the farmers. This has resulted in huge post-harvest losses of agricultural produce. Also, inadequate storage infrastructure forces farmers to resort to distress sales. Further, as a result of lack of storages facilities there is higher wastage in the supply chain. It has been reported that the range of post-harvest losses of cereals in India is 3.9 to 6 per cent, in pulses it is at 4.3 to 6.1 per cent while in the case of fruits and vegetable it is estimated at 5.8 to 18 per cent and 6.8 to 12.4 per cent respectively (DAC, 2013).

Despite the structural transformation in terms of its linkage with the international economy as well as the increased role of private players, the farmers' share in consumers' rupee is quite low. Long supply chains with a number of intermediaries have resulted in high marketing costs. The share of producers' price in consumer rupee is estimated to be to be 66 per cent, while it is as low as 20 per cent in the case of fruits and vegetables. This reflects the extent of inefficiencies existing in the agricultural marketing system of India (Gulati, 2009).

There is still a long way to go ahead in modernizing the agricultural markets in terms of developing state of art infrastructure, implementation of scientific grading and standardization methods, package and quality certification, product traceability, use of Information communication technology in disseminating the market information and intelligence. The recent initiatives of Gulbarga model of E-tendering in markets, proposed model of Unified Market Platform in agricultural marketing are important steps in revamping the agricultural marketing system under the Mandi Modernization Programme. These new initiatives are yet to be adopted on a large scale. The reluctance of traders in accepting such initiatives also highlights the importance of market extension system in the country.

An excellent example for the role of good marketing system in facilitating the spread of technology on the production front and enabling its gains to reach the farmers in terms of higher profitability is provided by the case of Bt Cotton in India, wherein, the increased production resulting from the introduction of Bt technology, led to increased gains from trade and farmers profitability (Gulati, 2009). In India, poor marketing linkages and infrastructure constraints have led to high and fluctuating consumer prices resulting in only a small share of consumer rupee reaching the farmer. In addition to this, the issues of poor produce handling, wastage of produce, lack of scientific grading and storage facilities have also affected the efficiency of agricultural marketing in India.

Importance of Agricultural Prices

There has been increasing emphasis in the recent past on assessing the impact of agricultural research in terms of its contribution towards efficiency, equity, sustainability and trade. Several researchers have assessed the gains from varietal research along with the improvement in research processes. Agricultural price situation on the other hand may further add or dilute such gains. The gains from positive price movements might significantly influence the farmer's well-being though their impacts on other section of the society may be negative.

Agricultural prices hold tremendous importance in Indian economy and have a significant influence on the decision making pattern of farmers and other stakeholders regarding the crop acreage as well as the marketing decisions. Agricultural prices create a significant impact on the well-being of famers and help in determining their income. The changes in terms of trade between agriculture and non- agricultural sectors affect the transfer of income to the farmers. Hence, agricultural price policy of the country helps in achieving the growth and equity in the Indian economy. The main objective of agricultural price policy is to ensure remunerative pries to the farmers for their produce. The Commission for Agricultural Costs and Prices (CACP) has been entrusted with the responsibility of fixing the Minimum Support Prices (MSP) of agricultural commodities in India. Cost of production (CoP) is one of the important factors in the determination of MSP of mandated crops; the Commission considers other important factors such as demand and supply, price trends in the domestic and international markets, inter-crop price parity and terms of trade between agricultural and non-agricultural sectors, the likely impact of MSPs on consumers, in addition to ensuring rational utilization of natural resources like land and water (Government of India, 2015).

Agricultural prices provide signals for allocation of resources across the various enterprises and different crops at farm level. Changes in relative prices of various agricultural commodities over a long period of time might have drastic impact on the cropping pattern and cropping system of various typologies. Agricultural prices usually follow a seasonal pattern and exhibit different trends during the crop growing season and off-season. As observed, monsoon failures often generate strong inflationary pressures on the prices due to shortage in supply and thereby reduced quantity of arrivals and many times the effect may spillover to others seasons as well.

Price Indications at the Macro Level

The indicative trends in agricultural prices at the macro level are reflected through the wholesale price indices compiled and released at the national level by the Office of the Economic Adviser (OAE), Ministry of Industry on weekly basis. The WPI series, at present, covers 676 commodities and is available with the latest base year 2004-05. These commodities covered under the WPI series are divided into three broad sectors mainly primary, secondary and territory sectors. The primary sector covers agricultural commodities (food and non-food) along with minerals. At present, primary commodities have been assigned the weight of 20.12; one may derive the WPI series for agricultural sector by deducting the series of minerals from the WPI series of primary commodities.

Recently, the prices of many agricultural commodities have shown a high degree of volatility caused by time lags between production decisions and delivery to the market. There is enough evidence to show that prices of agricultural commodities are more volatile than those of the non-farm commodities (Chand and Parappurathu, 2012). In the recent years the issue of high price volatility in agricultural commodities in domestic as well as international market has assumed critical importance. Figure 10.1 depicts the trends in inflation for all commodities, food commodities and non-.food commodities. As indicated earlier, food commodities have been highly

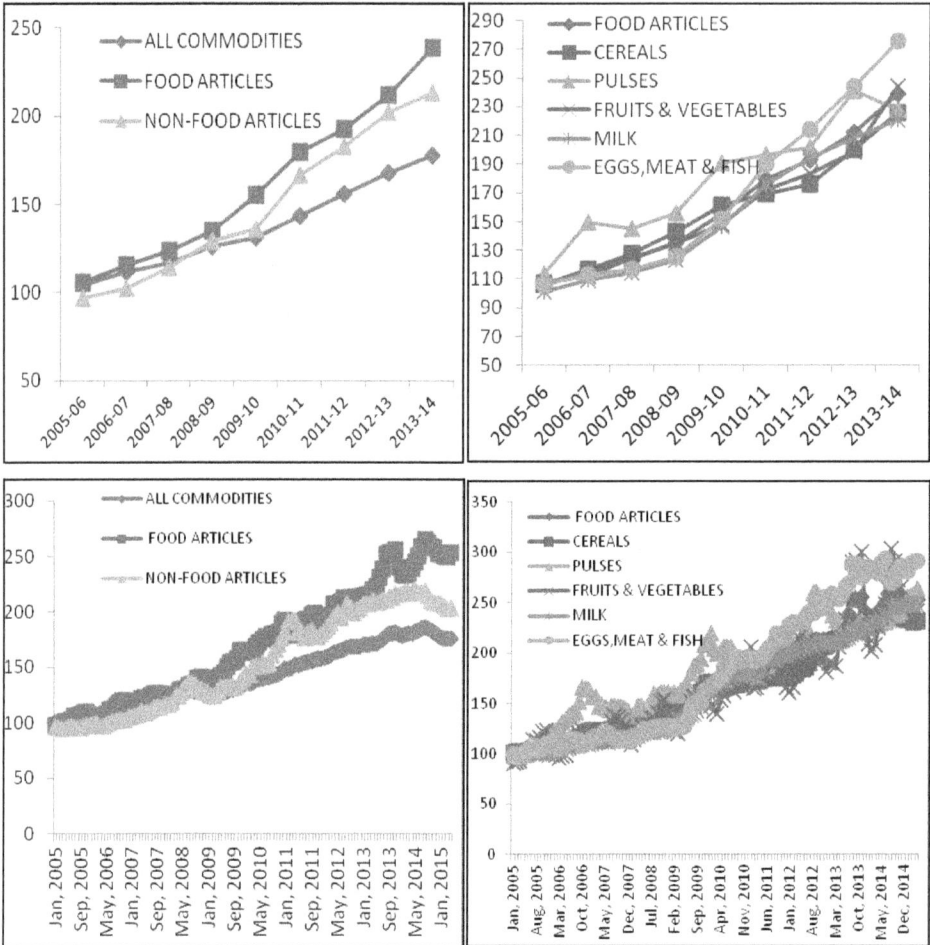

**Figure 10.1: Trends in the Wholesale Price Indices of
Food and Non-food Commodities.**

volatile during the recent years. An attempt has been made to reflect the changes separately. The changes have been depicted on the basis of both annual series as well as monthly series of WPI.

The annual series reflect smooth pattern in the WPI series of various categories. However, the monthly series capture the price volatility more precisely as agricultural commodities are seasonal in nature. Fruits and vegetables seem to exhibit highest price volatility among all agricultural commodities. Some commodities in this category, like onion, have created crisis situation in the economy many a times due to the extreme volatility in their prices. Onion is a highly sensitive commodity in the fruits and vegetables category, whose WPI has touched the highest peaks of 619 in January, 2011 and 846 in September, 2013.

The wholesale price indices may be treated as the index of price received by the farmers. However, if one has to analyze the changes in price paid by the farmers, the input price series published by the office of economic advisor may be examined. On the other hand, consumer price index for agricultural labor (CPIAL) published by the labor bureau indicates the changes in prices of various consumption goods expended by the agricultural labor segment.

The Labour Bureau of India has been compiling the Consumer Price Index for Agricultural Labourers (CPIAL) since September, 1964; the existing series is available with 1986-87 as the base year. For compilation of these index numbers, the Field Operations Division (FOD) of the National Sample Survey Organisation (NSSO) collects the monthly price data from 600 sample villages selected from 20 States with a well-structured price collection schedule. The consumer expenditure data collected by the NSSO during 38th round of National Sample Survey (NSS, 1983) formed the basis for the state level weights diagrams for the series (Labour Bureau). The rural labour households, who derive 50 per cent or more of their total income from wage paid for manual labour in agricultural activities, are treated as agricultural labour households. As per the methodology given by the Labour Bureau, the rural retail prices utilised in WPI and CPI index numbers are the same, but the weighting patterns used for compiling these indices are different.

The all-India index is worked out as a weighted average of the indices of 20 States, weights being the estimated consumption expenditure of all rural and agricultural labour households in each state as a proportion of corresponding expenditure for all-India. All-India group indices are also compiled by using the state weights in the particular group, derived as a proportion of corresponding expenditure at all-India level (Labour Bureau).

Volatility in Agricultural Prices

Indian agriculture is going through a phase transformations such as growing commercialization and diversification towards high value agricultural commodities, increasing liberalization and global interfaces, increase in foreign direct investments etc. Several institutional and policy initiatives have been taken to support these transformations. However, prices of agricultural commodities play a dominant role in determining farm profitability and distribution of income. A remunerative and stable price environment is considered to be very important for providing incentives to farmers for increasing agricultural production and productivity. Strong indications are emerging in India and at the global level that, in future, price increases will drive supply growth rather than supply growth resulting in a fall in prices (Chand and Parappurathu, 2012).

The prices of food and agricultural commodity in India are primarily determined by domestic market forces along with the domestic price policy. The imperfections in agricultural markets also influence the prices and price transmissions. Price rise of agricultural commodities has become a major concern for policy makers in India. A notable turnaround was observed in terms of trade after 2004-05, which was attributed to faster growth in agricultural prices (around 30 per cent higher) than those of non-farm commodities (Chand and Parappurathu, 2012).

In recent years, the agricultural prices have suffered from very high volatility. The issue of high price volatility in agricultural commodities in domestic as well as international market has assumed critical importance in the changing context of trade liberalisation. The volatility in the agricultural prices has catastrophic effect on all the stakeholders involved in the production, marketing and consumption of the food commodities (Sekhar, 2004). This has increased the risk faced by farming community.

Besides temporal volatility, there also exists wide spatial variability in the prices of agricultural commodities. Varying climatic conditions and differences in resource endowments result in regional specialization of the agricultural commodities which are marketed through alternate marketing channels to consumers spread across the country. The interplay of the available supply along with the demand determines the prevailing price in a region. Further, agricultural prices are influenced by variety of socio, economic, policy and inefficiency factors prevailing in the region. This necessitates regional/state level analysis to understand the causes and impact of agricultural prices.

Market Intelligence: Need and Implementation

Considering the fluctuations in agricultural price scenario, proper understanding of agricultural price mechanism and their forecasts would help farmers to plan and decide about the production portfolio and to take up appropriate marketing decisions for improved farm profit. Timely and reliable forecast information on future agricultural prices enables the farmer to decide on allocation of land across the various crops based on the information provided on expected prices during the pre-sowing period. Prior to the harvest such information provides guidance as to whether there is a scope for delayed harvest, whether immediate sale of the produce is desirable or if it would be remunerative for the farmer to store the produce and sell the produce later. This would also help the traders to understand the market trend and the Government to timely and apt policies that augment the welfare of producers and consumers. Sufficient information about the prices would strengthen the otherwise weak linkage between production and marketing in the country.

Market Intelligence is the process of collecting relevant statistics and information related to the existing market prices, domestic and global agricultural supply and demand conditions, weather parameters, policy environment and other relevant factors; and processing these information to through scientific modelling exercises to obtain the forecasts on probable future prices of the commodities. Such model based forecasts may be complemented with the surveys on stakeholders' perceptions to improvise the forecast range by capturing the qualitative dynamic factors of the market conditions. The forecasts, thus obtained, are disseminated through effective means so that informed and effective decisions can be taken by the farmers and other stakeholders. This entire process involves the conversion of market data into usable information and then to market intelligence. The purpose of this analysis is to derive meaning inferences based on the historic behavior of commodity prices which can be used by the stakeholders. In other words, market intelligence is the information, gathered and analyzed specifically for the purpose of accurate and confident decision making for determining the market opportunities and utilizing them in an effective manner.

The initial efforts on market intelligence started as early as 1954, when on the recommendation of the Agricultural Prices Enquiry Committee, (1954), the Directorate of Economics and Statistics, Ministry of Agriculture (DESMOA) set up 14 Market Intelligence Units (MIU) in the capitals of Andhra Pradesh, Assam, Bihar, Delhi, Gujarat, Karnataka, Kerala, Madhya Pradesh, Maharashtra, Orissa, Rajasthan, Tamil Nadu, Uttar Pradesh, and West Bengal (Government of India, 2010). The market intelligence units were intended to help the DESMOA in the formulation, implementation and review of the agricultural price policy relating to procurement, marketing, storage, transportation, import, export and credit, etc; the units were also required to give their appraisal of production of various kharif and rabi crops at regular intervals to help preparation of crop forecasts (Government of India, 2010).

AGMARKNET was the mega initiative launched by Government of India through a network of directorate of Marketing and Inspection, Department of Agriculture and Cooperation and National Informatics Centre. The initiative connected all major agricultural markets of the country and provided the current price information to the beneficiaries. The daily information is compiled by the regulated markets and provided to NIC for sharing on the web portal. Besides the commodity wise price and arrival information, the portal has been enriched over a period of time in terms of providing other useful information related to Government policies, regulations, subsidies etc. Based on the temporal trends, the information is useful for the academic and research organizations for making future predictions regarding the price behavior.

In this direction a Network Project on Market Intelligence was initiated by the Indian Council of Agricultural Research (ICAR) in 2013 to provide reliable and timely price forecasts to farmers for selected agricultural commodities in order to enable them to make informed production and marketing decisions, which in turn could lead to higher profitability. The project is implemented through a network of State agricultural universities and other ICAR and non-ICAR agricultural research organisations focussing on the regionally important commodities. The commodities have been selected based on a number of parameters like supply conditions, arrival pattern, global linkages etc which have important bearing on the prices of these commodities. Appropriate forecast models are developed to capture the unique behaviour of each commodity; forecasts are developed based on modelling framework along with the consideration of qualitative expectations of farmers and traders.

The forecasts are disseminated to farmers and other stakeholders through newspapers, mobile based voice messages, websites, television, radio, information bulletins etc. Stringent efforts are also being made to personally disseminate the price forecasts to the farmers before sowing and before harvesting of selected commodities. Some of the network centres have also used innovative dissemination modes such as facebook and whatsapp to reach a section of the farming society who are technology friendly. Excepting the case of few volatile horticultural commodities such as potatoes and onions, the centres have been developing regular pre-sowing and pre-harvest price forecasts with desired accuracy. Apart from this, case studies on agricultural marketing issues in the different study locales are being conducted to examine and understand recent developments and issues in agricultural marketing.

References

Acharya, S.S. (2003). Analytical framework for review of agricultural marketing institutions. In: Institutional Change in Indian Agriculture, Eds: Suresh Pal, Mruthyunjaya, P.K. Joshi and Raka Saxena, NCAP, New Delhi.

Acharya, S.S. (2006). Agricultural marketing and rural credit for strengthening Indian agriculture. *INRM Policy Brief No. 3,* The Asian Development Bank, India Resident Mission (INRM), New Delhi.

AGMARKNET (2014). Directorate of Marketing and Inspection, Government of India, http://www.agmarknet.nic.in/RMS2014.pdf [14 September, 2015].

Chand, R. (2012). Development policies and agricultural markets. *Economic and Political Weekly,* 47(52): 53-63.

Chand, R. and Parappurathu, S. (2012). Temporal and spatial variations in agricultural growth and its determinants. *Economic and Political Weekly,* 47 (26-27): 55-64.

Government of India (2010). Manual on Agricultural Prices and Marketing, Central Statistics Office, Ministry of Statistics and Programme Implementation, New Delhi. [14 September, 2015].

Government of India (2014). Agricultural statistics at a glance. http://eands.dacnet. nic.in/PDF/Agricultural-Statistics-At-Glance2014.pdf [2 September, 2015].

Government of India, Consumer price index numbers for agricultural and rural labourers, Labour Bureau, Chandigarh. http://labourbureau.nic.in/CPI per cent 20ALRL per cent 202K6-7 per cent 20Method.htm [4 October, 2015].

Gulati, A. (2009). Emerging trends in Indian agriculture: What can we learn from these? *Agricultural Economics Research Review,* 22:171-184.

Saxena, Raka, Pavithra S, Ranjit K Paul, Sanjay Chayal and Shikha Chaurasia (2015). A Manual on Price Forecasting Techniques, ICAR-National Institute of Agricultural Economics and Policy Research, New Delhi.

Sekhar, C.S.C. (2004). Agricultural price volatility in international and Indian markets. *Economic and Political Weekly,* 39(43): 4729-4736.

Chapter 11

Spatial Market Integration: A Case of Indian Milk and Ghee Markets

Sunil Kumar Singh[1], Balwant Singh Chandel[1]
and Shiv Kumar[2]

[1]Division of Dairy Economics, Statistics and Management,
ICAR- NDRI, Karnal-132 001
[2]ICAR- NIAP, New Delhi – 110 012

ABSTRACT

India is the largest milk producer in the world with 127.9 million tonnes but its share in world trade in dairy products is very small (0.3-0.4 per cent). Inter-regional differences in milk production in India are due to the inter-regional differences in processing and marketing infrastructure and other facilities for milk in India. The prices of milk and milk products differ widely from one region to other. But, with the improvement in marketing infrastructures and intelligence over time, price differences between different regions have been narrowed down. To assess whether there is any linkage among the markets of dairy products, co-integration method developed by Johansen (1991, 1995) has been used. The results have confirmed the existence of long-run co-integration among selected markets of milk at wholesale and retail price levels and ghee at wholesale level. The study concludes that markets strong in basics of production, processing, logistics and marketing infrastructure are more stable and requires less extended intervention for smooth conduct of market.

Keywords: Milk, Ghee, Wholesale, Retail, Price, Johansen co-integration test.

The dairy sector has been an important source of employment and income to the rural women besides enriching the protein in diet of the vegetarian population. There are significant regional differences in the consumption of milk largely due to its scarcity in some regions and surpluses in others. For example, the per capita milk consumption as well as production is the lowest in the eastern region and the highest in the northern region (Kumar and Birthal 2004). Such regional imbalances in demand and supply indicate a considerable scope for inter-regional trade in milk and milk products and growth of dairy sector. Until recently, dairy cooperatives provided much needed market support to dairy farmers. The cooperatives were protected from external and internal competition. Therefore, linkage between markets of dairy products is of significant importance in such a situation to the stakeholders of dairy sectors. If markets are well integrated, free flow of information between markets exists, reduce price volatility and encourage farmers to improve production efficiency, adopt best production practices and optimize their production portfolioes based on comparative advantage. While lack of market integration encourages arbitrages and unwarranted trade practices, in case of both excess demand and supply situations.

External trade in dairy products was regulated through licensing and tariffs. Internally, the entry of the private processors in the dairy industry was restricted through regulations. However, some notable changes have taken place in the dairy policy since the initiation of economic reforms programme in 1991. After such reforms, any change in the world market has direct effect on the domestic markets. Even if world prices do not directly influence the domestic prices, there are going to be indirect effects in terms of improvement in quality, pattern of product-mix, efficient marketing system, reduction in subsidy, etc. Accompanied by Information Technology (IT) developments, domestic dairy market without any exception is going to observe the law of one price in the near future.

Empirical evidence on integration of markets in India is scanty and scattered for agricultural commodities in general and dairy products in specific. Sekhar (2012) reported that the markets of commodities with less inter-state or inter-regional movement restrictions are likely to be well integrated. The study on integration of milk (Kumar et al., 2011) and milk products (Sharma and Ram, 1998) markets indicate that there exists integration among markets. Though the study on market integration of dairy products have been conducted by some researchers but either they have used very old technique which suffers from several limitations (Sharma and Ram, 1998) or they have covered only liquid milk market (Kumar et al., 2011) not any other manufactured dairy products. Therefore, studying the integration condition of manufactured dairy products' markets is necessary to understand whether the markets of manufactured dairy products are more strongly co-integrated or degree of their co-integration is similar to the liquid milk markets.

Indian Dairy Sector

Dairy sector is an important driver of agricultural growth in specific and Indian economy as a whole in general. India ranks first in the world in milk production, which went up from 17 million tonnes in 1950-51 to 127.9 million tonnes in 2011-

12. The per capita availability of milk has also increased from 112 grams per day in 1968-69 to 290 grams in 2011-12. Dairying has become an important secondary source of income for millions of rural families and has assumed an important role in providing employment and income-generating opportunities. Nearly two-thirds of the farm households are associated with dairy production and it contributes around 24 per cent of the total agricultural gross domestic product (DAHD and F). During 1980–81 to 2005–06, milk production grew at an annual rate of 4.5 per cent as compared to a growth rate of 2.9 per cent in the agricultural gross domestic product (Birthal and Taneja, 2006) providing a cushion to agricultural growth and livelihood of the farmers against income shocks of crop failure. The demand for dairy products is increasing due to rise in per capita income and rapid urbanization. Between 1983 and 1999 per capita milk consumption increased by 71 per cent (Kumar and Birthal 2004) and the demand for milk is expected to increase to around 140 million tonnes (Delgado *et al.,* 2001) or even more (Hazell and Bhalla, 1998) by 2020.

With appropriate policies in place the organized sector, cooperatives and private processors could procure 17 per cent of the total milk produced in 2005–06, up from 10 per cent in 1994– 95. During this period, the share of private sector in the organized milk market went up from 40 to 55 per cent (Candler and Kumar 1998, Birthal 2008). In anticipation of further increase in the share of private sector, milk markets are conjectured to move towards strong integration.

Materials and Methods

Data on prices of milk and milk products are very scanty in India and available only for limited markets. Even those markets for which price data is available, the data period is not uniform. The paucity of data on prices of dairy products also reflects from the fact that the number of markets differed from one product to other and for type of prices *i.e.* wholesale and retail prices. Moreover, the period of data available for different markets of milk and milk products were also not uniform. The study is based on secondary data of MMP prices. Monthly time series data on wholesale and retail prices of milk and ghee for important markets in the India were collected for the period of January, 1988 to December, 2007 from various issues of Agricultural Prices in India published by Directorate of Economics and Statistics, Department of Agriculture and Cooperation, Ministry of Agriculture, Government of India, New Delhi. The markets for which price data were available for entire period under study as per type of prices are given below.

Name of Product	Name of Market (State/UT)/Type of Prices
Wholesale Price	
Milk	Chennai (Tamil Nadu), Delhi, Kanpur (Uttar Pradesh) and Kolkata (West Bengal)
Ghee	Chennai (Tamil Nadu), Darbhanga (Bihar), Kanpur (Uttar Pradesh), Kolkata (West Bengal) and Rohtak (Haryana)
Retail Price	
Milk	Chennai (Tamil Nadu), Delhi, Kanpur (Uttar Pradesh), Kolkata (West Bengal) and Mumbai (Maharashtra)

Spatial market integration refers to a situation in which prices of a commodity in spatially separated markets move together and price signals are transmitted smoothly across the markets (Ghosh, 2000). Empirical testing of market integration has evolved over time from the early stages of using bivariate correlation coefficients to the more recent techniques that take into account non-stationarity, common trends and endogeneity of prices. With the advances in time-series and econometric techniques, recent studies in the Indian context have started using the co-integration methodology (Behura and Pradhan, 1998; Wilson, 2001; Kumar and Sharma, 2003).

Logarithmically transformed monthly wholesale and retail prices of milk and ghee were used for studying the market co-integration. We have used co-integration technique developed by Johansen (1991, 1995) to study the co-integration among the markets of milk (wholesale and retail) and ghee (wholesale) during 1988-2007. While studying the market co-integration, it was hypothesized that, with the improvement of market infrastructure and intelligence, the price volatility would reduce over the time period and lead to market integration where prices in one market are effectively transmitted to other market. As the Granger and Newbold, (1974) pointed out, the regression of a non stationary time series on another non-stationary time series may produce a spurious regression. Thus, the stationarity of time series on prices was ascertained using ADF test of the following nature.

$$\Delta P_t = a + \beta t + b P_{t-1} + \alpha_i \sum_{i=1}^{n} \Delta P_{t-j} + e_t$$

where,

$$\Delta P_t = P_t - P_{t-1}$$
$$\Delta P_{t-j} = P_{t-j} - P_{t-(j+1)}$$
$$j = \text{Number of time lags}, j = 1, 2, \ldots, n$$

A time series was stationary if null hypothesis (H_0: b = 0) was rejected as against the alternate hypothesis (H_1: b < 0).

The Schwarz Information Criterion (**SIC**) was employed to determine the optimum lag length for market integration test. The **SIC** is defined as:

$$SIC = n^{k/n} RSS/n \text{ or } SIC = n^{k/n} \Sigma u^2/n$$

where,

k is the number of regressors (including the intercept) and **n** is the number of observations.

The lag length at which **SIC** value was lowest has been selected for studying the co-integration.

Co-integration test is used to determine whether a group of non-stationary series is co-integrated or not. Johansen co-integration test involves the running VAR-based co-integration tests of following nature:

$$y_t = A_1 y_{t-1} + \ldots\ldots\ldots + A_p y_{t-p} + u_t \tag{1}$$

where,

y_t = Vector of non-stationary variables,

u_t = Vector of innovations.

P = Number of lags

The above VAR model may be written as:

$$\Delta Y_t = \pi Y_{t-1} + \sum_{i=1}^{p-1} \Gamma \Delta Y_{t-i} + u_t$$

where,

$$\pi = \sum_{i=1}^{P} A_i - I, \qquad \Gamma_i = -\sum_{j=i+1}^{P} A_j$$

The rank of π determines the number of co-integrating relations. Further, if the coefficient matrix π has reduced rank $r < k$, then there exist $r \times k$ matrices α and β each with rank r such that $\pi = \alpha\beta'$ and $\beta'y_t$ is **I(0)**. r is the number of co-integrating relations (the co-integrating rank) and each column of β is the co-integrating vector. The elements of π are known as the adjustment parameters or speed of adjustment. Likelihood ratio trace test statistics has been used to determine the number of co-integrating vectors with the null hypothesis of at most r co-integrating vectors against an alternative hypothesis of k co-integrating vectors, where k is the number of endogenous variables, for $r = 0, 1, ..., k-1$. The trace statistic for the null hypothesis of r co-integrating relations is computed as:

$$LR_{tr}\left(\frac{r}{k}\right) = -T \sum_{i=r+1}^{k} \ln(1-\lambda_i)$$

where,

T is the number of usable observations and λ is the calculated ordered characteristic root of the π matrix.

Maximum Eigenvalue statistic, which tests the null hypothesis of r co-integrating relations against the alternative of $r+1$ co-integrating relations, is computed as:

$$LR_{max}\left(\frac{r}{r+1}\right) = -T \ln(1-\lambda_{r+1})$$

$$= LR_{tr}\left(\frac{r}{k}\right) - LR_{tr}\left(r+\frac{1}{r}\right)$$

The co-integrating series do not move independent of each other and there is a systematic co-movement of the series in the long-run. However, in the short-run, if there is any deviation from the long-run equilibrium path, then some error correction process will bring the system back onto path defined by the equilibrium. A vector error correction (VEC) model is a restricted VAR designed for use with non-stationary series that are known to be co-integrated. The VEC has co-integration relations built into the specification so that it restricts the long-run behavior of the endogenous variables to converge to their co-integrating relationships while allowing for short-run adjustment dynamics. The co-integration term is known as the *error correction* term since the deviation from long-run equilibrium is corrected gradually through a series of partial short-run adjustments.

Let the co-integrating equation for two variable systems with one co-integrating equation and no lagged difference terms be given by:

$$Y_{2't} = \beta Y_{1't}$$

The VEC model corresponding to the above equation may be given as follows:

$$\Delta y_{1't} = \alpha_1 (y_{2't-1} - \beta y_{1't-1}) + e_{1,t}$$

$$\Delta y_{2't} = \alpha_2 (y_{2't-1} - \beta y_{1't-1}) + e_{2,t}$$

where,

y_1 and y_2 are the price of first product and second product,

α and β = Estimated coefficient,

e_1 and e_2 = Error terms

$t = 1, 2, ..., n$

In the above VEC model, the right-hand side variable is the error correction term. In long-run equilibrium, this term is zero. However, if y_1 and y_2 deviate from the long-run equilibrium, the error correction term will be non-zero and each variable adjusts to partially restore the equilibrium relation. The coefficient α_i measures the speed of adjustment of the ith endogenous variable towards the equilibrium.

Results and Discussion

The ADF test indicated that all the price series of selected dairy products and markets were found non-stationary at level data. However, at first difference, the entire wholesale and retail price series were found stationary (Appendix). Thus, the wholesale and retail price series of the selected dairy products and markets were integrated of order one *i.e.* I(1). This explains the existence of long-run equilibrium relationship among the markets. In the short-run, markets can, however, deviate from the long-run equilibrium path due to various exogenous shocks. The original long-run equilibrium path is reinstated only when some error correction process begins.

Wholesale Price

Milk

The selected markets of milk at wholesale prices are integrated in long term with one co-integrating relation (Table 11.1A) similar to finding of Kumar *et al.*, 2011. After knowing that markets are integrated in long-run, VEC model was estimated to obtain co-integration elasticities and the speed of adjustment over short-run shocks. Using information presented in Table 11.1B, the co-integrating equations with long-run elasticities normalized by the elasticity in Delhi market is written as:

Table 11.1A: Trace Statistics for Rank of Ordered Root Matrix

Ordered Root	Estimated π	Trace Statistic	Critical Value		Hypothesized No. of CE(s)
			1 per cent	5 per cent	
π^1	0.1000	53.217	54.682	47.856	None*
π^2	0.0720	28.240	35.458	29.797	At most 1
π^3	0.0432	10.507	19.937	15.495	At most 2
π^4	0.0001	0.0328	6.635	3.8415	At most 3

Table 11.1B: Long-run Elasticities and Speed of Adjustment

	Delhi	Kanpur	Kolkata	Chennai	Constant Term
Co-integrating Vectors	1.000	−0.517 (0.100)	−0.243 (0.076)	−0.644 (0.132)	289.341
Speed of adjustment	−0.264** [-5.084]	0.022 [0.552]	0.278** [2.572]	0.0182 [1.068]	

**: Significant at 1 per cent level; *: Significant at 5 per cent level.

Value in ( ) indicates standard error and value in [ ] indicates t value.

Delhi = -289.341; Kanpur +0.517; Kolkata +0.243; Chennai -0.644

The above equation suggested that milk prices in Delhi market were positively related to the milk prices in Chennai while it was negatively related to the milk prices in Kanpur and Kolkata markets as appears from the sign of estimates of co-integrating vectors. It could be interpreted as, in the long-run 1 per cent increase in wholesale prices of milk in Chennai market has led to increase in the prices of milk in Delhi market by about 0.64 per cent, while 1 per cent increase in wholesale price of milk in Kanpur and Kolkata markets has led to decrease in the prices of milk in Delhi market by about 0.52 per cent and 0.24 per cent, respectively. A comparison of the speed of adjustment in Delhi (-0.264) and Kolkata (0.278) markets reveals that the milk prices in Kolkata market took lesser time to correct the short–run deviation than milk prices in Delhi market. Any short-run deviation from this long-run relationship would be corrected by error correction process with speed of adjustment. The speed of adjustment in Kanpur and Chennai milk markets was not significantly different from zero at 5 per cent level of probability. This suggested that Kanpur and Chennai milk markets were weakly exogenous and there was likelihood that milk prices in these markets did not deviate much in short-run from the long-run equilibrium. In other words, the short-run milk prices in Kanpur and Chennai markets were less affected by the change in prices in Delhi and Kolkata milk markets. On the other hand, the speed of adjustment in Delhi and Kolkata markets was significantly different from zero, indicating that prices in these markets were sensitive to price change in Kanpur and Chennai markets. This implies that the long-run equilibrium in Indian wholesale milk market, if disturbed by any exogenous shock would primarily be reinstated by corrective measures in Delhi and Kolkata markets. The estimated speed of adjustment and together with its significance for different markets suggests that if there was a short-run positive deviation from the long-run relationship, the system would respond with decrease in milk prices in Delhi markets and increase in milk prices in Kolkata market. However, weak exogeneity in Kanpur and Chennai markets indicated that these markets were more stable and less prone to external shocks in the short-run.

Ghee

All the selected ghee markets are also integrated at wholesale prices with three co-integrating relations and there exists a long-run relationship among ghee prices in these markets (Table 11.2A). The co-integrating equation with long-run elasticities, normalized by the elasticity in Kanpur market is written as:

$$\text{Kanpur} = 5239.097; \text{Rohtak} +3.53; \text{Dharbhanga} +0.49;$$
$$\text{Kolkata} -0.35; \text{Chennai} -1.93$$

As implied by above long-run co-integrating equation, ghee prices in Kanpur market were positively related to the ghee prices in Rohtak and Dharbhanga markets while it was negatively related to the ghee prices in Kolkata and Chennai markets (Table 11.2B). This means, in the long-run, 1 per cent increase in wholesale price of ghee in Rohtak and Dharbhanga markets have led to increase the prices of ghee in Kanpur market by about 3.53 per cent and 0.49 per cent, respectively while 1 per cent increase in wholesale ghee price in Kolkata and Chennai ghee markets have led to decrease the prices of ghee in Kanpur market by about 0.35 per cent and 1.93 per cent, respectively. A comparison of the speed of adjustment in Kanpur (-0.121), Dharbhanga (0.251) and Kolkata (0.134) markets reveals that the ghee price in Dharbhanga market took lesser time to correct the short–run deviation than ghee prices in Kanpur and Kolkata markets. Any short-run deviation from this long-run relationship would be corrected by error correction process with speed of adjustment. The speed of adjustment in Rohtak and Chennai markets was not significantly different from zero at 5 per cent level of probability. This suggests that Rohtak and Chennai markets were weakly exogenous and there was likelihood that ghee prices in these markets did not deviate much in short-run from the long-run equilibrium. In other words, in short-run, ghee prices in Rohtak and Chennai markets were less affected by the changes in prices in Kanpur, Dharbhanga and Kolkata markets. The speed of adjustment in Kanpur, Darbhanga and Kolkata markets were significantly different from zero at 1 per cent level indicating that prices in these markets were sensitive to price changes in Rohtak and Chennai markets. This implies that the long-run equilibrium in ghee markets, if disturbed by any exogenous shock would primarily be reinstated by corrective measures in Kanpur, Darbhanga and Kolkata markets. The estimated speed of adjustment and together with its significance for different markets suggests that if there was a short-run positive deviation from the long-run relationship, then system would respond with a decrease in ghee prices in Kanpur market and increase in ghee prices in Darbhanga and Kolkata markets. However, weak exogeneity of Rohtak and Chennai markets indicates that these markets were more stable and less prone to external shocks in the short-run.

Table 11.2A: Trace Statistics for Rank of Ordered Root Matrix

Ordered Root	Estimated π	Trace Statistic	Critical Value		Hypothesized No. of CE(s)
			1 per cent	5 per cent	
π^1	0.275	171.722	77.819	69.819	None **
π^2	0.205	95.0866	54.682	47.856	At most 1 **
π^3	0.101	40.423	35.458	29.798	At most 2 **
π^4	0.061	14.968	19.937	15.495	At most 3
π^5	0.00003	0.009	6.635	3.841	At most 4

Table 11.2B: Long-run Elasticities and Speed of Adjustment

	Kanpur	Rohtak	Dharbhanga	Kolkata	Chennai	Constant Term
Co-integrating Vectors	1.000	−3.526 (0.432)	−0.493 (0.274)	0.346 (0.248)	1.931 (0.288)	−5239.097
Speed of adjustment	−0.121** [-3.917]	0.074 [1.542]	0.281** [5.593]	0.134** [3.808]	0.022 [0.468]	−

**: Significant at 1 per cent level.

Value in ( ) indicates standard error and value in [ ] indicates t value.

Retail Price

Milk

The trace statistics of co-integration indicate that all the milk markets at retail price are integrated in long-run with a single co-integrating relation (Table 11.3A). The presence of co-integrating equation signifies that there exists a long-run relationship among milk prices in these markets. The co-integrating equations with long-run elasticities, normalized by the elasticity in Delhi market may be written as:

Delhi = -10.825; Kanpur -0.607; Kolkata +2.607;
Mumbai -0.114; Chennai -0.079

The above equation suggested that milk prices in Delhi market was positively related to the milk prices in Kanpur, Mumbai and Chennai markets and it was negatively related to the prices in Kolkata market as indicated by the sign of coefficients of co-integrating vector (Table 11.3B). In other words, in the long-run 1 per cent increase in retail prices of milk in Kanpur, Mumbai and Chennai markets have increased the prices of milk in Delhi market by about 0.61, 0.11 and 0.08 per cent, respectively while 1 per cent increase in retail prices of milk in Kolkata has decreased the retail prices of milk in Delhi market by about 2.61 per cent. Any short-run deviation from this long-run relationship would be corrected by error correction process with the speed of adjustment. A comparison of the speed of adjustment in Kolkata (0.151) and Chennai (-0.009) markets showed that the milk price in Kolkata market took lesser time to correct the short–run deviation than milk prices in Chennai market. The speed of adjustment in Delhi, Kanpur and Mumbai retail milk markets were not significantly different from zero at 5 per cent level of probability. This suggests that Delhi, Mumbai and Kanpur milk markets were weakly exogenous and there was likelihood that milk prices in these markets did not deviate much in short-run from the long-run equilibrium. It also means that in short-run, milk prices in Delhi, Kanpur and Mumbai retail milk markets were less affected by the changes in prices of Kolkata and Chennai milk markets. On the other hand, the speed of adjustment in Kolkata and Chennai markets were significantly different from zero at least at 5 per cent level of probability, indicating that prices in these markets were sensitive to price changes in Delhi, Kanpur and Mumbai milk markets. It implies that the long-run equilibrium in retail milk market, if disturbed by any exogenous shock would primarily be reinstated by corrective measures in Kolkata and Chennai retail milk markets. The estimated speed of adjustment and together with its significance for different markets suggests that if there was a short-run positive deviation from the long-run relationship, then the system would respond with increase in milk prices in Kolkata and decrease in prices in Chennai market. However, weak exogeneity in Delhi, Mumbai and Kanpur milk markets indicated that these markets were more stable and less prone to external shocks in the short-run.

Table 11.3A: Trace Statistics for Rank of Ordered Root Matrix

Ordered Root	Estimated π	Trace Statistic	Critical Value		Hypothesized No. of CE(s)
			1 per cent	5 per cent	
π^1	0.2126	86.489	77.819	69.819	None **
π^2	0.0637	29.597	54.682	47.856	At most 1
π^3	0.0429	13.944	35.458	29.797	At most 2
π^4	0.0146	3.5152	19.937	15.495	At most 3
π^5	0.0001	0.0244	6.6349	3.8415	At most 4

Table 11.3B: Long-run Elasticities and Speed of Adjustment

	Delhi	Kanpur	Kolkata	Mumbai	Chennai	Constant Term
Co-integrating vector	1.000	0.607 (0.430)	−2.607 (0.313)	0.114 (0.287)	0.079 (0.530)	10.825
Speed of adjustment	−0.014 [-1.849]	0.0006 [-0.095]	0.151** [6.625]	−0.016 [-1.348]	−0.009* [-2.355]	–

**: Significant at 1 per cent level; *: Significant at 5 per cent level.

Value in ( ) indicates standard error and value in [ ] indicates t value.

Conclusions

Despite regional differences in milk production, consumption and marketing infrastructure, all the milk markets at wholesale and retail prices and ghee markets at wholesale price are co-integrated in long- run. Although, there is short-run deviation from long-run equilibrium but long-run equilibrium is restored after some error correction process. Our results highlight that markets of processed dairy products like ghee is more strongly integrated than markets of liquid milk and that may be due to fact that ghee can be stored for longer time and easily transported from one place to another. Moreover, any short-run deviation is corrected more quickly in case of ghee while milk prices require longer time to correct short-run deviation. The existence of long-run equilibrium among the markets of milk and ghee proved that our hypothesis about the impact of improvement of market infrastructure and intelligence hold true *i.e.,* with improvement of market infrastructure and intelligence have led to the co-integration of distance markets spread over different regions of India. Markets with strong production and well developed processing and market infrastructure are proving to be more stable. This also hints at positive development in marketing of dairy products in spite of the fact that the products are highly perishable. The integration of the distant markets could have been possible due to fast exchange of information besides better infrastructure and other marketing facilities like transportation, processing, storage etc., which enables producers/manufacturers to transport milk and milk products from one market to other in response of price change due to the change in demand or supply of dairy products. The policy implication of the study is that the markets which are affected weakly by exogenous forces have gathered strength and removes all sets of imperfections in market with their inherent forces and requires less intervention by government machinery to conduct the efficient functioning of the market.

References

Behura D. and Pradhan D.C. 1998. Co-integration and market integration – An application to the marine fish markets in Orissa. *Indian Journal of Agricultural Economics* **53** (3): 319-350.

Bhalla G S and Hazell P. 1998. Food grains demand in India to 2020 - A preliminary exercise. *Economic and Political Weekly* **32** (52): A150-164.

Birthal P S and Taneja V K. 2006. Livestock Sector in India: Opportunities and Challenges for Smallholders. Smallholder Livestock Production in India: Opportunities and Challenge. National Centre for Agricultural Economics and Policy Research, New Delhi, and International Livestock Research Institute, Nairobi.

Birthal P S. 2008. Linking Smallholder Livestock Producers to Markets: Issues and Approaches. *Indian Journal of Agricultural Economics* **63** (1): 19–37.

Candler W and Kumar N. 1998. India: The Dairy Revolution. The World Bank, Washington, D. C.

Delgado C, Rosegrant M. W. and Meijer S. 2001. Livestock to 2020: The revolution continues. Paper Presented at the Annual Meeting of the International Trade Research Consortium (IARTC), Auckland, New Zealand, January 18–19. (Retrieved from: http://www.ilri.org/ILRI_Dev-pdf/delgado.pdf.).

Dickey D. A. and Fuller W. A. 1981. Likelihood ratio statistics for autoregressive time series with a unit root. *Econometrica* **49**: 1057–1072.

Ghosh M. 2000. Co-integration tests and spatial integration of rice markets in India. *Indian Journal of Agricultural Economics* **55** (4): 616-626.

Government of India. 2012. Basic Animal Husbandry Statistics. Ministry of Agriculture, Department of Animal Husbandry, Dairying and Fisheries (DAHD and F). New Delhi (www.dahd.nic.in/).

Granger C .W. J. and Newbold P. 1974. Spurious Regressions in Econometrics. *Journal of Econometrics* **2** (2): 111-120.

Johansen S. 1991. Estimation and hypothesis testing of co-integration vectors in Gaussian vector autoregressive models. *Econometrica* **59**: 1551-1580.

Johansen S. 1995. Likelihood-based inference in co-integrated vector auto-regressions. In Advanced Texts in Econometrics, Oxford: Oxford University Press.

Kumar S, Birthal P. S. and Chaudhary K. R. 2011. Integration of food markets in India: A case of milk markets. *Indian Journal of Animal Sciences* **81** (5): 75-79.

Kumar P. and Birthal P. S. 2004. Changes in demand for livestock and poultry products in India. *Indian Journal of Agricultural Marketing* **18** (3): 110–123.

Kumar P. and Sharma R. K. 2003. Spatial price integration and pricing efficiency at the farm level: A study of paddy in Haryana. *Indian Journal of Agricultural Economics* **58** (2):201-217.

Sharma A. K. and Ram K. 1998. A study of inter-market integration in milk and milk products in India. *Indian Journal of Dairy Science* **51**(3): 168-171.

Sekhar C. S. C. 2012. Agricultural market integration in India: An analysis of select commodities. *Food Policy* **37**: 309–322.

Wilson E. J. 2001. Testing Agricultural Market Integration: Further Conceptual and Empirical Considerations Using Indian Wholesale Prices, Examining ten years of economic reforms in India, ANU, Canberra, Australia.

Appendix: Results of Unit Roots Tests

Markets	ADF Test at	Lag Length	ADF Test Statistics	Series Stationary
Milk wholesale				
Chennai	Level	0	−0.223	No
	First difference	0	−13.948	Yes
Delhi	Level	10	−0.237	No
	First difference	9	−8.843	Yes
Kolkata	Level	3	−1.301	No
	First difference	2	−12.841	Yes
Kanpur	Level	12	−1.297	No
	First difference	12	−4.023	Yes
Ghee wholesale				
Chennai	Level	12	0.065	No
	First difference	11	−4.072	Yes
Kolkata	Level	0	−1.440	No
	First difference	0	−14.756	Yes
Darbhanga	Level	13	0.046	No
	First difference	12	−5.108	Yes
Rohatak	Level	12	−0.442	No
	First difference	11	−4.161	Yes
Kanpur	Level	0	−1.065	No
	First difference	0	−16.594	Yes
Milk retail				
Kolkata	Level	12	−1.072	No
	First difference	11	−6.195	Yes
Delhi	Level	1	−0.868	No
	First difference	0	−20.091	Yes
Mumbai	Level	0	−0.844	No
	First difference	0	−16.641	Yes
Chennai	Level	0	0.065	No
	First difference	0	−16.969	Yes
Kanpur	Level	0	0.154	No
	First difference	0	−16.704	Yes

Note: The critical values for ADF test at 1 per cent and 5 per cent level of probability are -3.45763 and -2.87344, respectively.

Chapter 12

Decision Making Pattern of Potato Farmers in India

Rajesh K. Rana

Principal Scientist,
ICAR-NIAP, New Delhi – 110 012

Potato cultivation is a high risk-high returns crop enterprise. Cost A_1 of potato cultivation under reasonably good crop husbandry practices in different parts of the country varies from Rs. 69000 to Rs. 88000 per hectare while the Cost C ranges between Rs. 92000 to 122000 per hectare which is quite high compared to most of widely grown crops. Table 12.1 gives a glance of cost of potato cultivation under an average situation in the country. However, long term potato growers are generally found richer than other farmers in the locality. Prosperity of such potato growers creates temptation to other growers and even non-growers (with hired-in land) to go for potato cultivation. Such tendency increased during the years following those years during which potato farmers earn extra-ordinary profits. With the result potato area in India grew by 15-20 per cent during 2014-15 as potato farmers earned hefty profits during 2013-14. Such cycles of fluctuating potato supplies and prices keep on repeating in potato which is an indication that farmers are consistently taking some wrong decision on selection of crop.

Further, potato cultivation is highly technical affair and lack of precision and timeliness in performing various crop husbandry operations may lead to heavy crop and financial losses to the farmers. Potato yield responds to planting time, weed management, insect-pest (especially late blight) management, irrigation management and nutrient management is a big way. In addition to all this invariably the quality of seed potato is the most important factor responsible for potato yield performance.

Table 12.1: Average Cost of Potato Cultivation (Rs./ha unless specified)

Particulars	Overall
Costs components	
Seed potato$	48903
Farm yard manure	5789
Fertilizers	9625
Irrigation charges@@	4223
Bullock labour	4232
Tractor charges	7113
Hired human labour	8684
Plant protection chemicals	3767
Miscellaneous cost	2081
Interest on working capital	1886
Total Cost A₁	**96303**
Imputed rental value of own land@	10416
Cost B	**106719**
Imputed value of family labour	6410
Cost C	113130

$:   Seed potato prices may vary from year to year and therefore cost of seed in total potato cultivation may vary from Rs. 32000 to Rs. 59000 per hectare.

@@:   Irrigation charges may vary from place to place depending upon the ground water depth and availability in addition to quality of electricity supply and policies of the local state government in order to subsidize electricity or micro-irrigation systems.

@:   Imputed value of own land also varies from place to place depending upon land productivity.

Seed Potato

As heavy load of pathogens is transmitted from one generation to the next one in vegitatively propagated crops the importance is healthy seed become much more important in such crops. Hence, management of healthy seed potato is the most important function of a potato farmers (Figure 12.1). As agro-climatic conditions suitable for producing healthy seed potato exist only in Punjab and Western UP the availability of quality seed in distant states like West Bengal, North Eastern and Southern states becomes highly expensive. Potato farmers of the regions affected by abiotic and biotic stresses *e.g.* Hassan and Chickmagalur districts of Karnataka adopt unique cultivation model where they compromise with quality of seed and yield just to bet on higher market prices for their off season produce (Sharma *et al.*, 2013; Rana *et al.*, 2014). On the other hand farmers of West Bengal and Gujarat use good quality seed potato in order to achieve higher potato yield and sell at competitive prices in the main season. Taking expenditure on seed potato as the proxy for quality of seed in a study farmers were divided in two halves. The first half having lesser expenditure on seed potato has more or less every physical and

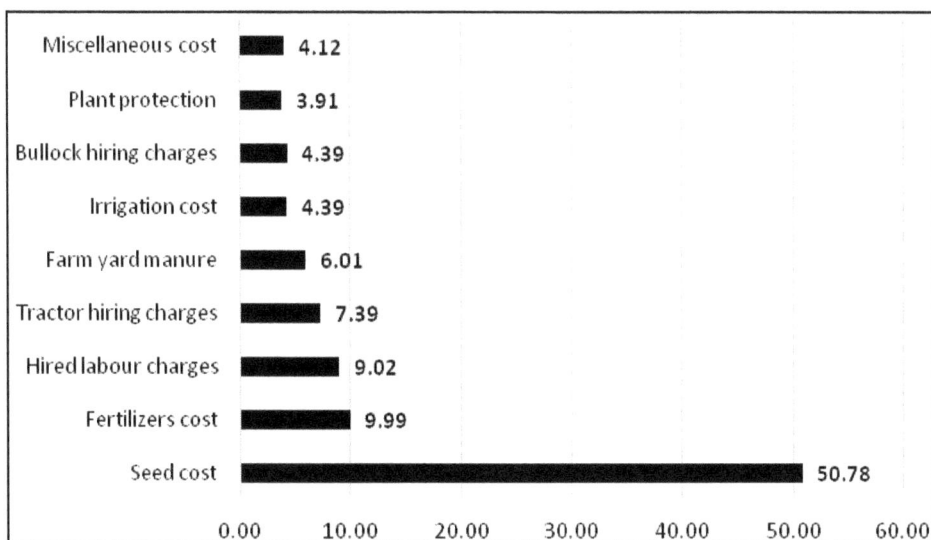

Figure 12.1: Components of Average Cost A₁ of Cultivation (Per cent).

financial indicator of potato cultivation lower than the second half spending higher on seed potato (Table 12.2).

Table 12.2: Profitability Analysis in UP and Punjab based on Seed Potato Expenditure

Attributes	Overall	
	Lower 50 per cent	Higher 50 per cent
Yield	21.58	23.88
Price	6543	7285
Cost of cultivation	80200	89834
Income	141202	173931
Net income	61002	84097
B-C ratio	1.76	1.94

Seed Replacement

In a vegetatively propagated crop like potato very high load of pathogens is transferred from one generation to the other hence quality of seed degenerates very fast. Hence maintaining quality/health of seed is one of the most important tasks of an entrepreneur. Those who can't efficiently maintain the quality of seed at their farms have to opt for quicker seed potato replacement for healthy returns from its cultivation. Seed potato producing farmers of Punjab and Western UP generally replace their seed after 5-7 years while general table purpose potato growers in these areas go for replacement of their seed after 3-4 years. Seed potato replacement is generally done in sequential or relay fashion where farmers keep on adding and replacing seed every year so that the intended cycle is maintained. In states unsuitable for multiplication of seed potato *e.g.* West Bengal, Maharashtra, Karnataka and Tamil Nadu etc. the seed replacement cycle is much shorter of every year or every alternate year. Table 12.3 provides an example of seed sources and seed replacement rate adopted by potato farmers in Punjab and UP state of India.

Table 12.3: Source of Seed Potato and Replacement Rate in Punjab and U.P. (Per cent)

Farm Saved	Other Farmers	Breeder Seed	State Farm	Private Companies	Traders	Replacement Rate	
						A	B
80.65	9.40	1.14	3.61	2.44	2.76	19.35	9.95

A: Other than own farm seed *i.e.* including seed purchased from other farmers in the region.

B: Seed duly sold as seed potato or the truthfully labelled seed potato.

Cold Storage

Cold storage of potatoes is an important marketing function as more than 90 per cent of the potatoes in India are produced during rabi season. However, cold storage needs significant financial and physical input. Transporting potatoes from farm to cold store (including loading and unloading charges), paying cold storage charges (Rs. 125 to 150/quintal); losses during sorting and grading after cold storage in addition to shrinkage; and finally transporting to market place after paying loading, unloading and repacking charges are completed by paying Rs. 250 to 275 per quintal. In order to save this big cost some of the farmers avoid cold storing potatoes and try to sell at field or storing them in heaps for a brief period of 2-3 months. UP followed by West Bengal, Punjab, Gujarat and MP are the states where cold storage industry has a big business. Despite being third largest potato producing state in the country, Bihar cold storage industry is in bad shape due to erratic electricity supply.

Fertilizers Application

Potato crop responds to nutrients in a big way. Potato growers tend to use very high doses of fertilizers in order to harvest higher yields. However, provision of subsidy on a particular fertilizer leads farmers to use extra doses of that fertilizers. Sometimes farmers use complex fertilizers for delivering a particular nutrient and waste unrequired nutrients in the process. Punjab is considered to be the leading state in respect of adoption of scientific package of practices. However, farmers in the state use much expensive and imported DAP in order to make sustained supply of nitrogen nutrient. In this process they oversupply phosphorus nutrient as soils in the region are quite rich in phosphorus. Injudicious use of fertilizers has been found more or less every part of the country in potato cultivation.

Irrigation

Potato being is water loving plant, the importance of timely and adequate irrigation is very important in its cultivation. However, under-irrigation in water scarce areas like plateau and over-irrigation in water rich areas like northern Indian Gangetic plains is frequent. Traditionally farmers used to provide furrow irrigation to potato crop, however, in the recent past role of micro-irrigation systems such as drip and sprinkler have acquired high importance in its cultivation. Micro-irrigation especially the drip irrigation has been found increasing potato yield by 30 per cent and saving water by more than 50 per cent when compared to the tradition furrow irrigation. Moreover, drip irrigated potato crop produces better quality tubers in terms of dry matter, distribution of dry matter and overall attractiveness of the tubers. With the result farmers get better price for drip irrigated potato produce. Higher incidence of late blight infestation in sprinkler irrigated potato crop is discouraging potato farmers to consider this system of irrigation a preferred option.

Micro-irrigation systems being expensive (approximately Rs. 2 lakh/ha for drip irrigation and Rs. 1.2 lakh/ha for sprinkler irrigation) farmers are unable to adopt these modern systems of irrigation at their own. Taking impending threat of water scarcity due to higher per capita use and uncertain availability under the realm of climate change, policy makers and implementers have been quite proactive in this area. Different states have very high proportion of subsidy on installing such systems and micro-irrigation systems have created success stories in the states of Gujarat, Maharashtra and MP. Other states like Karnataka and AP are also following the trend. Despite being tedious in maintenance and technical in operations, farmers are satisfied with this technology. In the states like Rajasthan the subsidy pattern is quite attractive but overall budget for this scheme being less the proportion of accepted farmers' requests is very less. In states like Punjab and Western UP farmers are not proactive to adopt this technology as large number of drugs addict persons in the region steal away components of micro-irrigation system and sell at throw away prices in order to earn money for their next dose of drugs. In the states like Bihar and West Bengal ground water level is so favourable that farmers are satisfied with the traditional method *i.e.* furrow irrigation.

Determination of Area Under Potato

Acreage response to previous year's prices/profitability is very strong in case of potato cultivation. In-spite of several advisory communications, the farmers (mostly the irregular potato farmers) fail to resist their temptation and tendency to gamble for earning higher profits on the analogy of previous year. Same is true when farmers stop growing potato crop as prices/profits during previous year were quite low. Herd mentality and irrational behaviour is quite common among potato farmers especially the small/marginal and non-regular ones. It is largely due to this tendency that the potato prices are fluctuating so vigorously over the years. However, large and regular potato farmers understand this phenomenon with a higher degree of precision and remain careful.

Selection of Potato Varieties

Selection of potato varieties in an area is largely governed by performance of the varieties in that area and availability of seed. More than 95 per cent of potato area in an area invariably remains under the same potato varieties its very small proportion of area on which farmers try new varieties. Cultivation of processing varieties of potato has been a major diversification in the recent past. Sustained seed supply of new varieties becomes principal reason for farmers' decision to discontinue their cultivation. It was found that a lack of mechanism to have precise feedback on desirable attributes in new potato varieties for breeders many of the varieties are not adopted in the field (Rana *et al.*, 2013)

Crop Insurance

Crop insurance has never been a highly preferred option among potato farmers. Only non-significant proportion of potato farmers tend to adopt crop insurance willingly while majority has to adopt under compulsion as insurance has been linked to farm credit in the form of KCCs or simple crop loans. Potato farmers have largely been unsatisfied the way crop insurance companies manage this business.

Contract Farming

In the beginning there were several apprehensions about success of contract farming in potato cultivation (Singh, 2002). However, highly specific requirements of potato processing industry for procuring processing grade potatoes put pressure on such companies to deliver value to potato farmers and make contract farming successful in various parts of the country. Later on seed-potato producing companies also made use of this business tool for seed potato multiplication. At this point of time potato farmers comfortably go for contract farming on an average on 20-25 per cent of their land holding. This strategy is adopted in order to avoid price risk after harvest of the crop. PepsiCo is the largest contractor for potato growing on farmers' fields in India. They have devised a contract farming model especially for small/marginal, resource poor and illiterate potato farmers (Figure 12.2). The salient features of this model have been the supply of quality seed-potato, assured technical support, monitoring of crop health, facilitation of farm credit and crop insurance to the contracted farmers in addition to the pre-fixed price (Chaturvedi, 2007; Singh *et al.*, 2011; Pandit *et al.*, 2015).

Selling

Taking right decision on selling the produce is the one of the most important and crucial decisions affecting profitability of the farmers in general and potato farmers in particular. There are two big groups of potato farmers in terms of selling decision. One is comprised of those who sell without cold storing and the other is comprised by those who sell after cold storing their produce. The former is predominantly a group of small and marginal farmers while the latter is composed by medium and large potato farmers. The first group take two types of decision for selling their produce; the first decision is to sell on the farm to the agent of commission agent or wholesaler and avoid the hassle of grading, arranging packaging material, packing and transportation. The second decision by the farmers who don't cold store their produce is to store in heaps and wait for suitable price during next two to three months as produce can't be stored for longer time in heaps. Those who opt for cold storing their produce have much longer span of time for making selling decision. Unless there is some financial obligation, such farmers wait for suitable

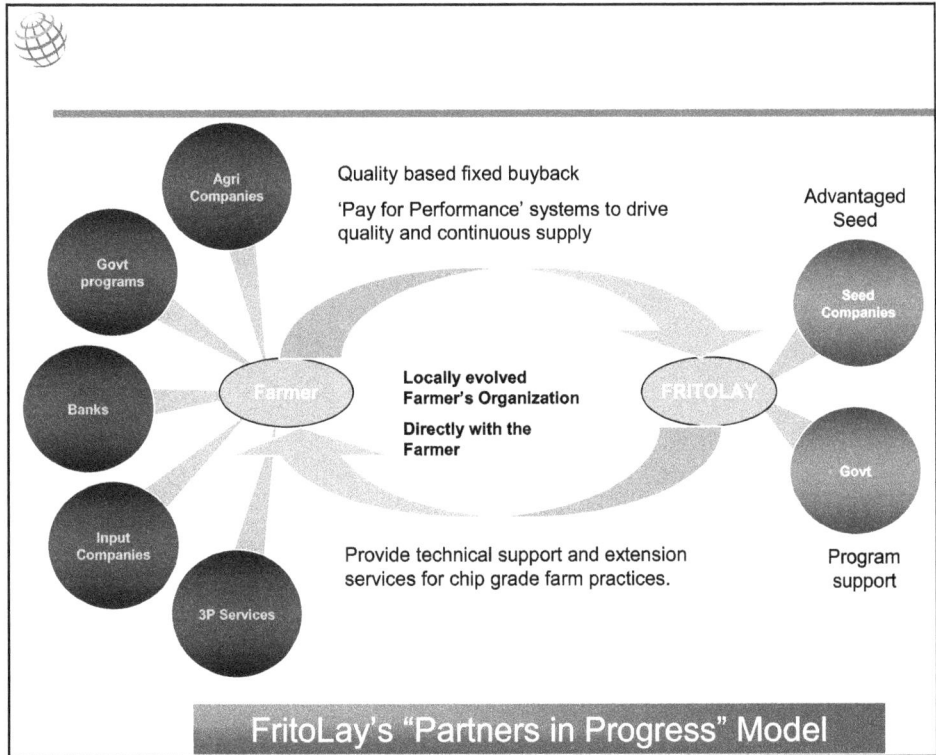

Figure 12.2: "Partners in Progress" Contract Farming Model Adopted by PepsiCo.

price and start selling their produce in the month of July and may go upto October. However, some of these farmers develop speculation tendency and start supporting speculators in the future markets and end up losing money just by playing the wrong role. In fact farmers should play the role of a hedger in the future markets in order to maximize their profit.

References

Chaturvedi, R. (2007). Contract farming and FritoLay's model of contract farming for potato. *Potato Journal* **34**(1-2): 16-19.

Pandit, Arun, Barsati Lal, Rajesh K. Rana (2015). An assessment of potato contract farming in West Bengal state, India. *Potato Research* **58**: 1-14.

Rana, Rajesh K., Neeraj Sharma, S. Arya, BP Singh, M.S. Kadian, Rahul Chaturvedi and S.K. Pandey (2013). Tackling moisture stress with drought-tolerant potato (*Solanum tuberosum*) varieties: Perception of Karnataka farmers. *Indian Journal of Agricultural Sciences* **83**(2): 216–22.

Rana, Rajesh K., Neeraj Sharma, S. Arya, M.S. Kadian, B.P. Singh and S.K. Pandey (2014). Status of potato husbandry and farmers' socio-economic profile in moisture and heat prone Karnataka, India. *Pakistan Journal of Agricultural Sciences* **51**(1): 7-16.

Sharma, Neeraj, Rajesh K. Rana, S. Arya, M. S. Kadian and B. P. Singh (2013). Dynamics of seed potato utilization in high temperature conditions under semi-arid ecosystem. *International Journal of Agricultural and Statistical Sciences* **9**(2): 619-26.

Singh, S. (2002). Contracting out solutions: political economy of contract farming in the Indian Punjab. *World Development* **30**(9): 1621-1638.

Singh, B.P., Rana Rajesh, K. and Manoj Kumar (2011). Technology infusion through contact farming: success story of potato. *Indian Horticulture* **56**(3): 49-52.

Chapter 13

Supply Side Constraints in Raising Pulses Production

A. Amarender Reddy

Principal Scientist (Agricultural Economics)
ICAR-IARI, New Delhi – 110 012

ABSTRACT

The United Nation declared 2016 as international year of pulses, given its importance in food and nutrition security and source of income and employment to small and marginal farmers in developing countries. Historically India is the largest producer, consumer and importer of pulses. Pulses production in India is about 19 million tonnes, every year India is importing about 3-4 million tonnes of pulses to meet its annual demand of 22-23 million tonnes. Even though there is a significant increase in pulses production in the last decade from 15 million tonnes to 18-19 million tonnes due to the implementation of National Food Security Mission (NFSM), Accelerated Pulses Production Programme (APPP) and Rastria Krishi Vikas Yojana (RKVY), there is little improvement in production of kharif pulses. There is a lot of scope of expansion in area under rice fallows in eastern and southern India and crop diversification from rice-wheat to cereal-pulse based cropping systems in northern India. The paper discusses strategies followed to increase pulses production in the last decade and the way forward to sustain the increased production. There are some isolated success stories like chickpea revolution in Andhra Pradesh and spring moong/urad in irrigated areas, expansion of area under pigeonpea in eastern India in the last decade. However, for effective upscale of these isolated success stories, there is a need for an integrated approach through strengthening NFSM and APPP along with policy prescription to strengthen entire value chain from production, procurement and distribution through public-private partnerships. The two policy instruments, Minimum Support Price and adjustments to tariff rates needs to be used judiciously to bridge the gap between demand and supply, to provide proper inceptive to farmers to increase production at the same to reduce spikes in open market prices to safeguard consumers.

Introduction

United Nations declared 2016 as international year of pulses. Pulses, also known as grain legumes, are a group of 12 crops that includes chickpeas, pigeonpea, urad, moong, lentils, khesari, beans and peas. They are high in protein, fibre, and various vitamins, provide amino acids, and are hearty crops. They are most popular in developing countries, but are increasingly becoming recognized as an excellent part of a healthy diet throughout the world. Because of its high protein content pulse crops are one of the most sustainable crops a farmer can grow. It takes just 359 litres of water to produce one kg of pulses, compared with 1802 for soybeans and 3071 for groundnut. They also contribute to soil quality by fixing nitrogen in the soil. Though India is the largest producer and consumer of pulses, the yield levels are too low (750 kg/ha), there is a massive yield gap between India and other developed countries and also within India, between research station yield and farmers yields. With the introduction of improved varieties, promotion of better management techniques and development of inclusive marketing channels, pulse crops can overcome the lower yields and make good profits to farmers in India (International Year of Pulses, 2016). This paper is aimed at examining the current status of pulses and suggests policy options to increase pulses production.

Trends in Production, Supply and Demand

With the stagnation in pulses production at below 15 MT until 2009-10 and steep rise prices pulses, government of India introduced many programmes and policy instruments targeted to increase pulses production and yield. Due to all these efforts, India achieved a record pulses production at 19.8 MT in 2013-14 with an all-time high production achieved in chickpea (9.53 MT). However, with the population of 1282 million, as per the Indian Council of Medical Research (ICMR) Recommended Dietary Intake (RDI) of 80 gm/capita/day, India needs to produce 36.9 million tonnes of pulses. This indicates that there is a deficit of 17.1 MT. However, some other studies projected a moderate demand of 25.39 MT by 2025 with the assumption of the current scenario of high prices continue and unaffordable to many of low income consumers. Almost every year, India is importing 3-4 MT of pulses to meet its annual demand of 21-22 MT at existing higher prices. The demand and production of pulses in the country along with the net imports during 2007-08 to 2014-15 is given in Table 13.1. The figures shows that even though, there is increased production from 14 MT to 19 MT, the net imports were increased given the increased population and purchasing power of the consumers.

Further, pulses demand is highly price elastic (consumers demand more pulses if the prices comes down) and income elastic (as income increases, consumer demand more pulses), we can reasonably predict that the demand will increase anywhere between 26 to 36 MT in the near future, if prices are reasonably low due to the reduction in the cost of production with the wider adoption of improved technology (as it happened in the case of chickpea during the past decade especially in southern states like Andhra Pradesh and Karnataka). In fact some econometric estimates of the income elasticity of demand of pulses range from 1.5 to 2.0. This would mean that with an increase of around 6.5 per cent annual in per capita income demand for pulses would increase around ten percent annually (Alagh, 2011).

Table 13.1: Projected Demand and Supply of Pulses (Million Tonnes)

Year	Production	Net Imports	Total Availability
2007-08	14.8	2.0	16.8
2008-09	14.6	2.9	17.5
2009-10	14.7	3.6	18.3
2010-11	18.2	2.6	20.8
2011-12	17.2	3.3	20.5
2012-13	18.3	3.8	22.2
2013-14	19.8	2.7	22.5
2014-15 (E)	17.38	5.0	22.38

Source: Department of Economics and Statistics (2015): net imports= imports-exports: total availability= production+ net imports.

State-wise Trends Area and Production of Pulses

Madhya Pradesh is the largest producer of pulses followed by Maharashtra, Rajasthan, Uttar Pradesh, Andhra Pradesh and Karnataka. These six states together contribute 79 per cent of pulses area and 80 per cent of pulses production. The area under chickpea is shifted from north India to south and central India during the last decade (Reddy, 2013). Area and production share of rabi pulses also increased compared to kharif pulses.

Table 13.2: Area and Production of Pulses (TE 2014)

State	Area (1000 ha)	Share in Total Area (per cent)	Production (1000 ha)	Share in Total Production (per cent)	Yield (kg/ha)
Madhya Pradesh	5310	22	4807	26	905
Maharashtra	3489	14	2565	14	735
Rajasthan	3967	16	2286	13	576
Uttar Pradesh	2365	10	2148	12	908
Andhra Pradesh	1850	8	1468	8	794
Karnataka	2345	10	1286	7	549
Others	4990	21	3674	20	736
All India	24315	100	18234	100	750

Some Isolated Success Stories

There are some success stories emerged during the last decade in respect of area and yield increase. There is significant progress in the chickpea production which has increased from 5.6 MT to 8.9 MT, due to the development of high yielding varieties like JG-11, which are drought tolerant and suitable for mechanized cultivation. The yield levels have increased in rabi pulses (chickpeas, lentil) and spring moong/urad compared to kharif pulses (like pigeonpea, kharif moong and urad). The greater challenge is how we can upscale this success in few crops in isolated places (especially for rabi pulses) to other pulses (kharif) and in to new locations. Between triennium ending (TE) 2006 to TE 2015, urad production increased by 71.8 per cent, chickpeas by 58.6 per cent and moong by 42.4 per cent mostly contributed by rabi season (Table 13.3). Now chickpeas contributes about 47 per cent of total pulses production. The past experience of yellow revolution shows most of the success is short lived if we don't improve our production technology in the long run (Reddy, 2009).

Table 13.3: Crop-wise Progress in Production (Million Tonnes) of Pulses

Crop	TE 2006	TE 2014-15	Per cent Increase
Pigeonpea	2.48 (18.0)	3.0 (15.8)	20.2
Chickpeas	5.6 (40.6)	8.9 (47.1)	58.6
Urad	1.02 (7.4)	1.8 (9.3)	71.8
Moong	0.98 (7.1)	1.4 (7.4)	42.4
Other Pulses	3.74 (27.1)	3.8(20.4)	2.7
Total	**13.81 (100)**	**18.9 (100)**	**36.5**

Source: Ministry of Agriculture, Government of India: figures in parenthesis per cent to total pulses production.

Distribution of districts based on yield levels (below 0.5t/ha; 0.5 to 1t/ha and more than 1t/ha) is given in Table 13.4. It is interesting to see that the districts with more than 1t/ha yield increased from 19 per cent to 66 per cent in case of chickpea. There was significant increase of high productivity districts in case of lentil also from 13 per cent to 18 per cent between 1999 and 2012. Whereas high productivity districts decreased from 37 per cent to 22 per cent for pigeonpea. Percentage of districts with less than 0.5t/ha yield decreased in all crops except in pigeonpea. However, still large number of districts are in below 0.5 t/ha category in case of moong and urad. These figures are indicating that most of the technological development and diffusion concentrated only in chickpea. For all other pulse crops there is a long way to go in spreading the new technology to have an impact on yields.

Table 13.4: Distribution of Districts by Level of Yield
(Per cent to total districts growing the crops)

Yield Level	Chickpea		Pigeonpea		Lentil		Moong		Urad	
	1999	2012	1999	2012	1999	2012	1999	2012	1999	2012
Less than 0.5t/ha	13	3	17	27	14	35	74	67	77	47
0.5 to 1t/ha	68	31	46	51	73	48	26	32	28	51
More than 1t/ha	19	66	37	22	13	18	0	1	0.7	2.1
Total	100	100	100	100	100	100	100	100	100	100

International Trade in Pulses

India's exports are exclusively dominated by chickpeas (98.5 per cent of total exports of pulses), while import basket is quite diversified although share of yellow peas(37.9 per cent) is much higher followed by moong/urad (17.8 per cent), lentils (17 per cent), chickpeas (13.7 per cent) and pigeonpeas(13.6 per cent) (Table 13.5). Chickpeas are mostly exported to Pakistan, Turkey, Algeria, Srilanka and United Arab Emirates. Peas are imported from Canada and Russia; moong/urad from Myanmar; lentils from Canada and USA; chickpeas from Australia and Russia and pigeonpes from Myanmar and Tanzania, Mozambique (Table 13.6).

Table 13.5. India's imports and exports (average of 2012-13 and 2013-14)

Pulses	Exports (1000 tonnes)	Share in Total Pulses Exports (Per cent)	Imports (1000 tonnes)	Share in Total Pulses Imports (Per cent)
Peas	0.7	0.3	1350.6	37.9
Chickpeas	264.4	98.5	486.9	13.7
Moong/Urad	1.6	0.6	633.5	17.8
Lentils	0.9	0.3	607.5	17.0
Pigeonpeas	0.8	0.3	486.0	13.6
Total	**268**	**100.0**	**3564.5**	**100.0**

Table 13.6: India's Trade Destinations of Major Pulses for 2013-14

Pulses	Top 5 Export Destinations	Top 5 Import Sources
Peas	Myanmar (84.70 per cent), Pakistan (7.37 per cent), Nepal (5 per cent), Sri Lanka DSR (2.82 per cent), Malaysia (0.04 per cent)	Canada (70.59 per cent), Russia (11.06 per cent), USA (8.37 per cent), Australia (6.19 per cent), France (1.74 per cent)
Chickpeas	Pakistan (29.93 per cent), Turkey (18.11 per cent), Algeria (17.24 per cent), Sri Lanka (5.34 per cent), U Arab EMTS (4.43 per cent)	Australia (61.43 per cent), Russia (22.77 per cent), Tanzania (7.84 per cent), Myanmar (6.40 per cent), USA (0.47 per cent)
Moong/urad	USA (49.69 per cent), Unspecified (10.21 per cent), Sri Lanka (7 per cent), Canada (7.72 per cent), Kenya (4.29 per cent)	Myanmar (82.83 per cent), Tanzania (4.23 per cent), Kenya (3.55 per cent), Australia (3.05 per cent), Mozambique (1.61 per cent)
Lentils	Myanmar (35.16 per cent), USA (25.17 per cent), Kuwait (7.17 per cent), Bhutan (6.55 per cent), Singapore (5.92 per cent)	Canada (79.33 per cent), USA (10.70 per cent), Australia (9.85 per cent), Uzbekistan (0.01 per cent), Turkey (0.01 per cent)
Pigeonpeas	Nepal (78.79 per cent), Canada (19.19 per cent), Israel (1.92 per cent), Korea (0.09 per cent)	Myanmar (51.37 per cent), Tanzania (27.44 per cent), Mozambique (14.69 per cent), Malawi (4.53 per cent), Kenya (1.79 per cent)

Long Run Inelastic Supply Reason for High Prices

Since 1966, pulse crops have been neglected with agricultural policy environment favouring spread of green revolution technology in few crops like paddy and wheat for food security reasons in many developing countries including India. This input-intensive technology further enhanced already exiting yield gap between major cereals and pulses. Due to prolonged neglect for several decades, yield levels of pulse crops are stagnant (increased only by 12.2 per cent from 1966 to 2009 as against 162.6 per cent increase in yield of wheat). Table 13.6 depicts the changes in real prices between TE 1969 and TE 2009 for pulses and competing crops. The real price steeply increased for pulses by 42 per cent compared to a decline for wheat (-10.2 per cent), maize (-18.9 per cent) and millets (-17.4 per cent), mainly due to low supply response of pulse crops (Table 13.7).

Table 13.7: Trends in Real Prices (Rs/quintal)

Crop	TE 1970	TE 2013	Per cent Change in Real Prices
Millet	1947	1609	−17.4
Wheat	2585	2321	−10.2
Maize	2101	1705	−18.9
Pigeonpea	2800	3977	42.0

Source: FAOSTAT accessed on 31st July 2011; prices were deflated by CPI for agricultural labourer with 1986/87 base year.

As a result of widened gap between yields of pulses and major cereals (the yield of wheat increased from 1.6 times that of pulses in 1969 to 3.8 times in 2009) the relative profitability and competitiveness of pulse crops reduced even though prices increased due to shortage of supply (due to inelastic supply). Another important reason for decreased preference for pulses by farmers is continued high instability in yields of pulse crops (instability is 16.5 per cent during 1989-2009, as against instability in wheat at 5.1 per cent) than major cereal crops.

Reasons for Long Run Inelastic Supply

The growth in production has not responded to increase in prices in case of pulses (especially in pigeonpea, moong, urad) is mainly due to (i) area stagnation: The main reason for stagnation in area under pulses has been differential impact of technology and relative profitability leading to shifting of area under pulses to more remunerative crops (ii) expansion of irrigation: Uncontrolled water flows (flooding) common in canal systems is incompatible with large scale area under pulses (iii) High risk in productivity and farm income. There is a significant decline in instability of yield of paddy and wheat from the onset of Green Revolution. Instability in productivity of chickpea remained much higher than of wheat: in pigeonpea, much higher than paddy. Pulses grown under unirrigated rainfed conditions, in marginal lands suffered instability, (iv) there is no major technological breakthroughs in India compared to countries like Canada and others achieving averages of around two tonnes per hectare in pulses productivity (v) technology breakthroughs in the difficult regions and adverse farming conditions (rainfed regions, the ghats and hill regions) was just not there on a large scale (Alagh, 2011). (vi) scattered and thin distribution of various types of pulse crops cultivated mostly on marginal lands, with each crop contributing a small share in total pulses area – the biggest hurdle for all stakeholders (researchers/extension/development/credit/market support agencies in both the public and private sectors) to provide input and output services and other institutional support (vii) indeterminate plant type of pulse crops with low yield potential and low response to input management. (v) near stagnation in yield and technology and hence profitability of pulse crops relative to other competing crops (vi) high frequency of crop failure and yield instability due to pests and diseases and drought and floods (vii) low priority by policy makers due to marginal importance of pulses at local level to have significant impact to farmers income (Materne and Reddy, 2007). As a result area under paddy and wheat increased in high –productive zones along with high doses of inputs like fertilizer and pesticides and pulse crops shifted to marginalized lands with little inputs even though prices are high. Still more than 90 per cent of the pulses growing districts are with less than 1 t/ha yield, although production risk is reduced slightly in recent years due to the development of abiotic and biotic stress tolerant varieties.

Spike in Prices in Recent Past

Prices of pulses consistently increased from 2005 to 2010, then after there is downward movement of pulses except chickpeas upto 2012, but chickpea prices steeply decreased after 2012-13 before recent rise again (Figure 13.1). While prices of moong and urad showed upward trends after 2013. Price indices of chickpeas

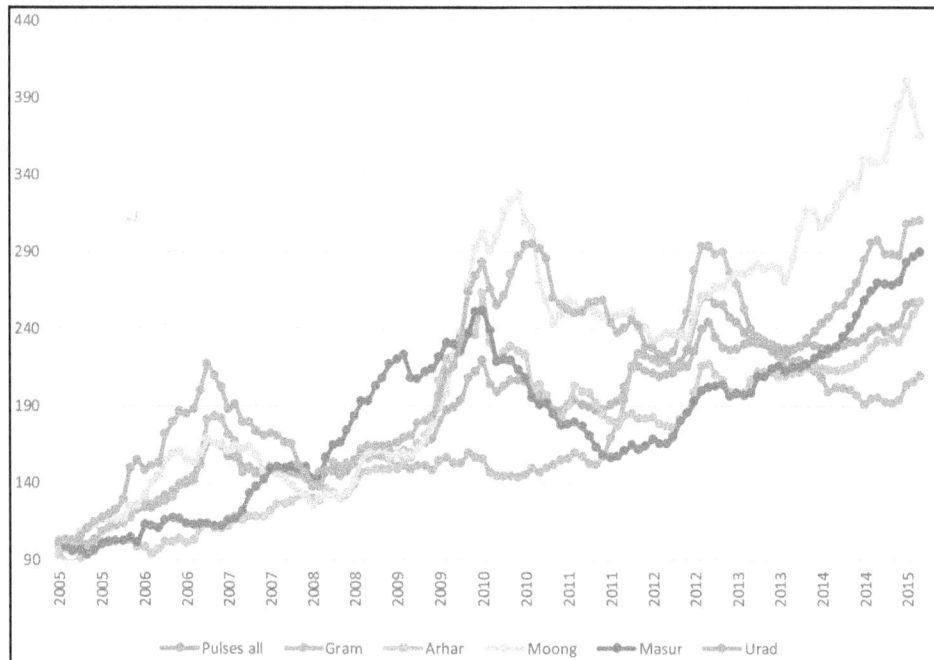

Figure 13.1: Index Number of Wholesale Prices (2004-05=100).

are always moderate compared to other pulse crops throughout the period, except between 2012 and 2013. The spike in the chickpea prices during the 2012 is mainly due to the higher world prices up to August 2012, then after domestic prices were higher than world prices due to short supply and higher MSP, although overall both domestic and world prices moderated after 2012. Pigeonpea, moong and urad showed rising trend in prices with less fluctuation, while lentil showed higher fluctuation in prices with overall upward trend.

Short-Term Measures to Manage Spike in Prices

The wholesale price index of pulses (2004-05=100) peaked in the year 2010 as a result of stagnant production (production is stagnate at below 15 MT (in 2007-08 only 14.8 MT; in 2008-09 14.6 MT and in 2009-10 14.7 MT), and rise in demand. Imports peaked in the year 2009-10 to 3.6 MT. Given that the India is a major importer in the world markets, whenever there is shortage in domestic production and India goes for importing from the world markets, world pulses prices increased steeply and invariably India has to import pulses at higher prices. As a result of high import prices, domestic prices raised further. The open market prices reached Rs.90/kg for pigeonpea, Rs.70 for moong and uard in the late 2010. In response to the higher prices, government of India has taken a number of policy initiatives to increase free imports, curtail speculative activities by traders, streamlining the distribution and supply chain through market intervention as mentioned below.

1. Reduced import duties to zero - for pulses up to 31.3.2011 (extended further)
2. Banned export of pulses (except kabuli chana) up to 31.3.2011.
3. Enabled imposition of stock limit orders by State governments in the case of pulses upto 30.9.2011 (extended further)
4. Publicity campaigns have been undertaken to popularise consumption of yellow peas.
5. There is a scheme for supply of imported pulses by Public Sector Undertakings to state Governments for distribution through Public Distribution System, @1 kg per family per month at a subsidy of Rs. 10 per kg.
6. The supply of imported pulses at subsidized rate helped increase the domestic availability. This helped in moderating the prices of pulses.

However, these measures can only be effective in controlling higher prices in the short run, as they are targeted to reduce prices through a mixture of trade policies (free imports and ban on exports) and demand management (like distribution of pulses through PDS) and not targeted increase production over long period. To reduce prices in the long run, India has to encourage domestic production at lower cost. Given India's large consumption needs and very limited international supply, it cannot depend on the world markets for pulses supply year after year, which will expose India's pulses consumers and producers to higher fluctuations in international markets.

Factors Contributed to Recent Increase in Production

In the past decade, pulses production increased by 36.5 per cent mostly contributed by chickpea, moong and urad. However, India needs to increase pulses production from 19 MT to anywhere between 25.39 MT and 36.9 MT to meet its deficit. Still the yield levels of most of the pulse crops remain very low compared to the potential as well as the world average except chickpeas. With the increased pulses imports year after year and higher prices, government of India initiated a combination of technology and market interventions. The recent break from the stagnant pulses production is attributed to proper implementation of various government programmes, larger increase in minimum support price (MSP), good monsoon, increase in area under rabi/spring pulses (especially chickpeas in non-traditional areas), strong technology back-up and timely availability of seeds in the market. To give a boost to pulses production, the government has been implementing National Food Security Mission-Pulses since rabi 2008 in all major pulses producing states covering about 97.5 per cent pulses area in the country. India has also launched Accelerated Pulses Production Programme (A3P) since Kharif, 2010 as a part of NFSM-Pulses for demonstration of production and protection technologies in village level compact blocks. Assistance is also being provided to the farmers under other crop development programmes such as special initiative for pulses in dryland area of 60,000 villages under Rashtriya Krishi Vikas Yojana (RKVY) since 2010-11, Integrated Development of 60000 Pulses villages in Rainfed Areas 2011-12, Special Plan to achieve 19+ million tonnes of Pulses production during Kharif 2012-13, Additional area coverage of Pulses Rabi/Summer under NFSM-Pulses for additional Rabi/Summer production during 2012-13, Macro Management of Agriculture (MMA) and Bringing Green Revolution to Eastern India (BGEI) in rain fed areas across the country for increasing crop productivity and strengthening market linking. In addition, 15 districts of Jharkhand and 10 districts of Assam have also been included under NFSM-Pulses based on their potential for pulses development. The Minimum Support Prices (MSPs) of Kharif Pulses (pigeonpea, moong and Urad) have been increased compared to the competing crops to induce farmers to take up pulses in kharif season. For example, the annual compound growth rate of MSP between 2001 and 2015 is 10.6 per cent for pigeonpea, 11.3 per cent for moong and 10.8 per cent for Urad, which is far higher than the competing crops (Table 13.8). NAFED procured the market arrivals whenever the prices falls below MSP. The substantial increase in the MSPs of pulses is to incentivise farmers to increase their area and production, to adopt high cost inputs like improved seed (which will increase seed replacement rate), fertilizers and irrigation for increasing productivity. All these efforts resulted in record production. However, still productivity of pulses in India (750 kg/ha) is lesser than the advanced countries including China (1567 kg/ha) (FAOSTAT, 2014).

Marketing Channels

Almost more than 95 per cent of the pulses produced in India go through private channels as mentioned below

(i) Producer – Dal Miller – Consumer,

(ii) Producer – Village Trader –Dal Miller – Wholesaler – Retailer – Consumer,

Table 13.8: The MSPs (Rs/quintal) of Pulses and Competing Crops

Year	Paddy	Maize	Wheat	Chickpeas	Pigeonpea	Moong	Urad
2000-01	510	445	610	1100	1200	1200	1200
2001-02	530	485	620	1200	1320	1320	1320
2002-03	530	485	620	1220	1320	1330	1330
2003-04	550	505	630	1400	1360	1370	1370
2004-05	560	515	640	1425	1390	1410	1410
2005-06	570	525	650	1435	1400	1520	1520
2006-07	580	540	750	1445	1410	1520	1520
2007-08	645	600	1000	1600	1550	1700	1700
2008-09	900	840	1080	1730	2000	2520	2520
2009-10	1000	840	1100	1760	2300	2760	2520
2010-11	1000	880	1170	2100	3500	3670	3400
2011-12	1080	980	1285	2800	3700	4000	3800
2012-13	1250	1175	1350	3000	3850	4400	4300
2013-14	1310	1310	1400	3100	4300	4500	4300
2014-15	1360	1310	1450	3175	4350	4600	4350
ACGR (per cent)	8.1	8.4	7.5	7.9	10.6	11.3	10.8

Source: Ministry of Agriculture, Government of India.

(iii) Producer – Dal Miller -Retailer - Consumer,

(iv) Producer – Wholesaler – Dal Miller - Retailer –Consumer,

(v) Producer – Wholesaler – Dal Miller – Wholesaler - Retailer –Consumer,

(vi) Producer – Wholesaler – Retailer – Consumer (For whole Greengram),

(vii) Producer – Commission Agent – Dal Miller – Wholesaler –Retailer - Consumer.

Institutional: (i) Producer – Procuring Agency - Dal Miller – Consumer, (ii) Producer – Procuring Agency – Dal Miller – Wholesaler – Retailer - Consumer, and (iii) Producer – Procuring Agency – Dal Miller – Retailer – Consumer.

For imported pulses, the channel will be Exporting country –

Importing country – Private/Government Agencies – Wholesaler/Cooperative

Societies – Retailer/Village Societies – Consumer

Resuming to Liberal Export and Import Policy

After recognition of the export potential of some of the pulse crops with recent increase in production especially *kabuli* chickpeas, stringent ban on exports is slowly withdrawn. Under the advance authorization scheme, import of pulses is allowed after domestic processing and value addition. The prohibition of export of pulses is not applied to exports of Kabuli chickpeas and a limited quantity of organic pulses. Export to neighboring countries like Bhutan and Maldives are allowed. Although statutory import duty is 50 per cent, applied duty is kept at zero for all pulses and import of pulses are free without any quantitative restrictions. However, free imports will not have any perceptible impact on the quantity imported and domestic prices, as there is no big difference between domestic and international prices, many times international prices are high than domestic prices except yellow peas.

Yield, Cost Structure and Profitability of Pulse Crops across Farm Size Groups

We have examined the plot level data of cost of cultivation scheme, government of India to work out profitability for the year triennium ending (TE) 2002 and 2010. Average crop yields have increased from 8.9 to 11.4 quintal in pigeonpea, from 9.3 to 9.7 quintal in chickpea, from 8.5 to 9.1 quintal in lentil, from 3.3 to 4.0 in moong and from stagnant at 5.2 quintal in urad between TE 2002 and TE 2010 among sample farmers (Table 13.9). In general marginal plots have higher yield per ha, compared to large plots, but there is no significant difference in yields among marginal, small and medium plots.

Table 13.9: Yield (Quintal/ha) among different Plot Sizes

	Year	Marginal	Small	Medium	Large	All
Pigeonpea	TE 2002	9.1	7.1	6.4	6.7	8.9
	TE 2010	11.8	9.1	7.5	7.1	11.4
Chickpeas	TE 2002	9.4	9.3	9.1	5.5	9.3
	TE 2010	9.6	10.0	10.1	7.6	9.7
Lentil	TE 2002	8.6	8.2	7.3	6.0	8.5
	TE 2010	9.3	8.0	9.1	7.5	9.1
Moong	TE 2002	3.3	3.4	5.3	3.5	3.3
	TE 2010	3.9	4.7	4.7	4.2	4.0
Urad	TE 2002	5.0	5.9	6.5	7.2	5.2
	TE 2010	4.9	6.4	7.4	4.4	5.2

Source: Cost of cultivation scheme unit level data: marginal < 1 ha; small 1-2 ha; medium 2-4 ha; large > 4 ha.

The changes in cost structure (share of different cost items in total cost) among different crops are given in Table 13.10. It indicates that the human labour contributes to about 37 per cent (chickpea) to 53 per cent (moong) in 2010. In general, share of casual labour is less compared to family labour except in moong. Further share of casual labour increased and family labour decreased. Share of animal labour is higher in pigeonpea (16 per cent) and lower in urad (6 per cent) and lentil (7 per cent) mostly contributed by own animals. Share of machine labour is higher in lentil (22 per cent), followed by chickpea (20 per cent) and least in moong (12 per cent) and pigeonpea (13 per cent). Share of all labour (human, animal and machine together) is contributing to 78 per cent in moong and 65 per cent in chickpea. Given that the labour scarcity is increased in the villages and wage rates have increased in the last decade, there was increase in farm mechanization across all the crops and states.

Table 13.10: Cost Structure (Per cent of total cost) in TE 2002 and TE 2010 of Major Pulse Crops

Crop	Pigeonpea		Chickpea		Lentil		Moong		Urad	
Cost Item	2002	2010	2002	2010	2002	2010	2002	2010	2002	2010
Family labour	21	18	22	17	17	17	24	27	17	17
Attached labour	2.4	2.4	1.1	1.1	1.1	0.7	2.9	1.9	2.1	1.0
Casual labour	21	27	12	18	21	23	20	23	31	32
Total human labour	44	47	35	37	39	40	47	53	50	50
Hired animal	4.3	4.1	0.9	1.9	0.8	1.0	2.7	1.9	2.2	0.7
Owned animal	18	12	8	6	12	6	21	12	14	5
Total animal labour	23	16	9	8	13	7	24	14	16	6
Hired machine	8	12	15	18	21	20	6	11	10	15
Own machine	0.8	0.7	2.2	1.9	1.7	2.6	0.6	1.0	0.7	1.1
Total machine labour	8	13	17	20	22	22	7	12	10	17
Labour (human, animal and machine)	75	76	60	65	74	69	77	78	76	73
Seed value	6	6	25	20	16	21	14	14	14	17
Fertilizer	8	7	7	7	8	7	6	4	5	3
Manure	2.5	2.2	0.1	0.3	0.3	0.2	2.2	2.7	1.5	1.1
Insecticides	7.6	7.6	1.1	4.6	0.9	1.3	1.1	1.2	3.3	5.7
Irrigation charges	0.9	0.7	7.1	3.6	1.2	1.2	0.3	0.3	0.5	0.9
Miscellaneous Cost	0.1	0.0	0.0	0.1	0.0	0.0	0.0	0.1	0.1	0.1
Total	100	100	100	100	100	100	100	100	100	100

Source: Cost of cultivation scheme unit level data.

Share of seed is higher in chickpea and lentils (about 20 per cent). Share of fertilizer contributes not more than 8 per cent in many pulse crops. Share of insecticide is higher in pigeonpea and uard.

In triennium ending 2010, profitability (gross returns-cost) of lentil was higher (Rs. 9000/ha), followed by pigeonpea (Rs.5000/ha), chickpea (Rs. 4000/ha), whereas for moong and urad profit is negligible (Table 13.11). In general profitability is much higher among medium (2-4 ha plots) and large (more than 4 ha) plots compared to marginal (< 1ha) and small (1-2 ha) plots. The trend is more or less similar in TE 2002 also. Overall, even though yields are higher among marginal plots, the profitability is low due to high overhead costs (indivisible costs like farm machinery, tractors, threshers and harvesters, supervision and management cost which is becoming very high given the increased wages), there is a need for development and diffusion of machinery suitable for marginal farmers to increase labour productivity (less than 1 ha). Low profitability of marginal and small plots shows the requirement of consolidation of marginal holdings for higher profits.

Pigeonpea profitability is higher in Karnataka (Rs. 10,000/ha), followed by UP and MP (Rs.8000) in TE 2010 (Table 13.12). The interstate differences are mainly explained by the differences in the cost per hectare. Even though gross returns are higher in Maharashtra (Rs.54,000), profitability is low in Maharashtra (only Rs.2000) is due to high cost of cultivation (Rs.52,000/ha). In Karnataka, profitability is high (Rs.10,000) due to low cost of cultivation (Rs.17000) even though gross returns are low (Rs.27000). Overall, cost of cultivation in chickpea is low compared to pigeonpea. Cost of cultivation ranged between Rs.14000 and 15 000 per ha in MP, Rajasthan and Karnataka, but a little higher in AP (Rs.24000) and UP (Rs.29,000). Profits were higher in Rajasthan and AP. Lentils also exhibit similar cost benefits as that of chickpeas due to similarity in agronomic practices and both are rabi crops. Again moong and urad exhibit similarity in costs and benefits with comparatively low costs and benefits compared to chickpea and lentil. For urad farmers incurred losses in both 2002 and even in 2010 in many states except in AP and MP. Over all, results shows that, cost reduction should be the main strategy to increase profitability, which can be done through judicious use of inputs and especially labour.

Role of Technology

Among various factors contributing to higher production (18 to 19 million tonnes) of pulses in recent years, availability of quality seeds of high yielding varieties (like JG-11 of chickpea which revolutionized pulses production in Andhra Pradesh and Karnataka which are non-traditional areas for pulses cultivation) played a major role. Due to wider adoption of JG-11 and other improved varieties, yield level of chickpea in Andhra Pradesh (about 2t/ha) is highest compared to any other major chickpea growing country. National Agricultural Research System(NARS) has made several efforts in producing required quantity of breeder seeds of major pulse crops during last decade. ICAR Institutes *viz.*, Indian Institute of Pulses Research (IIPR), Indian Agricultural Research Institute (IARI), State Agricultural Universities (SAUs) together with State Farm Corporation of India (SFCI) have produced sufficient quantity of breeder seed of major pulses which was subsequently

Table 13.11: Gross Returns, Total Cost and Profitability (Rs.1000/ha) among different Plot Size among Sample Farmers

		TE 2002					TE 2010				
		Marginal	Small	Medium	Large	All	Marginal	Small	Medium	Large	All
Pigeonpea	Gross returns	15	11	10	10	14	45	32	28	26	43
	Costs	13	8	6	6	13	41	19	14	10	38
	Profit	1	3	4	4	1	4	14	14	16	5
Chickpea	Gross returns	15	14	13	8	15	23	22	23	17	22
	Costs	13	8	7	0	11	21	14	12	9	18
	Profit	2	6	7	8	4	2	8	10	8	4
Lentil	Gross returns	13	12	10	9	13	30	25	29	24	29
	Costs	12	8	6	5	11	21	14	15	8	20
	Profit	1	4	4	5	2	9	11	14	16	9
Moong	Gross returns	6	6	9	6	6	15	17	16	15	15
	Costs	9	5	6	1	8	15	11	8	3	15
	Profit	–2	1	3	5	–2	0	6	8	12	0
Urad	Gross returns	9	10	11	13	9	18	24	28	18	19
	Costs	10	7	7	7	9	19	14	16	10	18
	Profit	–1	3	4	5	0	0	10	12	7	1

Source: Cost of cultivation scheme unit level data.

Note: costs does not include family labour; marginal < 1 ha; small 1-2 ha; medium 2-4 ha; large > 4 ha.

used in producing foundation and certified seeds and made available to farmers. However, due to administrative delays, procedures, lack of transparent and timely communication among different stakeholders in the seed supply chain (from block/ mandal level agricultural office to the state department of agriculture, National Seed Corporation, ICAR institute), the seed replacement ratio is still low. Most of the times, seed reached the villages after sowing season. Another major problem is that even though new improved varieties are recommended by the ICAR, many government departments are still procuring outdated varieties with low potential yield for distribution among the farmers. There is no competitive environment in pulses seed market as there is few or no private players.

Table 13.12: State-wise Changes in Profitability of different Pulse Crops (Rs.1000/ha)

		TE 2002			TE 2010		
		Gross Returns	Cost	Profit	Gross Returns	Cost	Profit
Pigeonpea	MP	9	9	0	26	18	8
	Maharashtra	16	15	2	54	52	2
	UP	16	14	2	36	28	8
	AP	11	15	−3	34	30	4
	Karnataka	9	9	0	27	17	10
Chickpea	MP	14	10	4	22	15	7
	Maharashtra	13	12	1	20	21	−2
	Rajasthan	13	9	5	22	14	8
	UP	18	16	2	30	29	1
	AP				31	24	7
	Karnataka				18	15	3
Lentil	MP	11	8	3	24	14	10
	UP	13	15	−2	30	28	3
Moong	Maharashtra	7	9	−2	19	29	−10
	Rajasthan	8	11	−2	19	19	0
	AP	11	8	3	28	19	9
	Karnataka				13	10	2
Urad	MP	8	7	1	18	13	5
	Maharashtra	7	9	−2	19	29	−10
	Rajasthan	8	11	−2	19	19	0
	UP	11	11	0	16	20	−5
	AP	11	8	3	28	19	9

Source: Cost of cultivation scheme unit level data. Marginal < 1 ha; small 1-2 ha; medium 2-4 ha; large > 4 ha.

Technology Demonstrations

Conduct of technology demonstrations on various pulse crops in different states were undertaken under the aegis of the ICAR with technology back up by Indian Institute of Pulses Research. Krishi Vigyan Kendra (KVKs) at district level and All India coordinated projects in different centres were given the responsibility of organizing these demonstrations. Demonstrations on high yielding varieties along with package technology showed that moong yield can be enhanced by 46.7 per cent with average grain yield of 1100 kg/ha and with profit of Rs. 35700 per ha with short duration crop maturing in less than 65 days. This has encouraged farmers to cultivate summer moong. Similarly, encouraging incremental yield achieved during kharif from short duration pulse crops like urad and pigeonpea showed that popularization of high yielding and disease resistant varieties along with matching package technology can enhance the yield levels by 34-47 per cent from the present low levels. The results of successful technology demonstrations at ICRISAT and IIPR, Kanpur provided enough confidence on the potential of the existing technologies to upscale on farmers fields. There is a need for development of model extension strategy for pulse crops in collaboration with state department of agriculture, KVKs, SAUs and ICAR at district level to reduce yield gaps between lab and land.

Opportunities for Expanding Pulses Area

The recent task force on pulses headed by Alagh identified the areas/states which have the potential for increasing pulses area *viz.* (i) identification of additional area having potential for pulse crops by utilization of rice fallow lands (3 to 4 million ha) largely in Eastern India and can yield around 2.5 million tones, (ii) diversification of about 5 lakh ha area of upland rice, 4.5 lakh ha area of millets and 3 lakh ha area under barley, mustard and wheat, currently giving low yields can be brought under kharif/rabi pulses (iii) about 16.5 lakh ha area vacated by wheat, peas, potato and sugarcane can be used for raising 60-65 day summer moong crop in the UP, Punjab, Haryana, Bihar, Gujarat, and West Bengal where adequate irrigation facilities exist and the menace of blue bull is contained and (iv) similarly pigeon pea on rice bunds and intercropping in specific agro climatic regimes is identified.

Strategies for Streamlining Production, Procurement and Distribution

Development of varieties, hybrids and GM crops which are high yielding as well as abiotic and biotic stress tolerant. The adoption of newly released promising varieties, integrated crop management (with components of integrated nutrient management, integrated pest management) and life saving irrigation for rabi crops. However, scientific and technological development without reaching farmers through proper distribution channels is not fruitful. Hence, the increased availability of quality seeds at the village level through innovative seed production and distribution mechanisms is important. Efforts need to be made to increase farm mechanization through varietal development and innovative custom hiring facilities to reduce peak season labour requirement. Mandatory procurement of pulses by the government agencies incase prices falls below MSP. Procurement centre with adequate storage facilities need to be established at district and block level in major pulse growing zones. There is a need to blend domestic price policy with tariff policy such that domestic price of pulses stabilize and assured profits to pulse producers are ensured. Import duties on pulses need to be calibrated in response to the demand and supply situation (Alagh, 2013). The policy instruments which are detrimental to free market such as stocking limit orders, trading movement controls, licensing requirements and other controls needs to be removed in a phased manner.

Conclusion

Apart from enhanced availability of newly released seeds of high yielding varieties recommended by ICAR, the strong field level extension, government procurement at enhanced minimum support prices in case of glut in markets and effective government programmes like NFSM, APPP and RKVY helped in enhancing pulses production especially in a few pockets in the country. This initial gains needs to be up- scaled and out-scaled through appropriate technology support, favourable Govt. policies and remunerative price backed by effective supply chain management. With this, India can reduce or eliminate the projected deficit (17 MT deficit projected based on recommended consumption requirements 80 gm/capita/day or to meet the 6 million tones deficit projected by IIPR, Kanpur by 2020 (Reddy, 2009 and Reddy *et al.*, 2013).

References

Alagh, Yoginder K. "The future of Indian agriculture." New Delhi, India: National Book Trust India (2013).

International Year of Pulses (2016). What Are Pulses and Why Are They Important? Downloaded on 16.4.2015 from http://www.iyop.net/.

Materne, M and Reddy, A. A (2007). Commercial cultivation and Profitability, (ed) Lentil, Yadav, Shyam S. McNeil, David L. and Stevenson, Philip C. Lentil, *Springer* Netherlands, pp. 173-186.

Reddy, A. A. (2013). Strategies for reducing mismatch between demand and supply of grain legumes. *Indian Journal of Agricultural Sciences*, 83(3), 243-59.

Reddy A A (2004). Consumption Pattern, Trade and Production Potential of Pulses, *Economic and Political Weekly*, Vol.39 (44) pp.4854-4860, 2004.

Reddy AA (2009). Pulses Production Technology: Status and Way Forward, *Economic and Political Weekly*, Vol. 44, No. 52, pp. 73-80, December 2009.

Reddy, A. A., Bantilan, M. C. S., and Mohan, G. (2013). Enabling pulses revolution in India, International Crops Research Institute for Semi-Arid Tropics (ICRISAT)-Hyderabad, Policy Brief no. 26.

Chapter 14

Volumetric Assessment of Groundwater Irrigation in Major Crops in Punjab*

S.K. Srivastava[1], Ramesh Chand[1], S.S. Raju[1], Rajni Jain[1],
I. Kingsly[1], Jatinder Sachdeva[2], Jaspal Singh[1]
and Amrit Pal Kaur[1]

[1]ICAR-NIAP, New Delhi-110 012
[2]Punjab Agricultural University (PAU), Ludhiana-141 004

Introduction

The groundwater irrigation has played a catalytic role in averting food crisis in India during mid-sixties. But, injudicious utilization and excessive reliance on this precious natural resource has resulted into emergence of a groundwater crisis, especially in North-West region of the country (Srivastava *et al.*, 2014a). Punjab, agriculturally the most advanced state, stands at an extreme end of over-exploitation of groundwater (Kulkarni and Shah, 2013). As per the Central Groundwater Board (CGWB) estimates, total annual draft of groundwater in Punjab is 72 per cent higher than the net annual replenishable level of 20 billion cubic metre (BCM).

* The paper is drawn from the ongoing ICAR network project on Regional Crop Planning for Improving Resource Use Efficiency and Sustainability. The authors acknowledge the PAU, nodal agency (Punjab) of cost of cultivation scheme for sharing unit-level data for the project.

Another version of paper is under-consideration for the IJAE conference, 2015 at PAU, Ludhiana.

Agriculture sector being the largest user of groundwater resources bears the prime responsibility in averting the groundwater crisis. Many studies have elucidated several hydrological, socio-economic, institutional and policy related aspects of groundwater management (Srivastava *et al.*, 2014b, Ghosh *et al.*, 2014), but without any systematic effort towards volumetric assessment of groundwater use in crop production in the farmer's field. CGWB, a nodal agency for monitoring groundwater resources, carries out periodic assessment of groundwater use for different sectors (irrigation, domestic, industry) of the country. But such estimates are not available for individual crops within agriculture sector. The present study attempts to fill this void and estimates volume of groundwater use for irrigating different crops in Punjab using unit-level cost of cultivation survey data of Directorate of Economics and Statistics (DES) and groundwater level data of CGWB.

Data and Methodology

The study is primarily based on plot-level data collected under "comprehensive scheme for cost of cultivation of principal crops" of Directorate of Economics and Statistics, Ministry of Agriculture. The cost of cultivation survey (CCS) has been collecting a rich source of representative and comparable data on different aspects of farming across different regions of the country since 1970-71. However, this wealth of data has remained grossly underutilized due to many administrative and non-administrative hurdles (Sen and Bhatia, 2004; Nawn, 2013). In the CCS, each sample household is surveyed consecutively for three years and the latest available data pertains to the period 2008-09 to 2010-11 (block year ending 2010-11). For Punjab, the plot-wise data was collected from the 300 representative households of 30 tehsils during each year of the block period (2008-09 to 2010-11) by the Punjab Agricultural University, Ludhiana, which is a nodal agency for this state. The data on groundwater level was collected from CGWB.

The volume of total groundwater for irrigating major crops (paddy, wheat, cotton, sugarcane, maize) in Punjab was estimated as the product of irrigation hours and per hour groundwater draft (cum/hr). The irrigation hours (hrs/ha) for each crop were taken from plot-wise CCS data. As CCS does not collect information on groundwater draft, it was estimated using the following formula (Srivastava *et al.*, 2014b);

$$\text{Groundwater draft} \left(\frac{\text{lit}}{\text{sec}} \right) = \frac{\text{Hp} \times 75 \times \text{Pump efficiency}}{\text{Total head (m)}}$$

The information on horse power (Hp) of the pumps owned by the farmers was extracted from CCS dataset. For the households purchasing groundwater, average Hp of the pumps (estimated separately for electric and diesel) in respective tehsil was taken into consideration. Total head was estimated as sum of groundwater table (m bgl) and friction loss (10 per cent of water table). For submersible pumps additional depth of 11 metre was added to the total head after discussion with the experts because these pumps are placed far below the groundwater table. Pump efficiency was assumed to be 40 per cent (Srivastava *et al.*, 2014b). As irrigation pumps vary in terms of type (centrifugal/submersible) and energy use (electric/

diesel), per unit (cum/hr) and thereafter total groundwater draft (cum/ha) was estimated for each category of pump separately. The summation of groundwater draft from each category of pumps gave total groundwater use (cum/ha) for each crop cultivated by the farmer.

The crop-wise groundwater footprints (cum/kg) was estimated by dividing total groundwater use with the respective crop yield. Similarly, groundwater productivity (Rs/cum) was estimated by dividing value of output (main + by product) with the groundwater use.

Results and Discussion

Within agriculture, the extent of groundwater use varies across different crops depending upon the pumping hours and average yield {cubic meter/hour (cum/hr)} of the pumps. The estimated per hour groundwater draft in the study area varied from 8.17 cum/hr to 349 cum/hr during TE 2010-11 depending upon the horse power of the pump used and heterogeneity in water level (Table 14.1). The groundwater draft of sample farmers' field was found to be comparable with CGWB estimates of ≤ 50 to ≥ 150 cum/hr in different aquifer zones of Punjab (Gupta, 2009).

Table 14.1: Summary Statistics of Variables for Estimating Groundwater Extraction in Punjab during TE 2010-11

Particulars	Mean	Minimum	Maximum	Standard Deviation
Hp: DoCP	9	2	15	1.4
Hp: EoCP	5	2	10	1.4
Hp: EoSP	10	2	20	2.6
Total head (m)	14.89	2.71	24.26	6.10
Groundwater draft (Cum/hr): DoCP	75.28	18.50	349.13	56.94
Groundwater draft (Cum/hr): EoCP	41.99	8.69	203.66	28.26
Groundwater draft (cum/hr): EoSP	47.14	8.17	87.39	17.28

DoCP: Diesel operated centrifugal pumps; EoCP: Electric operated centrifugal pump; EoSP: Electric operated submersible pumps.

The product of per hour groundwater draft and pumping hours produces estimates of total volume of groundwater extraction for different crops grown in the farmers' field. It was found that Punjab farmers run tubewell for 285 hours to cultivate one hectare of paddy followed by 170 hours for sugarcane, 60 hours for wheat, 53 hours for maize and 46 hours for cotton (Table 14.2). The pump wise decomposition further revealed that more than 50 per cent of the groundwater irrigation is given using submersible pumps except for cotton and sugarcane. The dominance of submersible pumps for major crops indicates a deeper water table in large part of the state. For cotton cultivation, submersible pumps were not used primarily because it is grown in water-logging and salinity affected south-western part of the state. Due to salinity problem, farmers prefer canal irrigation and use groundwater as a source of supplementary irrigation. About 88 per cent of the cotton area of the sample farmers was irrigated using "tubewell+canal" source

Table 14.2: Pattern of Groundwater Extraction in Punjab in TE 2010-11

Crops	Groundwater Irrigation Hours (hours/ha)				Share in Total Irrigation hours (per cent)			
	Diesel Pump	Electric Centrifugal	Electric Submersible	Total	Diesel Pump	Electric Centrifugal	Electric Submersible	
Paddy	11	124	150	285	4	43	53	
Non-basmati	12	131	141	283	4	46	50	
Basmati	9	98	183	290	3	34	63	
Wheat	4	23	33	60	6	39	55	
Cotton	22	21	3	46	48	46	6	
Sugarcane	8	118	44	170	4	69	26	
Maize	7	18	28	53	13	35	52	

Source: Authors' estimate based on unit level CCS data of DES.

of irrigation followed by canal (9.17 per cent) and tubewell alone (1.80 per cent) during TE 2010-11.

Among major crops, paddy was found to be the most water-guzzling crop with the groundwater use of 12151 cum/ha during TE 2010-11. The groundwater use for cultivation of other crops was only 12 (for maize) to 55 (for sugarcane) per cent of the groundwater use in paddy depending upon the crop duration and water requirement (Table 14.3). On an average, production of one kilogram of paddy in Punjab required 2053 litres groundwater and the estimated groundwater footprints for other crops (except cotton) were much less than for paddy. Due to substantially high groundwater use, groundwater productivity (Rs/cum) of paddy was also much lower than other crops. Technological and policy support during the green revolution period (1960s) brought a significant increase in area under paddy from 4 lakh ha during TE 1973 to 28 lakh ha during TE 2013. Presently, paddy occupies about 36 per cent of total gross cropped area and about 77 per cent of *kharif* area of the state. Thus, paddy a dominant crop in existing cropping pattern is ecologically misfit for Punjab and putting groundwater resources in a jeopardy situation.

Table 14.3: Crop-wise Groundwater Use in Punjab in TE 2010-11

Crops	Groundwater Draft (cum/ha)	Crop Yield (kg/ha)	Groundwater Footprints (Lit/kg)	Crop Value (Rs/ha)	Groundwater Productivity (Rs/cum)
Paddy	12151	5918	2053	69188	5.69
Non-basmati	12127	6569	1846	67035	5.53
Basmati	12237	3440	3557	77379	6.32
Wheat	2520	4224	597	53405	21.19
Cotton	3920	2112	1856	71635	18.27
Sugarcane	6735	72906	92	155324	23.06
Maize	1485	3674	404	34306	23.10

Source: Authors' estimate based on unit-level CCS data of DES.

The promotion of basmati variety over the common paddy is often suggested as an option to reduce the groundwater demand in the light of less water requirement* by the former (Hindustan time, 2014). But, the farm-level evidences showed that farmers use almost equal volume of groundwater for cultivation of basmati as well as common paddy in Punjab (Table 14.3). It is interesting to note that about 80 per cent of the total water requirement of paddy (including basmati) is met by groundwater even though it is grown in monsoon season. It is also indicative of the fact that Punjab farmers do not rely on arrival of monsoon for crop cultivation. In terms of per unit production, basmati variety consumed almost double (3557 lit/kg) volume of groundwater than the common paddy (1846 lit/kg) due to substantially lower yield in TE 2010-11. However, it is interesting to note that inspite of the lower yield, large price differential made basmati variety more remunerative than the

---

* Usually, basmati paddy in Punjab is transplanted in July which coincides with the onset of the monsoon, thus requiring less groundwater than common paddy.

common paddy. Therefore, it is imperative to say that replacement of common paddy with basmati may improve the farmers' income but without reducing the pressure on depleting groundwater resources in the state.

A shift in cropping pattern away from wheat-rice to a wheat-maize has been one of the suggestions to curb the groundwater depletion since Johl committee report in 1986 (Sarkar and Das, 2014). But the cropping pattern could not be altered. Again in March 2013, the government initiated crop diversification programme for diverting at least 5 per cent of area under paddy in identified over-exploited and critical blocks of Punjab, Haryana and Western Uttar Pradesh towards alternate crops (Government of India, 2013). However, under the prevailing conditions of electricity pricing and minimum support price, paddy will remain the most remunerative crop (Sarkar and Das, 2014) and farmer may not move towards diversification until incentivized by economically attractive alternatives.

Conclusions and Policy Implications

Among other crops, paddy was found to be the most water-guzzling crop. Punjab farmer were primarily dependent on groundwater even though paddy is a grown in monsoon season. The promotion of basmati variety over the common paddy is often suggested as an option to reduce the groundwater demand in the light of less water requirement. But empirical evidences indicate that replacement of common paddy with basmati may improve the farmers' income but without reducing the pressure on depleting groundwater resources in the state. Overall, paddy was found to be the ecologically misfit crop putting groundwater resources in a jeopardy situation. A shift in cropping pattern away from wheat-rice has been suggested since long but farmer may not move towards diversification until incentivized by economically attractive alternatives. Till then, the excess use of groundwater in paddy may be curtailed by, (1) increasing marginal cost of water through subsidy reduction, (2) reducing dependency on groundwater by promoting integrated water resources utilization and strictly monitoring the Punjab Preservation of Sub-Soil Water Act, 2009, and (3) promoting water saving methods of paddy cultivation such system of rice intensification (SRI), direct seeded rice, etc.

References

Ghosh, S., S. K. Srivastava, A. K. Nayak, D. K. Panda, P. Nanda and A. Kumar (2014). "Why Impacts of Irrigation on Agrarian Dynamism and Livelihoods are Contrasting? Evidence from Eastern India States", *Irrigation and Drainage*, Vol. 65 (3), pp. 573-583.

Government of India (2013). "Report of the High Level Expert Group on Water Logging in Punjab", Planning Commission, Government of India, New Delhi.

Gupta S. (2009). *"Groundwater Management in Alluvial Areas"*, Technical Paper in Special Session on Groundwater in the 5th Asian Regional Conference on INCID, December 9-11 at Vigyan Bhawan, New Delhi.

Hindustan times (2014). "Punjab Wants Farmers to Grow Basmati", October 2, http://www.hindustantimes.com/chandigarh/punjab-wants-farmers-to-grow-basmati/article1-1270997.aspx.

Kulkarni H. and M. Shah (2013). "Punjab Water Syndrome: Diagnostic and Prescriptions", *Economic and Political Weekly*, Vol. XLVIII (52), pp. 64-73.

Nawan, Nandan (2013). "Using Cost of Cultivation Survey Data: Changing Challenges for Researchers", *Economic and Political Weekly*, Vol. XLVIII, (26 and 27), pp. 139-147.

Sarkar A. and A. Das (2014). "Groundwater Irrigation – Electricity - Crop Diversification Nexus in Punjab: Trends, Turning Points and Policy Initiatives", *Economic and Political Weekly*, Vol. XLIX (52), pp. 64-73.

Sen, Abhijit and M S Bhatia (2004). "Cost of Cultivation and Farm Income", State of the Indian Farmer – A Millennium Study, Vol. 14 (New Delhi: Department of Agriculture and Cooperation, Ministry of Agriculture, Government of India, and Academic Foundation).

Srivastava, S. K., R. C. Srivastava, R. R. Sethi, A. Kumar and A.K. Nayak (2014b). "Accelerating Groundwater and Energy Use for Agricultural Growth in Odisha: Technological and Policy Issues", *Agricultural Economics Research Review*, Vol. 27 (2), pp. 259-270.

Srivastava, S.K., S. Ghosh, A. Kumar and PSB Anand (2014a). "Unravelling Spatio-Temporal Pattern of Irrigation Development and Its Impact on Indian Agriculture", *Irrigation and Drainage*, Vol. 63 (1), pp. 1-11.

Chapter 15

Various Elementary Concepts of Sample Surveys

Hukum Chandra

National Fellow
ICAR-IASRI, New Delhi – 110 012

Introduction

The prime objective of a sample survey is to obtain inferences about the characteristic of a population. Population is defined as a group of units defined according to the objectives of the survey. The population may consist of all the households in a village/locality, all the fields under a particular crop etc. We may also consider a population of persons, families, fields, animals in a region, or a population of trees, birds in a forest depending upon the nature of data required. The information that we seek about the population is normally, the total number of units, aggregate values of various characteristics, averages of these characteristics per unit, proportions of units possessing specified attributes etc. The data can be collected in two different ways. The first one is complete enumeration which means collection of data on the survey characteristics from each unit of the population. This type of method is used in censuses of population, agriculture, retail stores, industrial establishments etc. The other approach is based on the use of sampling methods and consists of collection of data on survey characteristics from selected units of the population. The first approach can be considered as its special case. A sampling method is a scientific and objective procedure of selecting units from the population and provides a sample that is expected to be representative of the population. A sampling method makes it possible to estimate the population parameters while reducing at the same time the size of survey operations. Some of the advantages of sample surveys as compared to complete enumeration are reduction in cost, greater speed, wider scope and higher accuracy. A function of the unit values of the sample is called an estimator. Various measures, like bias, mean square errors, variance etc. are used to assess the performance of the estimator.

The main problem in sample surveys is the choice of a proper sampling strategy, which essentially comprise of a sampling method and the estimation procedure. In the choice of a sampling method there are some methods of selection while some others are control measures which help in grouping the population before the selection process. Developed methods of sample selection from a finite population and of estimation that provide estimates of the unknown population parameters, generally population total or population mean, which are precise enough for our purpose. Survey samples can broadly be categorized into two types: probability samples and non-probability samples. Surveys based on probability samples are capable of providing mathematically sound statistical inferences about a larger target population. Inferences from probability-based surveys may, however, suffer from many types of bias. Surveys that are not based on probability sampling have no way of measuring their bias or sampling error. Surveys based on non-probability samples are not externally valid. They can only be said to be representative of the people that have actually completed the survey. Henceforth, a sample survey would always mean a probability sampling, unless otherwise stated. Sample survey methods, based on probability sampling, have more or less replaced complete survey (or census) methods on account of several well known advantages. It is well recognized that the introduction of probability sampling approach has played an important role in the development of survey techniques. The concept of representativeness through probability sampling techniques introduced by Neyman (1934) provided a sound base to the survey approach of data collection. One of the salient features of probability sampling is that besides providing an estimate of the population parameter, it also provides an idea about the precision of the estimate (sampling error). Throughout this lecture, the attention would be restricted to sample surveys and not the complete enumeration. For a detailed exposition to the concepts of sample survey, reference may be made to the texts of Cochran (1977), Murthy (1977), Sukhatme *et al.* (1984). In the methods of selection, schemes such as simple random sampling, systematic sampling and varying probability sampling are generally used. Among the control measures are procedures such as stratified sampling, cluster sampling and multi-stage sampling etc. A combination of control measures along with the method of selection is called the sampling scheme. We shall describe in brief the different sampling methods in the following sections:

Simple Random Sampling

Simple random sampling (SRS) is a method of selecting a sample of 'n' units out of population of 'N' units such that each one of the possible non-distinct samples has an equal chance of its being chosen. In practice, a simple way of obtaining a simple random sample is to draw the units one by one with a known probability of selection assigned to each unit of the population at the first and each subsequent draw. The successive draws may be made with or without replacing the units selected in the preceding draws. The former is called the procedure of sampling with replacement while the latter sampling without replacement.

The units in the population are numbered from 1 to N. A series of random numbers between 1 and N are then drawn either by means of a Table of random numbers or by means of a computer program that produces such a Table.

It can be seen that in simple random sampling without replacement (SRSWOR), the probability of selecting the units in the sample is equal for all the units. Let Y be the characteristic of interest. The N units that comprise the population are denoted

by $y_1, y_2, ..., y_N$. Let the population mean, $\overline{Y}_N = \dfrac{(y_1 + y_2 + \cdots + y_{N-1} + y_N)}{N} = \dfrac{1}{N}\sum_{i=1}^{N} y_i$, denote the parameter of interest.

Let us draw a simple random sample, without replacement, of size n. We denote

by $\overline{y}_n = \dfrac{(y_1 + y_2 + \cdots + y_i + \cdots + y_{n-1} + y_n)}{n} = \dfrac{1}{n}\sum_{i=1}^{n} y_i$, the sample mean, an unbiased estimator of the population mean $\overline{Y}_N$. In other words, the average value of $\overline{y}_n$ over all possible samples ($^N C_n$ in this case) is equal to $\overline{Y}_N$.

Also, the sampling variance of $\overline{y}_n$ is given by

$$V(\overline{y}_n) = (\frac{1}{n} - \frac{1}{N})S^2 \tag{1.1}$$

where, $S^2 = \dfrac{1}{N-1}\sum_{i=1}^{N}(y_i - \overline{Y}_N)^2$ is the population mean square.

An unbiased estimator of this sampling variance is given by

$$\hat{V}(\overline{y}_n) = (\frac{1}{n} - \frac{1}{N})s^2 \tag{1.2}$$

where, $s^2 = \dfrac{1}{n-1}\sum_{i=1}^{n}(y_i - \overline{y}_n)^2$ is the sample mean square.

Drawing Simple Random Samples using a Table of Random Numbers.

An easy way to select a SRS is to use a random number table, which is a table of digits 0,1,…,9, each digit having equal chance of being selected at each draw. To use this table in drawing a random sample of size n from a population of size N, we do the following:

☆ Label the units in the population from 0 to N - 1.

☆ Find r, the number of digits in N - 1. For example; if $N = 100$, then $r = 2$.

☆ Read r digits at a time across the columns or rows of a random number table.

☆ If the number in (3) corresponds to a number in (1), the corresponding unit of the population is included in the sample, otherwise the number is discarded and the next one is read.

☆ Continue until n units have been selected.

If the same unit in the population is selected more than once in the above process of selection, then the resulting sample is called a SRS with replacement; otherwise it is called a SRS without replacement. The observations in the sample are the enumeration or readings of the units selected.

Example 1

To draw a SRS, consider the data below as our population. In a study of wrap breakage during the weaving of fabric, one hundred pieces of yarn were tested. The number of cycles of strain to breakage was recorded for each yarn and the resulting data are given in the following table.

86	175	157	282	38	211	497	246	393	198
146	176	220	224	337	180	182	185	396	264
251	76	42	149	66	93	423	188	203	105
653	264	321	180	151	315	185	568	829	203
98	15	180	325	341	353	229	55	239	124
249	364	198	250	40	571	400	55	236	137
400	195	38	196	40	124	338	61	286	135
292	262	20	90	135	279	290	244	194	350
131	88	61	229	597	81	398	20	277	193
169	264	121	166	246	186	71	284	143	188

Here we have a population of size $N = 100$. To draw a simple random of size n=10 without replacement, we proceed as follows:

☆ Label the units in the population from 00 to 99.

☆ Find r, the number of digits in N. For example, if $N = 100$, then $r = 2$.

☆ Read 2 digits at a time across the columns or rows of a random number table.

Part of a Random Number Table

8571	7683	5118	7669	6126	3663	3059	7807	9219	4383	9021	7013	0233	3348	4077
0864	5055	8631	5770	0505	0386	9792	1690	4874	3084	0228	8539	9375	5046	8635
4753	1992	8182	2658	2914	4005	1577	1714	7862	7009	0252	3070	1563	3008	3716
1267	1063	4415	8496	6779	1563	7833	5351	2278	0674	1252	6813	4016	3961	6890
9497	0105	5626	0529	0602	4573	1499	7772	7759	9405	9502	3408	6931	7946	4655
6823	7365	6140	0357	7069	7715	9083	6180	1131	7059	9808	9803	7883	5943	6649
6532	4048	3044	8035	1045	8349	5422	0315	7470	7679	1726	1390	4997	5632	9033

8184	8336	5684	5846	7056	2847	4715	2869	2576	5373	8175	0384	5348	8232	8186
5605	0939	9380	1647	7307	5893	7569	7092	4437	2722	7807	5908	5425	9679	2348
4926	1561	7299	2195	5374	3664	8269	5241	4436	5265	7571	8299	6006	2142	2273
0933	6131	2406	0715	5069	1663	8015	9120	0667	4884	8601	3370	3449	7158	8950
7413	9526	9670	3075	8321	8295	6327	5475	5650	9061	7687	3849	2207	6910	4166

Suppose we read the first two digits of the first two columns of the above random number table to get the following numbers

85	71	76	83	51	18	76	69	61	26	36

Since the random digit 85 corresponds to a unit in (1), we select unit 85 of the population in the sample. If any random digit in (3) exceeds 99, the random digit is discarded and the next one is read. After selecting 6 random numbers of two digits, we find a random number 76 which is discarded for SRS without replacement as it appeared before.

Continue until $n = 10$ units have been selected. Thus we have the sample units:

85 71	76	83	51	18	69	61	26	36

so that the sample observations are:

81 262	290	229	368	396	135	195	234	185

A SRS with replacement in the above example would be:

81 262	290	229	368	396	290	135	195	234.

Example 2

We now take an example to illustrate the concepts of unbiasedness of sample mean ($\bar{y}_n$) and sample mean square (s^2). Suppose we have a population of $N = 5$ units, say U_1, U_2, U_3, U_4, U_5. The characteristic under study, Y is the yield in kg per plot. We want to estimate $\bar{Y}_N$, the population mean of Y on the basis of a sample of size $n = 2$ drawn by SRSWOR. The data and the analysis are as given in the Table below:

Units (U_i)	U_1	U_2	U_3	U_4	U_5	Total
Values of y_i (kg/plot)	32	28	25	30	35	150
Population Mean $(\bar{Y}_N) = \dfrac{(y_1 + y_2 + y_3 + y_4 + y_5)}{5} = \dfrac{32 + 28 + 25 + 30 + 35}{5} = \dfrac{150}{5} = 30$ kg						
y_i^2	1024	784	625	900	1225	4558

$$\text{Population Mean Square}(S^2) = \frac{\left(\sum_{i=1}^{N} Y_i^2 - N\overline{Y}_N^2\right)}{N-1}$$

$$= \frac{4558 - 5 \times 30 \times 30}{4} = \frac{4558 - 4500}{4} = \frac{58}{4} = 14.5$$

Units in the Sample	Sample Observations	Sample Mean $(\overline{y}_n)$	Sample Mean Square (s^2)
U_1, U_2	32, 28	30.0	8.0
U_1, U_3	32, 25	28.5	24.5
U_1, U_4	32, 30	31.0	2.0
U_1, U_5	32, 35	33.5	4.5
U_2, U_3	28, 25	26.5	4.5
U_2, U_4	28, 30	29.0	2.0
U_2, U_5	28, 35	31.5	24.5
U_3, U_4	25, 30	27.5	12.5
U_3, U_5	25, 35	30.0	50.0
U_4, U_5	30, 35	32.5	12.5
Average		300/10 = **30**	145.0/10 = **14.5**

A similar approach applies when sampling is with replacement (SRSWR). In this case, there are N^n possible samples. The estimator of population mean, sampling variance of the estimator, and estimator of the sampling variance are given as

$$\overline{y}_n = \frac{1}{n}\sum_{i=1}^{n} y_i \tag{1.3}$$

$$V(\overline{y}_n) = \frac{\sigma^2}{n} \tag{1.4}$$

and

$$\hat{V}(\overline{y}_n) = \frac{s^2}{n} \tag{1.5}$$

where, $\sigma^2 = \frac{1}{N}\sum_{i=1}^{N}(y_i - \overline{Y}_N)^2$ is the population variance and s^2 is the sample mean square.

Consider all possible samples of size N which can be drawn from a given population. In SRSWOR scheme, there will be in all $^N C_n$ possible samples. For each sample, one can compute a statistic, such as the mean, standard deviation etc., which will vary from sample to sample. In this manner, one can obtain a distribution of the statistic which is called its sampling distribution.

For estimating the population total $Y = \sum\limits_{i=1}^{N} y_i$, we have an estimator

$$\hat{Y} = N \sum\limits_{i=1}^{n} y_i / n = N.\bar{y}_n \qquad (1.6)$$

i.e., the population size N multiplied by the sample mean $\bar{y}_n$.

This estimator can be expressed as $\hat{Y} = \sum\limits_{i=1}^{n} w_i y_i = (N/n)\sum\limits_{i=1}^{n} y_i$, where $w_i = N/n$.

The constant N/n is the sampling weight and is the inverse of the sampling fraction n/N .

The estimator of sampling variance of $\hat{Y}$ is given by

$$\hat{V}(\hat{Y}) = \hat{V}(N.\bar{y}_n) = N^2.\hat{V}(\bar{y}_n) \qquad (1.7)$$

and the estimator of standard error of $\hat{Y}$ is given by

$$S\hat{E}(\hat{Y}) = S\hat{E}(N.\bar{y}_n) = N.S\hat{E}(\bar{y}_n) \qquad (1.8)$$

From the above, it is evident that under Simple Random Sampling With Replacement (SRSWR),

i) The sample mean $(\bar{y}_n)$ is unbiased for the population mean $(\bar{Y}_N)$,

ii) Sample mean square (s²) is unbiased for the population variance (σ^2), and

iii) $V(\bar{y}_n) = \dfrac{\sigma^2}{n}$.

Like-wise, under Simple Random Sampling Without Replacement (SRSWOR),

i) The sample mean $(\bar{y}_n)$ is unbiased for the population mean $(\bar{Y}_N)$,

ii) Sample mean square (s²) is unbiased for the population mean square (S^2) and

iii) $V(\bar{y}_n) = \left(\dfrac{1}{n} - \dfrac{1}{N}\right) S^2$

Estimation of Population Proportion

Sometimes, the units in the population are classified into two groups (i) having a particular characteristic and (ii) not having that characteristic. For example, a crop field may be irrigated or not irrigated. If it is irrigated, we say that it possesses the characteristic, 'irrigation'. If it is not irrigated, we say that it does not possess the particular characteristic of irrigation. If we are interested in estimating the proportion of irrigated fields, the population of N fields can be defined with variate y_i as having value 1 if the field is irrigated, a value 0, otherwise. If the total number of irrigated fields be N_1 out of N, then

$$\sum_{i=1}^{N} y_i = N_1 \tag{2.1}$$

Thus,

$$\bar{Y} = \frac{1}{N}\sum_{i=1}^{N} y_i = \frac{N_1}{N} = P = \text{proportion of irrigated fields in the population} \tag{2.2}$$

and

$$\sum_{i=1}^{N} y_i^2 = N_1 = N.P \tag{2.3}$$

Thus the problem of estimating a population proportion becomes that of estimating a population mean by defining the variate as above. If n_1 units out of a random sample of size n possess that characteristic, the proportion of irrigated fields in the sample is given by $p = \frac{n_1}{n}$.

Thus

$$\sum_{i=1}^{n} y_i = n_1 = \sum_{i=1}^{n} y_i^2 = n.p \tag{2.4}$$

Hence an unbiased estimator of P is given by

$$\hat{P} = (\frac{n_1}{n}) = p = \frac{1}{n}\sum_{i=1}^{n} y_i = \text{sample mean} \tag{2.5}$$

In sampling without replacement, the variance of p is given by

$$V(p) = \frac{(N-n)}{(N-1)}.\frac{P.Q}{n} \tag{2.6}$$

where $Q = 1 - P$.

In sampling with replacement, the variance of p is given by

$$V(p) = \frac{P.Q}{n} \qquad (2.7)$$

In sampling without replacement, an unbiased estimator of V(p) is given by

$$\hat{V}(p) = \frac{(N-n)}{N} \cdot \frac{p.q}{(n-1)} \qquad (2.8)$$

where $q = 1 - p$.

In sampling with replacement, an unbiased estimator of V(p) is given by

$$\hat{V}(p) = \frac{p.q}{(n-1)} \qquad (2.9)$$

Example 3

The data given below pertains to the average yield of sugarcane crop (in quintals) pertaining to 108 villages in a tehsil of a District in India.

Village Sl. Nos.	Yield (in quintals)									
1-10	20	21	32	41	55	22	64	42	28	35
11-20	25	25	24	32	75	28	29	38	19	19
21-30	16	28	30	29	29	19	37	34	31	35
31-40	29	19	27	42	39	11	26	21	45	61
41-50	16	29	32	40	63	30	21	35	28	18
51-60	24	32	23	8	35	27	35	25	29	29
61-70	25	31	38	31	43	21	36	30	37	47
71-80	15	19	32	19	50	10	27	36	28	43
81-90	28	25	31	6	4	22	24	39	71	44
91-100	24	34	18	28	10	70	20	32	42	47
101-108	16	28	30	29	29	19	37	34		

Select a random sample of size 10 by simple random sampling without replacement (SRSWOR) and estimate the average yield along with its standard error on the basis of selected sample units. Set up 95 per cent confidence interval for the population mean.

Solution

As the population size $N = 108$ is a three digit number, so for selecting a simple random sample of size $n = 10$, we shall select three-digit random numbers from the Random Number Table (from 000 to 972, which is the highest multiple of 108 up to 999) as follows:

Random Number	Sampling Unit Sl. No. (Remainder of Random Number/108)	Yield(q)
120	12	25
572	32	19
649	01	20
211	103	30
327	03	32
673	25	29
153	45	63
317	101	16
586	46	30
943	79	28

Estimate of Population Average yield = $\hat{Y}_N = \bar{y}_n = \dfrac{\sum_{i=1}^{n} y_i}{n} = \dfrac{292}{10} = 29.2$ q

Estimate of Population Total $= \hat{Y} = N \times \bar{y}_n = 108 \times 29.2 = 3153.6q$

The estimate of standard error of $\hat{Y}$ is given by

$$S\hat{E}\left(\hat{Y}\right) = S\hat{E}\left(N.\bar{y}_n\right) = N.S\hat{E}\left(\bar{y}_n\right)$$

where $S\hat{E}(\bar{y}_n) = \sqrt{\left(\dfrac{1}{n} - \dfrac{1}{N}\right)} . s$

where $s^2 = \dfrac{1}{n-1}\sum (y_i - \bar{y}_n)^2 = \dfrac{1}{10-1} \times 1533.6 = 170.4 \, q^2$

So, $s = \sqrt{170.4} = 13.0537 \, q$

Hence, $S\hat{E}(\bar{y}_n) = \sqrt{\left(\dfrac{1}{10} - \dfrac{1}{108}\right)} \times 13.0537 = 0.3012 \times 13.0537 = 3.9322$

ii) The 95 per cent confidence interval for population mean is given by

$\bar{y}_n \pm t_{0.05/(10-1=9)df} \times S\hat{E}(\bar{y}_n) = 29.2 \pm 2.262 \times 3.9322 = 29.2 \pm 8.89$

So, the 95 per cent confidence interval for population mean is (29.2 - 8.89 to 29.2 + 8.89) *i.e.* (20.31, 38.09). It can be clearly seen that the population mean

$\bar{Y}_N = \dfrac{3320}{108} = 30.74q$ is contained in this confidence interval. It may be mentioned here that out of total number of possible samples *i.e.* $^{108}C_{10}$, the population mean will be contained in such like confidence intervals corresponding to 95 per cent of the total number of samples.

Stratified Random Sampling

When sub-populations vary considerably, it is advantageous to sample each subpopulation (stratum) independently. **Stratification** is the process of grouping members of the population into relatively homogeneous subgroups before sampling. The strata should be mutually exclusive: every element in the population must be assigned to only one stratum. The strata should also be collectively exhaustive: no population element can be excluded. Then random or systematic sampling is applied within each stratum. This often improves the representativeness of the sample by reducing sampling error. It can produce a weighted mean that has less variability than the arithmetic mean of a simple random sample of the population.

There are several possible strategies:

1. Proportionate allocation uses a sampling fraction in each of the strata that is proportional to that of the total population. If the population consists of 60 per cent in the male stratum and 40 per cent in the female stratum, then the relative size of the two samples (one male, one female) should reflect this proportion.

2. Optimum allocation (or Disproportionate allocation) - Each stratum is proportionate to the standard deviation of the distribution of the variable. Larger samples are taken in the strata with the greatest variability to generate the least possible sampling variance.

A real-world example of using stratified sampling would be for a US political survey. If we wanted the respondents to reflect the diversity of the population of the United States, the researcher would specifically seek to include participants of various minority groups such as race or religion, based on their proportionality to the total population as mentioned above. A stratified survey could thus claim to be more representative of the US population than a survey of simple random sampling or systematic sampling.

Similarly, if population density varies greatly within a region, stratified sampling will insure that estimates can be made with equal accuracy in different parts of the region, and that comparisons of sub-regions can be made with equal statistical power. For example, in Ontario a survey taken throughout the province might use a larger sampling fraction in the less populated north, since the disparity in population between north and south is so great that a sampling fraction based on the provincial sample as a whole might result in the collection of only a handful of data from the north.

Advantages

☆ Focuses on important subpopulations but ignores irrelevant ones

☆ Improves the accuracy of estimation

☆ Efficient

☆ Sampling equal numbers from strata varying widely in size may be used to equate the statistical power of tests of differences between strata.

Disadvantages

☆ Can be difficult to select relevant stratification variables

☆ Not useful when there are no homogeneous subgroups

☆ Can be expensive

☆ Requires accurate information about the population, or introduces bias.

☆ Looks randomly within specific sub headings.

In case of SRSWOR, the sampling variance of the sample mean is

$$V(\bar{y}_n)=(\frac{1}{n}-\frac{1}{N})S^2$$

Clearly, the variance decreases as the sample size 'n' increases while the population variability S^2 decreases. Now one of the objectives of a good sampling technique is to reduce the sampling variance. So we have to either increase 'n' or decrease S^2. Apart from the sample size, therefore, the only way of increasing the precision of an estimate is to devise sampling procedure which will effectively reduce S^2 *i.e.* the heterogeneity in the population. In fact, S^2 is a population parameter and is inherent with the population, therefore, it cannot be decreased. Instead, the population may be divided into number of groups (called strata), thereby, controlling variability within each group. This procedure is known as stratification.

In stratified sampling, the population consisting of N units is first divided into K subpopulations of sizes $N_1, N_2,...,N_K$ units respectively. These subpopulations are nonoverlapping and together they comprise the whole of the population *i.e.* $\sum_{i=1}^{K} N_i = N$. These subpopulations are called strata. To obtain full benefit from stratification, the values of N_i's must be known. When the strata have been determined, a sample is drawn from each stratum, the drawings being made independently in different strata. If a simple random sample is taken in each stratum then the procedure is termed as stratified random sampling. As the sampling variance of the estimate of population mean or total depends on within strata variation, the stratification of population is done in such a way that strata are homogeneous within themselves with respect to the variable under study. However, in many practical situations, it is usually difficult to stratify with respect to the variable under consideration especially because of physical and cost consideration. Generally the stratification is done according to administrative groupings, geographical regions and on the basis of auxiliary characters correlated with the character under study.

Let $N_1, N_2,...,N_K$ denote the sizes of K strata, such that $\sum_{i=1}^{K} N_i = N$ (total number of units in the population).

Let y_{ij} denotes the jth observation in the ith stratum.

Denote $\overline{Y}_N = \frac{1}{N}\sum_{i=1}^{K}\sum_{j=1}^{N_i} y_{ij}$ as population mean.

Again,

$$S^2 = \frac{1}{N-1}\sum_{i=1}^{K}\sum_{j=1}^{N_i}(y_{ij} - \overline{Y}_N)^2 = \text{population mean square,}$$

$$S_i^2 = \frac{1}{N_i-1}\sum_{j=1}^{N_i}(y_{ij} - \overline{Y}_{N_i})^2 = \text{population mean square in the } i^{th} \text{ stratum,}$$

where $\overline{Y}_{N_i} = \frac{1}{N_i}\sum_{j=1}^{N_i} y_{ij} = \text{population mean for the } i^{th} \text{ stratum.}$

We select a simple random sample of size n_1 from the first stratum, of size n_2 from the second stratum,.., of size n_i from the ith stratum and so on such that

$n_1 + n_2 +.+ n_K = n$ (sample size).

The population mean $\overline{Y}_N$ can be written as

$$\overline{Y}_N = \frac{1}{N}\sum_{i=1}^{K} N_i \overline{Y}_{N_i} = \sum_{i=1}^{K} P_i \overline{Y}_{N_i} \qquad (4.1)$$

where $P_i = \dfrac{N_i}{N}$

.

Since within each stratum, the samples have been drawn by SRSWOR,

$\overline{y}_{n_i}\left(=\dfrac{1}{n_i}\sum_{j=1}^{n_i} y_{ij}\right)$ sample mean for the ith stratum is an unbiased estimator of $\overline{Y}_{N_i}$ and obviously

$$\overline{y}_s = \frac{1}{N}\sum_{i=1}^{K} N_i \overline{y}_{n_i} = \sum_{i=1}^{K} P_i \overline{y}_{n_i} \qquad (4.2)$$

The weighted mean of the strata sample means with strata sizes as the weights, will be an appropriate estimator of the population mean.

Clearly $\overline{y}_s$ is an unbiased estimator of $\overline{Y}_N$, since

$$E(\overline{y}_s) = E\left(\sum_{i=1}^{K} P_i \overline{y}_{n_i}\right) = \sum_{i=1}^{K} P_i E(\overline{y}_{n_i}) = \sum_{i=1}^{K} P_i \overline{Y}_{N_i} = \overline{Y}_N \qquad (4.3)$$

Since the sample in the ith stratum has been drawn by SRSWOR, so

$$V\left(\overline{y}_{n_i}\right) = \left(\frac{1}{n_i} - \frac{1}{N_i}\right) S_i^2$$

The sampling variance of $\overline{y}_{st}$ is given by

$$V(\overline{y}_s) = \sum_{i=1}^{K} P_i^2 V(\overline{y}_{n_i}) + \sum_{i=1}^{K}\sum_{i=1}^{K} P_i P_j Cov(\overline{y}_{n_i}, \overline{y}_{n_j}) \tag{4.4}$$

Since the samples have been drawn independently in each stratum, so

$$Cov(\overline{y}_{n_i}, \overline{y}_{n_j}) = 0 \ and \ so$$

$$V(\overline{y}_s) = \sum_{i=1}^{K} P_i^2 V(\overline{y}_{n_i}) = \sum_{i=1}^{K} P_i^2 (\frac{1}{n_i} - \frac{1}{N_i}) S_i^2 \tag{4.5}$$

Since the sample mean square for the ith stratum, $s_i^2 = \frac{1}{n_i - 1}\sum_{j=1}^{n_i}(y_j - \overline{y}_{n_i})^2$

unbiasedly estimates the population mean square for the ith stratum, S_i^2, it follows that an unbiased estimator of $V(\overline{y}_s)$ is given by

$$\hat{V}(\overline{y}_s) = \hat{V}(\overline{y}_s) = \sum P_i^2 (\frac{1}{n_i} - \frac{1}{N_i}) s_i^2 \tag{4.6}$$

From the above, we see that sampling variance of stratified sample mean depends on S_i's, variability within the strata which suggests that the smaller the S_i's, *i.e.* the more homogeneous the strata, greater will be the precision of the stratified sample.

Example 4

The data given below pertains to the total geographical area in 20 villages of a Block. Treating this as population of 20 units, stratify this population in three strata taking stratum sizes to be villages with geographical area, 50 ha or less, villages with geographical area in between 50 and 100 ha and villages having geographical area more than 100 ha. A sample of 6 villages is to be selected by taking 2 villages in each stratum. Compare the efficiency of stratified sampling with corresponding unstratified simple random sampling.

Village Sl.No.	:	01	02	03	04	05	06	07	08	09	10
Geographical Area (in ha.)	:	020	080	050	100	150	070	020	250	220	010
Village Sl.No.	:	11	12	13	14	15	16	17	18	19	20
Geographical Area (in ha)	:	050	140	080	020	050	030	070	090	100	220

Solution

Clearly $N = 20$, $n = 6$.

Population Mean
$$\overline{Y}_N = \frac{1}{20}\sum_{i=1}^{20} y_i = \frac{1820}{20} = 91\,ha$$

Population Mean Square
$$S^2 = \frac{1}{N-1}\sum_{i=1}^{N}(y_i - \overline{Y}_N)^2 = \frac{1}{N-1}(\sum_{i=1}^{N} y_i^2 - N\overline{Y}_N^2) = \frac{96180}{19} = 5062\,ha^2$$

Sampling Variance of Simple Random Sample Mean
$$V(\overline{y}_n) = (\frac{1}{n} - \frac{1}{N})S^2 = 590\,ha^2$$

Now stratify the population according to given strata sizes into following three strata:

Strata Sl. No. Units
I (less than 50 ha) 020 050 020 010 050 020 050 030
II (between 50 and 100 ha) 080 100 070 080 070 090 100
III (more than 100 ha) 150 250 220 140 220

Clearly, $N_1 = 8$, $\overline{Y}_{N_1} = 031.3$ ha, $S_1^2 = 0270$ ha^2

$N_2 = 7$, $\overline{Y}_{N_2} = 084.3$ ha, $S_2^2 = 0161$ ha^2

$N_3 = 5$, $\overline{Y}_{N_3} = 176.0$ ha, $S_3^2 = 2330$ ha^2

From each stratum, a sample of 2 villages has been taken so $n_1 = n_2 = n_3 = 2$.

Now,
$$V(\overline{y}_{st}) = \sum_{i=1}^{K} P_i^2 (\frac{1}{n_i} - \frac{1}{N_i})S_i^2 = 67\,ha^2$$

Obviously the stratification has reduced the sampling variance of the sample mean from 590 ha^2 (in case of SRSWOR) to 67 ha^2 (in case of stratified sampling) *i.e.* a reduction of about 89 per cent.

In stratified sampling, having decided the strata and the sample size, the next question which a survey sampling expert has to face is regarding the method of selection within each stratum and the allocation of sample to different strata. The expression for the variance of stratified sample mean shows that the precision of a stratified sample for given strata depends upon the n_i's which can be fixed at will. The guiding principle in the determination of the n_i's is to choose them in such a manner so as to provide an estimate of the population mean with the desired degree of precision for a minimum cost or to provide an estimate with maximum precision for a given cost, thus making the most effective use of the available resources. The allocation of the sample to different strata made according to this principle is called the principle of optimum allocation.

The cost of a survey is a function of strata sample sizes just as the variance. The manner in which cost will vary with total sample size and with its allocation among the different strata will depend upon the type of survey. In yield estimation surveys, the major item in the survey cost consists of labour charges for harvesting of produce and as such survey cost is found to be approximately proportional to the number of crop cutting experiments (CCEs). Cost per CCE may, however, vary in different strata depending upon labour availability. Under such situations, the total cost may be represented by $C = \sum_{i=1}^{K} c_i n_i$ where c_i is the cost per CCE in the ith stratum. When c_i is same from stratum to stratum, say c, the total cost of a survey is given by $C = cn$. The cost function will change in form, if travel cost, field staff salary, statistical analysis etc. are to be paid for.

To find optimum values of n_i (cost function being $C = \sum_{i=1}^{K} c_i n_i$), consider the function

$$\phi = V(\bar{y}_s) + \mu C \tag{4.7}$$

where μ is some constant.

Now, $V(\bar{y}_s) + \mu C = \sum_{i=1}^{K} P_i^2 (\frac{1}{n_i} - \frac{1}{N_i}) S_i^2 + \mu \sum_{i=1}^{K} c_i n_i$

$$= \sum_{i=1}^{K} \frac{1}{n_i} P_i^2 S_i^2 + \mu. \, c_i.n_i + \text{terms independent of } n_i$$

$$= \sum_{i=1}^{K} (P_i S_i / \sqrt{n_i} - \sqrt{\mu c_i n_i})^2 + \text{terms independent of } n_i$$

Clearly, $V(\bar{y}_{st})$ is minimum for fixed cost C, or cost of a survey is minimum for a fixed value of $V(\bar{y}_{st})$, when each of the square terms on right-hand side of the above equation is zero *i.e.*

$$\frac{P_i S_i}{\sqrt{n_i}} = \sqrt{\mu c_i n_i} \quad (i = 1,2,.,K)$$

or $n_i = \dfrac{P_i S_i}{\sqrt{\mu.c_i}} \quad (i = 1,2,.,K)$ \hfill (4.8)

From the above, one can easily infer that:

☆ the larger the stratum size, the larger should be the size of the sample to be selected from that stratum,

☆ the larger the stratum variability, the larger should be the size of the sample from that stratum, and

☆ the cheaper the cost per sampling unit in a stratum, the larger should be the sample from that stratum.

The exact value of n_i for maximizing precision for a fixed cost C_0 can be obtained by evaluating $1/\sqrt{\mu}$, the constant of proportionality as

$$n_i = \frac{P_i S_i}{\sqrt{c_i}} \frac{C_0}{\sum\limits_{i=1}^{K} P_i S_i \sqrt{c_i}}$$

(4.9)

and the total sample size as

$$n = \sum\limits_{i=1}^{K} n_i = \frac{C_0 \sum\limits_{i=1}^{K}(P_i S_i / \sqrt{c_i})}{\sum\limits_{i=1}^{K} P_i S_i \sqrt{c_i}}$$

(4.10)

The allocation of the sample size 'n' to different strata according to the above equation is known as optimum allocation.

When c_i is the same from stratum to stratum *i.e.* $c_i = c$ (say), the cost function takes the form $C = c.n$, or in other words, the cost of survey is proportional to the size of the sample, the optimum values of n_i's are given by

$$n_i = n \frac{P_i S_i}{\sum\limits_{i=1}^{K} P_i S_i}$$

(i= 1,2,.,K)

(4.11)

The allocation of the sample according to the above equation is known as Neyman Allocation. On substituting for n_i in V ($\bar{y}_{st}$) expression (4.5), we obtain

$$V_N(\bar{y}_s) = \frac{1}{n}(\sum\limits_{i=1}^{K} P_i S_i)^2 - \frac{1}{N}\sum\limits_{i=1}^{K} P_i S_i^2$$

(4.12)

where the subscript 'N' stands for stratification with Neyman Allocation.

Another logical approach of allocation appears to be to allocate larger sample sizes for larger strata *i.e.* $n_i \propto N_i$ or $n_i = n. \frac{N_i}{N}$ (i=1,2,.,K). The allocation of sample size 'n' according to this equation is known as proportional allocation and V($\bar{y}_{st}$) in this case becomes

$$V_P(\bar{y}_s) = (\frac{1}{n} - \frac{1}{N})\sum\limits_{i=1}^{K} P_i S_i^2$$

(4.13)

where the subscript 'P' indicates the stratification with proportional allocation.

Cluster Sampling

A cluster may be defined as a group of units. When the sampling units are clusters, the method of sampling is known as cluster sampling. Cluster sampling is used when the frame of units is not available or it is expensive to construct such a frame. Thus, a list of all the farms in the districts may not be available but information on the list of villages is easily available. For carrying out any district level survey aimed at estimating the yield of a crop, it is practically feasible to select villages first and then enumerating the elements (in this case farms) in the selected village. The method is operationally convenient, less time consuming and more importantly such a method is cost-wise efficient. Elements within a cluster should ideally be as homogeneous as possible. But there should be heterogeneity between clusters. Each cluster should be a small scale version of the total population. The clusters should be mutually exclusive and collectively exhaustive. A random sampling technique is then used on any relevant clusters to choose which clusters to include in the study. In single-stage cluster sampling, all the elements from each of the selected clusters are used. In two-stage cluster sampling, a random sampling technique is applied to the elements from each of the selected clusters.

The main difference between cluster sampling and stratified sampling is that In cluster sampling the cluster is treated as the sampling unit so analysis is done on a population of clusters (at least in the first stage). In stratified sampling, the analysis is done on elements within strata. In stratified sampling, a random sample is drawn from each of the strata, whereas in cluster sampling only the selected clusters are studied. The main objective of cluster sampling is to reduce costs by increasing sampling efficiency (This contrasts with stratified sampling where the main objective is to increase precision.). One version of cluster sampling is area sampling or geographical cluster sampling. Clusters consist of geographical areas. A geographically dispersed population can be expensive to survey. Greater economy than simple random sampling can be achieved by treating several respondents within a local area as a cluster. It is usually necessary to increase the total sample size to achieve equivalent precision in the estimators, but the savings in cost may make that feasible. The main disadvantage of cluster sampling is that it is less efficient than a method of sampling in which the units are selected individually. The efficiency of cluster sampling procedure increases as the heterogeneity between units belonging to same cluster increases. Cluster sampling becomes more efficient than element sampling if the units pertaining to same cluster are negatively correlated.

Let there be N clusters in the population. Further, let M be the size of each cluster. We denote by Y the character under study. We define

y_{ij} = value of the characteristic under study for j^{th} element, ($j=1,2,\ldots,M$) in the ith cluster, ($i=1,2,\ldots,N$)

$$\overline{Y}_{N.} = \frac{1}{N}\sum_{i=1}^{N} \overline{y}_{i.} \quad \text{the mean of the cluster means in the population,}$$

$$\overline{Y}_{..} = \frac{1}{NM}\sum_{i=1}^{N}\sum_{j=1}^{M} y_{ij} = \frac{1}{N}\sum_{i=1}^{N} \overline{y}_{i.} \quad \text{the mean per element in the population.}$$

It is clear that $\overline{Y}_{N.} = \overline{Y}_{..}$. This is so since the clusters are of equal size. If, however, the clusters vary in size, the two means will generally not be equal.

We denote by $\overline{y}_d$, the estimator of $\overline{Y}_{..}$ as

$$\overline{y}_{cl} = \frac{1}{n}\sum_{i=1}^{n} \overline{y}_{i.} = \frac{1}{nM}\sum_{i=1}^{n}\sum_{j=1}^{M} y_{ij} \quad \text{the mean of cluster means in a sample of } n \text{ clusters} \quad (5.1)$$

Clearly $\overline{y}_{cl}$ is an unbiased estimate of $\overline{Y}_{..}$ and its variance is given by

$$V(\overline{y}_d) = (\frac{1}{n} - \frac{1}{N}) S_b^2 \tag{5.2}$$

where,

$$S_b^2 = \frac{1}{N-1}\sum(\overline{y}_{i.} - \overline{Y}_{N.})^2 \quad \text{is the mean square between cluster means in the}$$
population.

The variance of the mean of n cluster means in terms of intra-class correlation ρ_c (intra-cluster correlation between elements belonging to the same cluster), if N is sufficiently large, is given by

$$V(\overline{y}_d) = \frac{S^2}{nM}\left[1+(M-1)\rho_c\right] \tag{5.3}$$

where,

$$S^2 = \frac{1}{NM-1}\sum_{i=1}^{N}\sum_{j=1}^{M}(y_{ij} - \overline{Y}_{..})^2 \quad \text{is the mean square between elements in the}$$
population.

If an equivalent sample of nM elements were selected from the population of NM elements by SRSWOR, the variance of the mean per element $\overline{y}_{nM}$ would be

$$V(\overline{y}_{nM}) = (\frac{1}{nM} - \frac{1}{NM}) S^2 \tag{5.4}$$

Accordingly, the relative efficiency of a cluster as the unit of sampling compared with that of an element is given by

$$R.E. = \frac{V(\overline{y}_{nM})}{V(\overline{y}_t)} = \frac{S^2}{MS_b^2} \tag{5.5}$$

Thus, the relative efficiency of cluster sampling increases with decrease in both S_b^2 and M.

Since relative efficiency of cluster sampling depends upon M, it is natural to determine the optimum size of the cluster. As in the case of stratified sampling, the optimum size of the cluster can be determined by minimizing variance for a fixed cost or vice-versa. A simple cost function can be

$$C = c_1 nM + c_2 d \tag{5.6}$$

where,

C = Total cost of survey operation,

c_1 = Cost of enumerating an element including the time spent and cost of transportation within clusters,

c_2 = Per unit cost of travelling a unit distance between clusters, and

d = The distance between the clusters.

By minimizing the variance subject to the above cost function, we obtain

$$M \alpha \frac{c_2^2}{c_1 C} \tag{5.7}$$

Thus, M will be smaller if c_1 and C are large and c_2 is small.

Multi-Stage Sampling

Generally, elements belonging to the same cluster are more homogeneous as compared to those elements which belong to different clusters. Therefore, a comparatively representative sample can be obtained by enumerating each cluster partially and distributing the entire sample over more clusters. This will increase the cost of the survey but the proportionate increase in cost vis-à-vis cluster sampling will be less as compared to increase in the precision. This process of first selecting clusters and then further sampling units within a cluster is called as two-stage sampling. The clusters in a two-stage sample are called as primary stage units (psu$_s$) and elements within a cluster are called as secondary stage units (ssu$_s$).

A two-stage sample has the advantage that after psu$_s$ are selected, the frame of the ssu$_s$ is required for the sampled psu$_s$ only. The procedure allows the flexibility of using different sampling design at the different stages of selection of sampling units. A two-stage sampling procedure can be easily generalized to multi-stage sampling designs. Such a sampling design is commonly used in large scale surveys. It is operationally convenient, provides reasonable degree of precision and is cost-wise efficient.

Systematic Sampling

In the method of systematic sampling, only the first unit is selected at random while rest of the units are selected according to a pre-determined pattern. Let N and n be the population size and sample size respectively. Further, N = n.k, where k is an integer. A random number 'i' is selected such that $1 < i < k$. Then the sample contains n units with serial number $i, i+k, i+2k,\ldots, i+(n-1)k$. Systematic sampling can be used in situations such as selection of kth strip in forest sampling, selection of corn fields every k^{th} kilometre apart for observation on incidence of borers, or the selection of every k^{th} time interval for observing the number of fishing crafts landing at a centre.

The method of systematic sampling is used on account of its low cost and simplicity in the selection of the sample. It makes control of field work easier. Since every k^{th} unit will be in the sample, the method is expected to provide an evenly balanced sample.

When N is not an exact multiple of n *i.e.* $N = nk + r$, a method of sampling called circular systematic sampling (given by Lahiri) is used to select the sample. This method consists of selecting a random number from 1 to N and thereafter selecting cyclically every k^{th} unit until n units have been chosen in the sample. Cyclic selection means assigning number (N+1) to 1st unit, (N+2) to 2nd unit and so on, in order to continue the selection procedure when the Nth unit has been reached. A drawback of systematic sampling is that it is not possible to get an unbiased estimate of the variance of the estimator. However, it is possible to get an unbiased estimator of the variance based on number of systematic samples.

Varying Probability Sampling

In SRSWOR, the selection probabilities are equal for all the units in the population. However, if the sampling units vary in size considerably, SRSWOR may not be appropriate as it does not take into account the possible importance of the larger units in the population. To give possible importance to larger units, there are various sampling methods in which this can be achieved. A simple method is of assigning unequal probabilities of selection to the different units in the population. Thus, when units vary in size and the variable under study is correlated with size, probabilities of selection may be assigned in proportion to the size of the unit *e.g.* villages having larger geographical areas are likely to have larger populations and larger areas under food crops. For estimating the crop production, it may be desirable to adopt a selection scheme in which villages are selected with probabilities proportional to their population sizes or to their geographical areas. A sampling procedure in which the units are selected with probabilities proportional to some measure of their size is known as sampling with probability proportional to size (pps). The units may be selected with or without replacement. In sampling with replacement, the probability of drawing a specified unit at a given draw is the same.

Procedure of Selecting a Sample with Varying Probabilities

i) Cumulative Total Method

To draw a sample of size n from a population of size N with ppswr, the procedure is as follows:

Let x_i be an integer proportional to size of the ith unit (i=1,2.,N), we make successive cumulative totals $x_1, x_1 + x_2, x_1 + x_2 + x_3, ..., x_1 + x_2 + x_3 + ... + x_N$, and

draw a random number R in between 1 and $\sum_{i=1}^{N} x_i$ from a random number Table. Select the ith unit in the population for which

$$x_1 + x_2 + x_3, ..., x_{i-1} \prec R \leq x_1 + x_2 + x_3 + ... + x_{i-1} + x_i$$

It is clear that this procedure of selection gives to the ith unit in the population, a probability of selection proportional to x_i. This procedure is to be repeated n times, if a sample of size n is required.

ii) Lahiri's Method

The main drawback of cumulative total method is that it involves writing down the successive cumulative totals which is time consuming and tedious especially if the number of units in the population is large. Lahiri (1951) had suggested an alternative procedure which avoids the necessity of writing down cumulative totals. It consists in selecting a pair of random numbers, say (i, j) such that $1 \leq i N$ and $1 \leq j \leq M$ where M is the maximum of the sizes of the N units in the population. If $j \leq x_i$, the ith unit is selected; otherwise it is rejected and another pair of random numbers is chosen. For selecting a sample of n units with ppswr, the procedure is to be repeated till n units are selected. It can be seen that the procedure leads to the required probabilities of selection.

Determination of Sample Size

In the planning of a sample survey, determination of sample size is an important decision which a survey statistician has to take while deciding the sampling plan. One has to be careful while deciding the sample size, because too large a sample implies waste of resources, and too small a sample diminishes the utility of the results. An efficient sampling plan should enable an optimum utilization of budgetary resources to provide the best estimators of the population parameters. As is well known, efficiency of an estimator is normally measured by inverse of mean square error (or variance in case of unbiased estimators). A desirable proposition would be to minimize the cost as well as variance simultaneously. But, unfortunately, it is not possible. With an increase in the sample size, normally the cost of the survey increases while the variance decreases, thereby increasing the efficiency. Thus for determination of sample size, a balance is required to be struck which is reasonable with respect to cost as well as efficiency. Sampling theory provides a framework within which the problem of determining sample size may be tackled reasonably.

We first consider the estimation of sample size in case of simple random sampling. The problem has been analyzed in a very elegant way by considering hypothetical example by Cochran (1977). We quote the example, "An Anthropologist is preparing to study the inhabitants of some island. Among other things, he wishes to estimate the percentage of inhabitants belonging to blood group O. Co-operation has been secured so that it is feasible to take a simple random sample. How large should the sample be?" This is just a typical example. In fact, in almost all the sampling investigations, one has to face such problems. An answer to the question is not straight forward. First of all, one must be very clear about the objective of the study. Or atleast, the user must know to what use their results are going to be put, so that he should be able to answer as to what is the margin of error he is going to tolerate in the results. In the above example, the Anthropologist should be able to answer as to how accurately does he wish to know the percentage of people with blood group O? In this case he is reported to be content with a 5 per cent margin in the sense that if the sample shows 43 per cent to have blood group O, the percentage for the whole island is sure to be between 38 and 48. Since a random sampling procedure has been used, every sample has got some chance of selection and the possibility of getting the estimates lying outside the above specified range cannot be ruled out. Aware of this fact, the Anthropologist is prepared to take a 1 in 20 chance of getting an unlucky sample with the estimate lying outside the above margin.

Principal Steps Involved in the Choise of a Sample Size

☆ A statement about the margin of error to be tolerated in the results.

☆ Choice of desired confidence level.

☆ Some equation that connects n with the desired precision of the sample should be found.

☆ This equation will contain, as parameters, certain unknown properties of the population. This must be estimated in order to give specific results.

☆ Usually in a sample survey, more than one characteristic is measured. Sometimes, the number of characteristics is large. If a desired degree of precision is prescribed for each characteristic, the calculation leads to a conflicting values of n, one for each characteristic. Some method must be found for reconciling these values.

☆ Finally, the chosen value of n must be appraised to see whether it is consistent with the resources available to take the sample. This demands an estimation of the cost, labour, time and material required to obtain the proposed size of sample. It sometimes becomes apparent that n will have to be drastically reduced. One has to choose whether to proceed with a much smaller sample size, thus reducing precision, or to abandon efforts until more resources can be found. Regarding the choice of a level for tolerable margin of error and the confidence level, the user normally has only a vague idea and it is only through the discussions and clarifications that a quantitative specific measures are obtained. It may be remarked that these measures are mainly subjective and depend largely on the judgment of the user regarding the importance, applicability and vulnerability of the results.

References

Cochran, W.G. (1977). Sampling Techniques. Third Edition. John Wiley and Sons.

Des Raj (1968). Sampling Theory. TATA McGRAW-HILL Publishing Co. Ltd.

Des Raj and Chandok, P. (1998). Sample Survey Theory. Narosa Publishing House.

Murthy, M.N. (1977). Sampling Theory and Methods. Statistical Publishing Society, Calcutta.

Singh, D. and Chaudhary, F.S. (1986). Theory and Analysis of Sample Survey Designs. Wiley Eastern Limited.

Singh, D., Singh, P. and Kumar, P. (1978). Handbook of Sampling Methods. I.A.S.R.I., New Delhi.

Singh, R. and Mangat, N.S. (1996). Elements of Survey Sampling, Kluwer Academic Publishers.

Sukhatme, P.V. and Sukhatme, B.V. (1970). Sampling Theory of Surveys with Application. Second Edition. Iowa State University Press, USA

Sukhatme, P. V., Sukhatme, B.V., Sukhatme, S. and Asok, C. (1984). Sampling Theory of Surveys with Applications. Third Revised Edition, Iowa State University Press, USA.

Chapter 16

Bioinformatics Application in Agricultural Research

A.K. Mishra, Amrender Kumar and A.K. Jain

ICAR–IARI, New Delhi – 110 012

Introduction

Bioinformatics is relatively a new field at the interface of the twentieth century revolutions in molecular biology and computers. Bioinformatics came into being after the invention of first protein sequence was that of bovine insulin in 1956, consisting of 51 residues. The development of protein-sequencing methods led to the sequencing of representatives of several of the more common protein families such as cytochromes from a variety of organisms. Margaret Dayhoff (1972, 1978) and her collaborators at the National Biomedical Research Foundation (NBRF), Washington, DC, were the first to assemble databases of these sequences into a protein sequence atlas in the 1960s, and their collection center eventually became known as the Protein Information Resource (PIR, formerly Protein Identification Resource). The Protein DataBank followed in 1972 with a collection of ten X-ray crystallographic protein structures, and the SWISSPROT protein sequence database began in 1987. DNA sequence databases were first assembled at Los Alamos National Laboratory (LANL), New Mexico, by Walter Goad and colleagues in the GenBank database and at the European Molecular Biology Laboratory (EMBL) in Heidelberg, Germany.

Translated DNA sequences were also included in the Protein Information Resource (PIR) database at the National Biomedical Research Foundation in Washington, DC. Goad had conceived of the GenBank prototype in 1979; LANL collected GenBank data from 1982 to 1992. GenBank is now under the auspices of the National Center for Biotechnology Information (NCBI). The EMBL Data Library was founded in 1980 (http://www.ebi.ac.uk). In 1984 the DNA DataBank of Japan

(DDBJ), Mishima, Japan, came into existence (http://www.ddbj.nig.ac.jp). GenBank, EMBL, and DDBJ have now formed the International Nucleotide Sequence Database Collaboration, which acts to facilitate exchange of data on a daily basis. PIR has made similar arrangements. The most common format used in various tools is the FASTA format.

A major challenge in Biology is to make sense of the enormous quantities of sequence data and structural data that are generated by genome sequencing projects, proteomics and other large scale molecular biology efforts. The tools of bioinformatics include computer programs that help to reveal fundamental mechanism underlying biological problem related to the structure and function of macromolecules, biochemical pathways, disease process and evolution It is one of the frontier and interdisciplinary area of research and development which has created interest among scientists from various disciplines like computer science, information technology, mathematics, statistics biotechnology and medical sciences.

The term bioinformatics was coined by Paulien Hogeweg and Ben Hesper in 1978 for the study of informatic processes in biotic systems. Its primary use since at least the late 1980s has been in genomics and genetics, particularly in those areas of genomics involving large-scale DNA sequencing. Bioinformatics involves close relation between biology and computers that influence each other and synergistically merging more than once. The variety of data from biology, mainly in the form of DNA, RNA, protein sequences is putting heavy demand in computer sciences and computational biology.

Emergence of Bioinformatics

Biological data are flooding in at an unprecedented rate. For example as of August 2000, the GenBank repository of nucleic acid sequences contained 8,214,000 entries and the SWISS-PROT database of protein sequences contained 88,166. On average, the amount of information stored in these databases is doubling every 15 months. In addition, since the publication of the *H. influenzae* genome, complete sequences for over 40 organisms have been released, ranging from 450 genes to over 100,000. Add to this the data from the myriad of related projects that study gene expression, determine the protein structures encoded by the genes, and detail how these products interact with one another, and we can begin to imagine the enormous quantity and variety of information that is being produced.

There are three important factors that facilitated the emergence of Bioinformatics which are as following:

1. First, an expanding collection of amino-acid sequences provided both a concourse of data and a set of interesting problems that were infeasible to solve without the number-crunching power of computers.

2. Second, the idea that macromolecules carry information became a central part of the conceptual framework of molecular biology. Although some historians and philosophers have questioned the theoretical significance of this idea for modern molecular biology5–7, it seems likely that thinking in terms of macromolecular information provided an important conceptual

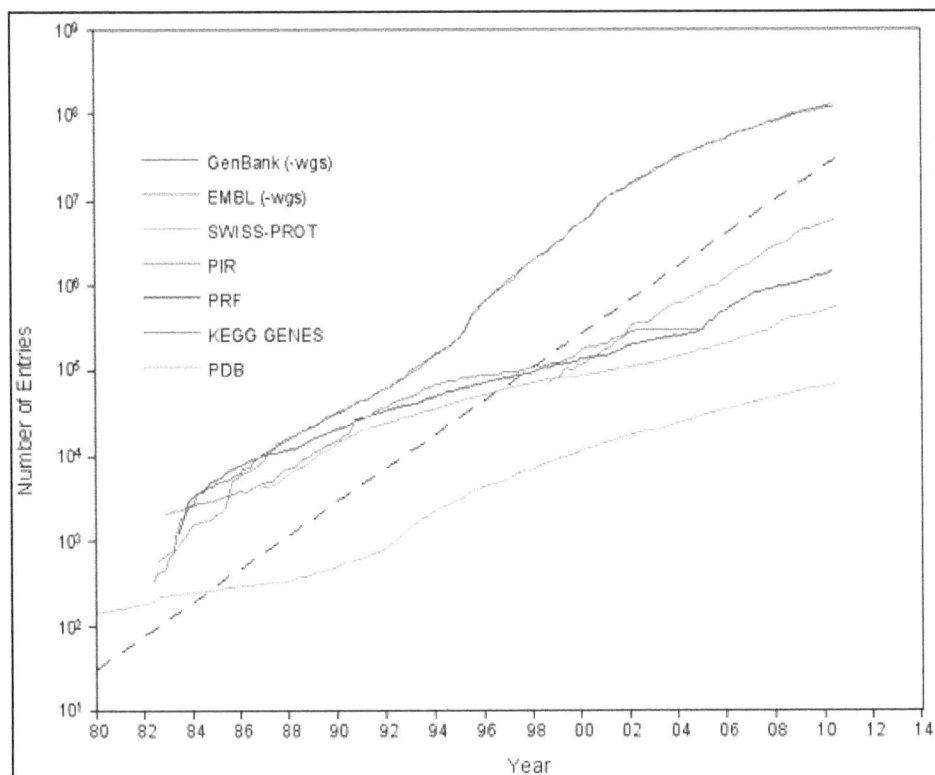

Figure 16.1: Growth of Biological data in Various Databases.
(*Source*: http://www.genome.jp/en/db_growth.html).

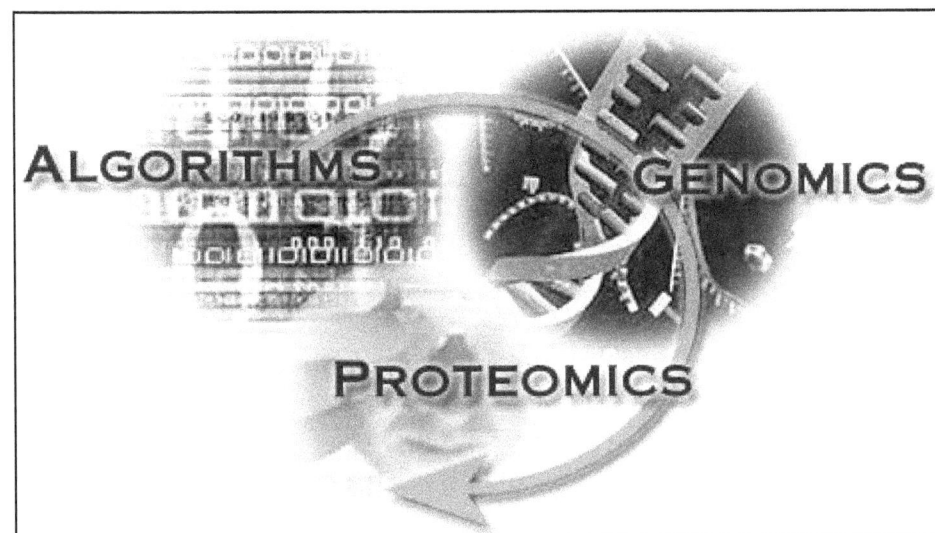

Figure 16.2: Basic Components of Bioinformatics.

link between molecular biology and the computer science from which formal information theory had arisen.

3. Third, high-speed digital computers, which had developed from weapons research programmes during the Second World War, finally became widely available to academic biologists. Not all biologists had – or wanted to have – access to these machines but, by 1960, scarcity of computers was no longer a serious stumbling block for the development of computational biology.

Aims of Bioinformatics

The aims of bioinformatics are three-fold.

1. First, at its simplest bioinformatics organises data in a way that allows researchers to access existing information and to submit new entries as they are produced, *e.g.* the Protein Data Bank for 3D macromolecular structures.

2. While data-curation is an essential task, the information stored in these databases is essentially useless until analysed. Thus the purpose of second aim is to develop tools and resources that aid in the analysis of data.

3. The third aim is to use these tools to analyze the data and interpret the results in a biologically meaningful manner.

Traditionally, biological studies examined individual systems in detail, and frequently compare them with a few that are related. In bioinformatics global

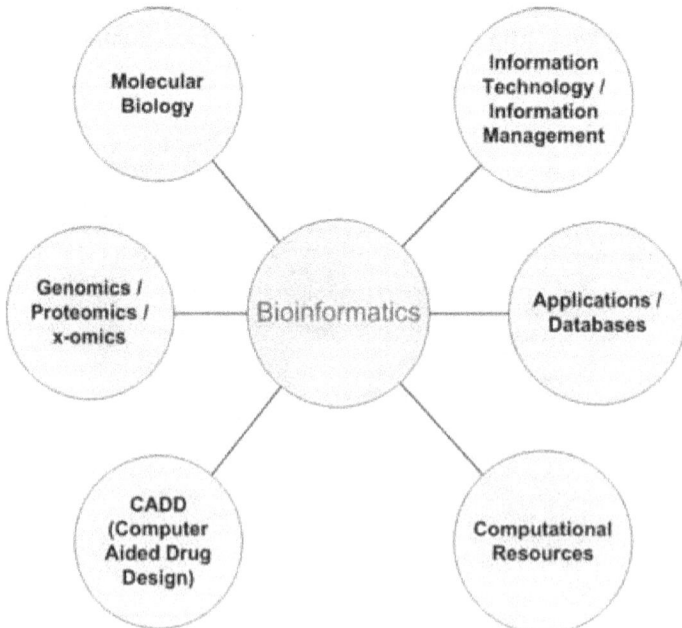

Figure 16.3: Various Research Areas in Bioinformatics.

analyses of all the available data with the aim of uncovering common principles that apply across many systems and highlight features that are unique to some.

Research Areas of Bioinformatics

Current research in bioinformatics can be classified into:

(i) **Genomics**: Genomics is the study of an organism's genome. This term is given by Thomas H. Roderick in 1987.

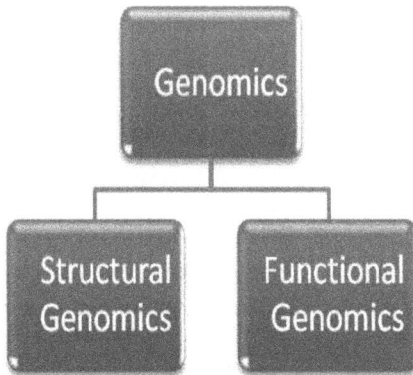

Figure 16.5: Areas of Proteomics.

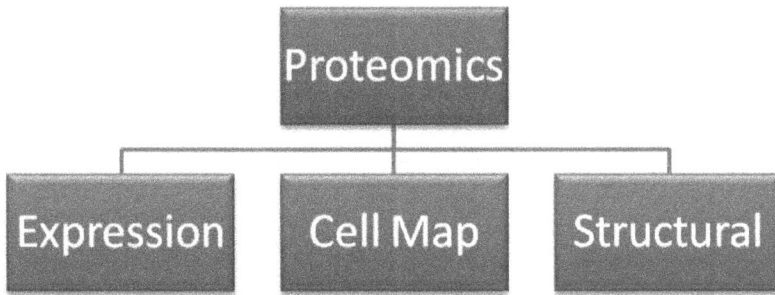

Figure 16.4: Areas of Genomics.

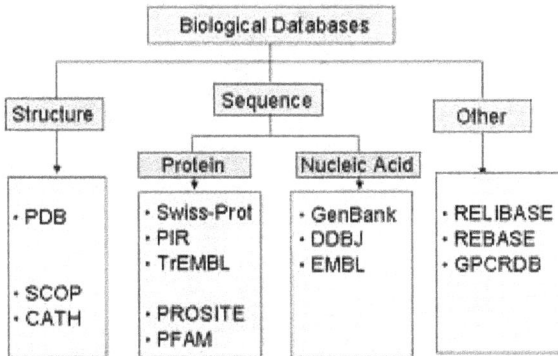

Figure 16.6: Study of Interaction of a Drug in Biological Environment.
(Source: http://www.mpi-inf.mpg.de/departments/d3/areas/docking.html)

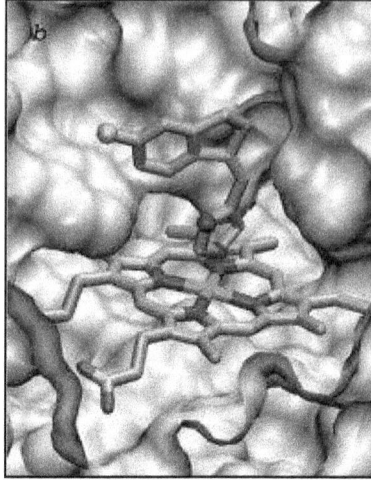

Figure 16.7: Types of Biological Databases.

(*Source*: http://www.mrc-lmb.cam.ac.uk/genomes/madanm/pres/biodb.htm)

(ii) **Proteomics**: it is defined as the study of the proteome. Proteome refers to the entire set of expressed proteins in a cell.

(iii) **Computer Aided Drug Designing:** Computer-Aided Drug Design (CADD) is a specialized discipline that uses computational methods to simulate drug-receptor interactions. CADD methods are heavily dependent on bioinformatics tools, applications and databases.

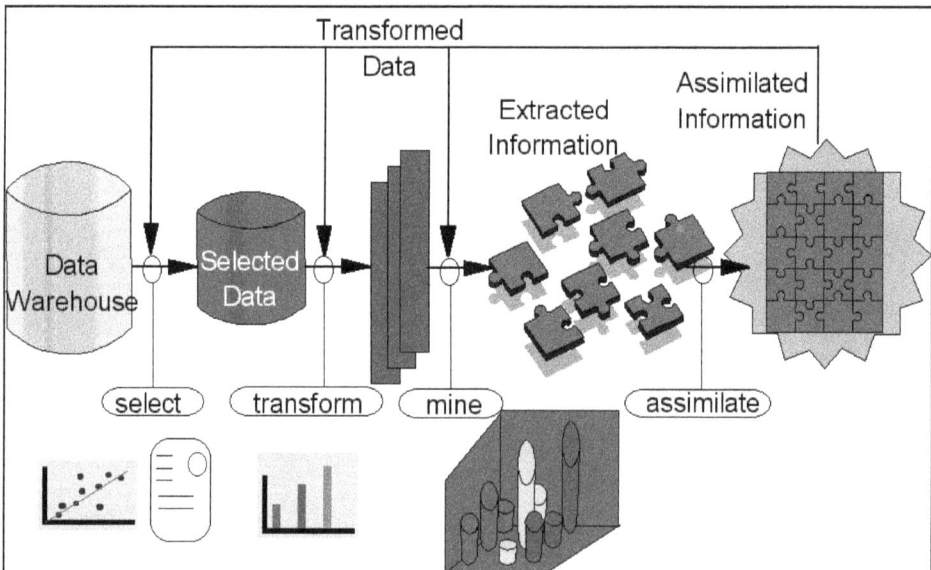

Figure 16.8: Various Steps Involved in Data Mining.

(Source: http://cs.salemstate.edu/hatfield/teaching/courses/DataMining/M.htm)

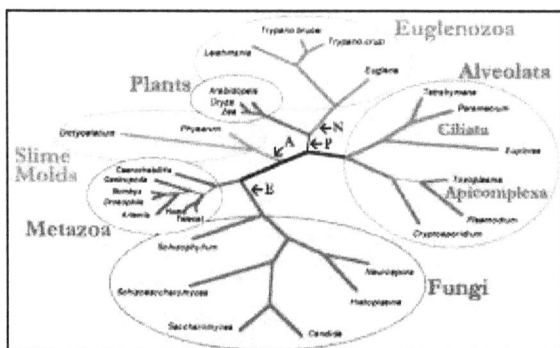

Figure 16.9: Phylogenetic Relation between Various Organisms.
(Source: http://www.tulane.edu/~wiser/protozoology/notes/tree.html).

(iii) **Biological database:** Biological databases are libraries of life sciences information, collected from scientific experiments, published literature, high-throughput experiment technology, and computational analyses. They contain information from research areas including genomics, proteomics, metabolomics, microarray gene expression, and phylogenetics. Information contained in biological databases includes gene function, structure, localization (both cellular and chromosomal), clinical effects of mutations as well as similarities of biological sequences and structures.

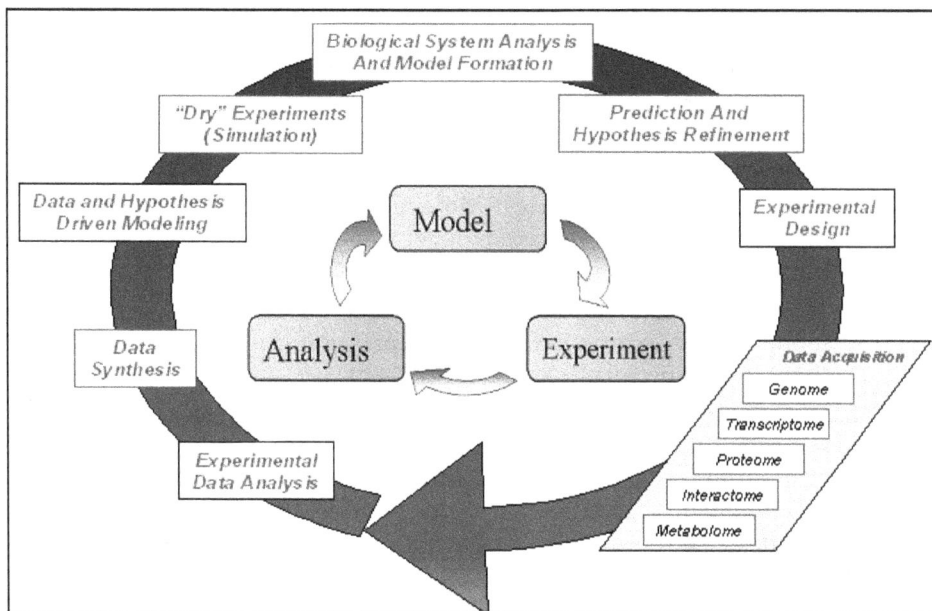

Figure 16.10: Principle of Microarray Analysis for Gene Expression.
(Source: http://www.accessexcellence.org/RC/VL/GG/microArray.php)

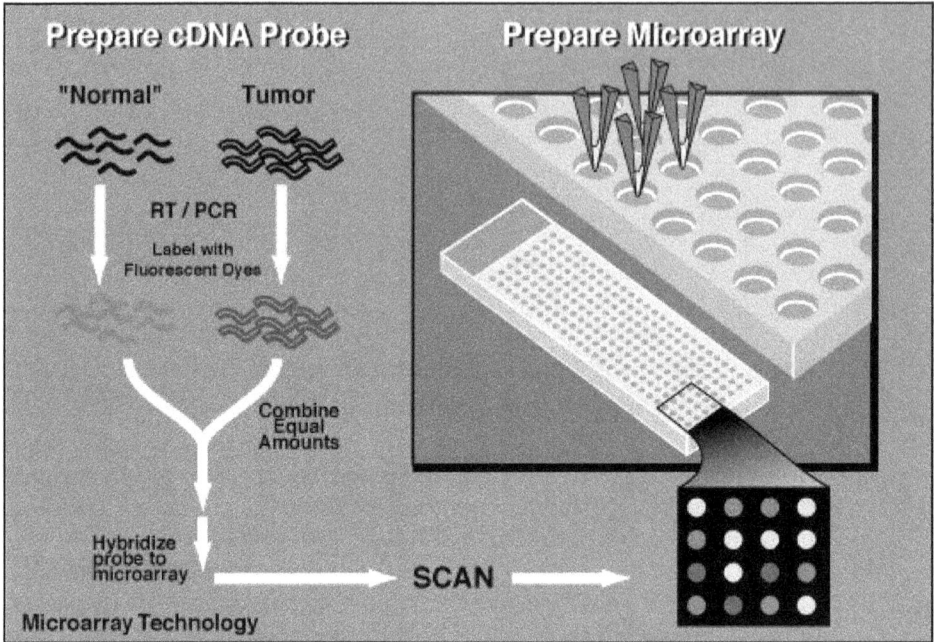

Figure 16.11: Modeling and System Biology.
(Source: http://kdbio.inesc-id.pt/~orlando/kdbio/software.html).

(iv) **Biological Data Mining:** Biological Data mining is the discovery of useful knowledge from biological databases. Data mining employs algorithms and techniques from statistics, machine learning, artificial intelligence, databases and data warehousing etc. Some of the most popular tasks are classification, clustering, association and sequence analysis, and regression. Clustering, association and sequence analysis, and regression.

(v) **Molecular Phylogenetics:** Molecular phylogenetics is the study of organisms on a molecular level to gather information about the phylogenetic relationships between different organisms.

(vi) **Microarray informatics:** Microarray Technology is a powerful tool to monitor gene expression or gene expression changes of hundreds or thousands of genes in a single experiment.

(vii) **System biology:** Systems biology studies biological systems by systematically perturbing them (biologically, genetically, or chemically); monitoring the gene, protein, and informational pathway responses; integrating these data; and ultimately, formulating mathematical models that describe the structure of the system and its response to individual perturbations.

(viii) **Agro-informatics:** Agricultural informatics concentrates on the aspects of Bioinformatics dealing with plant genomes. The term "Agri-Informatics" (AI) is coined to cover broadly for all types of development and

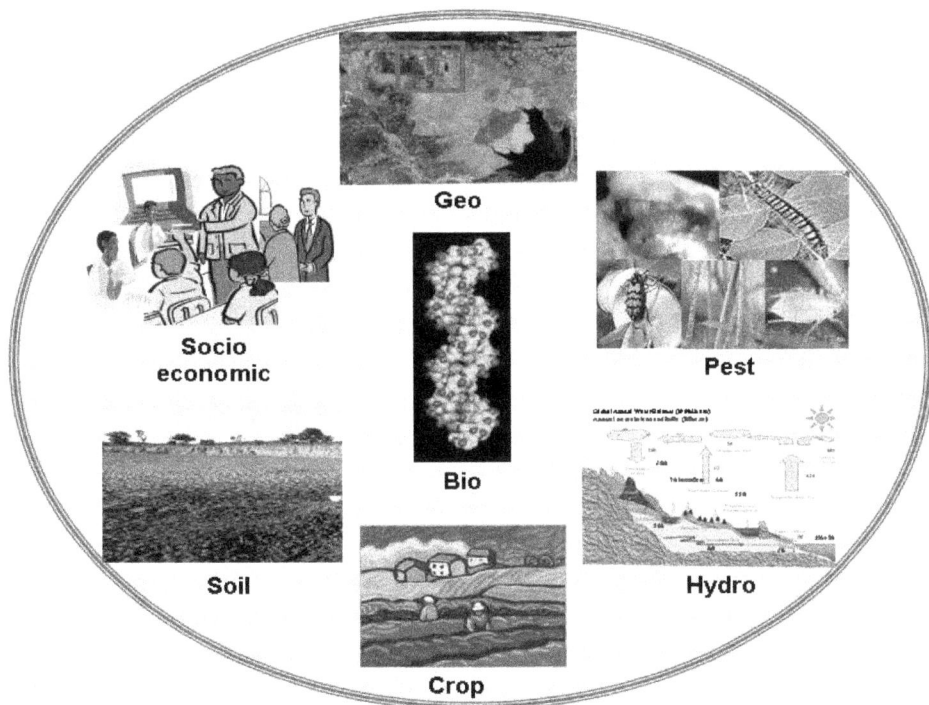

Figure 16.12: Agro-informatics Components.

applications of computerized information technology-based solutions for gathering, managing and analyzing data produced by agricultural systems and to develop models and forecasting systems.

References

Allen, J. E., *et al.* (2004). Computational gene prediction using multiple sources of evidence. *Genome Res.* 14, 142-148.

Altschul, S. F., Gish, W., Miller, W., Myers, E. W. and Lipman, D. J. (1990). Basic Local Alignment Search Tool. *J. Mol. Biol.* 215, 403-410.

Black, D. L. (2000). Protein diversity from alternative splicing: a challenge for bioinformatics and post-genome biology. *Cell* 103, 367–370.

Bork, P. and Koonin, E. V. (1998). Predicting function from protein sequence. Where are the bottlenecks? *Nature Genet* 13, 313-318.

Burge, C. and Carlin, S. (1998). Finding the genes in Genomic DNA. *Curr Opin. Struct. Biol.* 8, 346-354.

Burset, M. and Guigó, R. (1996). Evaluation of gene structure prediction programs. *Genomics.* 34, 353-367.

Durbin, R., Eddy, S., Krogh, A. and Mitchison, G. (1998). Biological sequence analysis. Cambridge University press.

Fickett, J. W. (1996). Finding genes by computer: The state of the art. *Trends in genetics* 12, 316–320.

Gish, W. and States, D. J. (1993). Identification of protein coding regions by database similarity search. *Nature Gen*et 3, 266–272.

Guigo, R., Knudsen, S., Drake, N. and Smith, T. (1992). Prediction of gene structure. *J. Mol. Biol.* 226, 141-157.

Murukami, K and Takagi, T. (1998). Gene recognition by combination of several gene finding programs. *Bioinformatics* 8, 665-675.

Synder, E. E. and Stormo, G. D. (1997). Identifying genes in genomic DNA sequences. In DNA and Protein sequence Analysis, M.J. Bishop and C. J. Rawlings, eds. (New York University Press), pp. 209-224.

Zhang, M. Q. (2002). in Current Topics in Computational Molecular Biology. Jiang, T., Xu, Y. and Zhang, M. Q. eds.

Chapter 17

Development of Pests Forewarning System in Crops

Amrender Kumar and A.K. Mishra

ICAR–IARI, New Delhi – 110 012

Introduction

Reliable and timely forecasts provide important and useful input for proper, foresighted and informed planning, more so, in agriculture which is full of uncertainties. Agriculture now-a-days has become highly input and cost intensive. Without judicious use of fertilizers and plant protection measures, agriculture no longer remains as profitable as before. Uncertainties of weather, production, policies, prices, etc. often lead to losses to the farmers. New pests and diseases are emerging as an added threat to the production. Under the changed scenario today, forecasting of various aspects relating to agriculture are becoming essential. But in-spite of strong need for reliable and timely forecasts, the current status is far from satisfactory. Various organisations in India and abroad are engaged in developing methodology for preharvest forecasts of crop yields/forewarning of pest and diseases.

Weather is an important factor, which affects the infestation of various pests and diseases in crops. There is considerable loss in the yield of the crop as well as quality of produce due to the infestation of various crop pests and diseases. Such losses can be reduced to a considerable extent if their occurrence is known in advance so that timely remedial measures may be taken up. To this end, one must have prior knowledge of the time and severity of the outbreak of these pests and diseases. There is thus a need to develop statistically sound objective forecasts of crop yield as well as forewarning pests/diseases on the basis of weather variables so that reliable forecasts can be obtained. In pests and diseases forewarning system, the variables of interest may be maximum pest population/disease severity, pest population/disease severity at most damaging stage of the crop, pest population/disease severity at different stages of crop growth or at various standard weeks, time of first appearance of pests/diseases, time of maximum pest population/disease severity, time of pest population/disease severity crossing threshold limit, extent of damage, weekly monitoring of pests and diseases progress, occurrence/non-occurrence of pests and diseases. If data are available at periodic interval for 15-20 years, the detailed study can be carried out for different variables of interest. However, depending upon the data availability, different types of models can be utilized for developing forewarning models. These developed models were converted into web-based forewarning system using 3-tier architecture. NetBeans 8.0.1 IDE (Integrated Development Environment), MS SQL Server, Java Server Pages (JSP) technologies have been used for the development of the web enabled forecasting of the two rice pests.

Development of Forewarning Models

The models could be of two types, 'Between year model' and 'Within year model'.

Between Year Models

These models are developed using previous years' data. An assumption is made that the present year is a part of the composite population of the previous years and accordingly the relationships developed on the basis of previous years' data will be applicable for the present year. The forecast for pests and diseases are obtained by substituting the current year data into the model developed upon the previous years. Various methods have been attempted when data are available in quantitative form. Some of the important techniques are discussed below:

Thumb Rule

This approach is the most common and extensively used. It is a simple system which describes the forecasting of the pests and diseases based on past experience. For example for potato late blight, a day is favorable if

- ☆ the 5 day temperature average is $< 25.5°C$
- ☆ the total rainfall for the last 10 days is > 3.0 cm
- ☆ the minimum temperature on that day is $> 7.2°$ C

When this situation arises, there is a possibility of potato late blight appearance.

Regression Model

The regression model taking pest/disease variable as dependent and suitable independent variables such as weather variables, crop stages, population of natural enemies/predators etc. is used. The form of the model is

$$Y = \beta_0 + \beta_1 X_1 + \beta_2 X_2 + \ldots\ldots\ldots + \beta_p X_p + e$$

where $\beta_0, \beta_1, \beta_2, \ldots\ldots\beta_p$ are regression coefficients, $X_1, X_2, \ldots\ldots, X_p$ are independent variables and e is error term. These variables are used in original scale or on a suitable transformed scale such as cos, log, exponential etc. (Coakley *et al.*, 1985; Trivedi *et al.*, 1999).

Growing Degree Day Approach

This method is based on the assumption that the pest becomes inactive below a certain temperature known as base temperature. Growing degree day is worked out as

GDD = Σ (mean temp. – base temp.)

GDD is used in the model as explanatory variable. This method requires proper knowledge of base temperature and initial time from which accumulation is to start.

Model Based on Weather Indices

The extent of weather influence on crop pests/diseases depends not only on the magnitude but also on the distribution pattern of weather variables over the crop season which, as such, calls for the necessity of dividing the whole crop season into fine intervals. This will increase number of variables in the model and in turn a large number of model parameters will have to be evaluated from the data. This will require a long series of data for precise estimation of parameters which may not be available in practice. Thus, a technique based on relatively smaller number of manageable variables and at the same time taking care of entire weather distribution, weather indices were obtained which were used as predictors for models development. In this type of model weekly weather data were utilized, for each weather variable two indices have been developed, one as simple total of values of weather parameter in different weeks and the other one as weighted total, weights being correlation coefficients between variable to forecast and weather variable in respective weeks. The first index will be representing the total amount of weather parameter received by the crop during the period under consideration while the other one will take care of distribution of weather parameter with special reference to its importance in different weeks in relation to the variable to forecast. On similar lines, composite indices were computed with products of weather variables (taken two at a time) for joint effects. The general form of the model was

$$Y = a_0 + \sum_{i=1}^{p} \sum_{j=0}^{1} a_{ij} Z_{ij} + \sum_{i \neq i'}^{p} \sum_{j=0}^{1} b_{i\,i'\,j} Z_{ii'\,j} + e$$

$$\text{where } Z_{ij} = \sum_{w=n_1}^{n_2} r^j_{iw} X_{iw}$$

$$Z_{ii'\,j} = \sum_{w=n_1}^{n_2} r^j_{ii'w} X_{iw} X_{i'w}$$

where,

$\quad Y$ = Variable to forecast

$\quad X_{iw}$ = Value of ith weather parameter in wth week

r_{iw} = Correlation coefficient between Y and i[th] weather parameter in wth week

r_{iiw} = Correlation coefficient between Y and product of X_i and $X_{i'}$ in wth week,

p = number of weather parameters

n_1 = initial week for which weather data were included in the model

n_2 = Final week for which weather data were included in the model

e = Error term

In some cases previous disease incidence/pest population (or their indices) and/or previous year's last population has also been included in the model. Stepwise regression technique was used for selecting important variables to be included in the model.

Using these models, reliable forewarnings are possible at least one week in advance. [Agrawal *et al.* (2004), Desai *et al.* (2004) Chattopadhyay *et al.* (2005-a), Chattopadhyay *et al.* (2005-b), and Dhar *et al.* (2007), Kumar (2013); Kumar *et al.* (2013); Agrawal *et al.* (2014)]. In general, the models fitted well for all the available data with all the coefficients of determination highly significant and forecasts comparing well with the observed values. If information on favourable weather conditions is known, subjective weights based on this information can also be used for constructing weather indices and these indices were used as independent variables in models developments.

Principal Component Regression

Forewarning models can be developed using the principal component technique as normally relevant weather variables are large in number and are expected to be highly correlated among themselves. Using the first few principal components of weather variables as independent variables forecast models can be developed.

Discriminant Function Analysis

Forewarning models of pests and diseases based on time series data on weather variables can be developed using the discriminant function analysis. For this analysis, a series of data for 25-30 years are required. Based on the pest and diseases variables, data can be divided into different groups – low, medium and high etc. and using weather data in these groups, linear or quadratic discriminant functions can be fitted which can be used to find discriminant scores. Considering these discriminant scores as independent variables and diseases/pest as a dependent variable, regression analysis can be performed. Johnson *et al.* (1996) used discriminant analysis for forecasting potato late blight.

Fuzzy Regression

In regression analysis, the unfitted errors between a regression model and observed data are generally assumed as observation error that is a random variable having a normal distribution, constant variance, and a zero mean. In fuzzy regression analysis, the same unfitted errors are viewed as the fuzziness. Fuzzy regression can be quite useful in estimating the relationship among variables where the availability data are imprecise and fuzzy. Fuzzy regression analysis gives a fuzzy functional relationship between dependent and independent variables where vagueness is present in some form. There are three situations where the fuzzy analysis can be viewed *viz.* Crisp parameters and fuzzy data, Fuzzy parameters and crisp data and Fuzzy parameters and fuzzy data. Fuzzy regression method is based on minimizing fuzziness as an optimal criterion, which can be achieved by linear programming procedures (Kumar *et al.*, 2014).

Complex Polynomial [Group Method of Data Handling (GMDH)]

The group method of data handling (GMDH) technique was developed by A.G. Ivaknenko in 1968. It provides complex polynomial in independent variables. It selects the structure of the model itself without prior information about relationship. Form of the model:

$$Y=a+\sum_{i=1}^{m} b_i X_i + \sum_{i=1}^{m} \sum_{j=1}^{m} c_{ij} X_i X_j + \sum_{i=1}^{m} \sum_{j=1}^{m} \sum_{k=1}^{m} d_{ijk} X_i X_j X_k + ...$$

The technique involves fitting of quadratic equations for all pairs of independent variables and identifying a few best performers in terms of predictive ability (using appropriate statistics); converting entire set of independent variables (called zero generation variables) to new variables (first generation variables) which are obtained as predicted values from these selected quadratic equations (of zero generation variables). The process of fitting and identifying best quadratic equations is repeated using first generation variables and second generation variables are obtained. The whole process is repeated with every new generation of variables till appropriate model is obtained (using certain criteria). At final stage, one best quadratic equation is selected as the final model. (Bahuguna *et al.*, 1992; Trivedi *et a.l* 1999).

Machine Learning Techniques

Machine learning techniques offer many methodologies like decision tree induction algorithms, genetic algorithms, neural networks, rough sets, fuzzy sets as well as many hybridized strategies for the classification ad prediction (Han and Kamber, 2001; Pujari, 2000; Komorowski *et al.*, 1999; Witten and Frank, 1999). Decision tree induction represents a simple and powerful method of classification that generates a tree and a set of rules, representing the model of different classes, from a given dataset. Decision Tree (DT) is a flow chart like tree structure, where each internal node denotes a test on an attribute, each branch represents an outcome of the test and each leaf node represents the class. The top most node in a tree is the root node. For decision tree ID3 algorithm and its successor C4.5 algorithm by Quinlan (1993) are widely used. One of the strengths of decision trees compared to other methods of induction is the ease with which they can be used for numeric as well as nonnumeric domains. Another advantage of decision tree is that it can be easily mapped to rules. Artificial Neural Networks (ANNs) is another attractive tool under machine learning techniques for forecasting and classification purposes. ANNs are data driven self-adaptive methods in that there are few apriori assumptions about the models for problems under study. These learn from examples and capture subtle functional relationships among the data even if the underlying relationships are unknown or hard to describe. After learning from the available data, ANNs can often correctly infer the unseen part of a population even if data contains noisy information. As forecasting is performed via prediction of future behaviour (unseen part) from examples of past behaviour, it is an ideal application area for ANNs, at least in principle. (Dewolf *et al.*, 1997, 2000; Laxmi and Kumar 2011a; Laxmi and Kumar 2011b; Kumar *et al.*, 2010). However, the technique requires a large data base.

Deviation Method

This method can be utilized when periodical data at different intervals during the crop season are available for only 5-6 years. The pest population at a given point of crop stage is assumed to be due to two reasons – natural cycle of the pest and weather. To identify the natural cycle, data at different intervals is averaged over years and a suitable model is fitted to these averaged data points. Then the entire data is converted as deviations from the predicted natural cycle. Appropriate model is fitted using these deviations as dependent and weather as independent variables.

Ordinal Logistic Model – Model for Qualitative Data

The timely control measures to prevent pest/disease outbreak can be taken even if the information on the extent of severity is not available but merely the epidemic status is accessible. This information could be obtained through modeling qualitative data. Such models have added advantage that these could be obtained even if the detailed and exact information on pest count/disease severity is not available but only the qualitative status such as epidemic or no epidemic/low, medium or high is known. Such a situation arises quite often in pest/disease data. In such cases, the data are classified as 0/1 (2 categories); 0,1,2 (three categories). The logistic regression is used for obtaining probabilities of different categories. For example, for two categories, the model is of the form:

$$P(E=1) = \frac{1}{1 + \exp(-z)} + e$$

where z is a function of weather variables.

Forecast/Prediction rule:

If P ≥.5 more chance of occurrence of epidemic

If P <.5 probability of occurrence of epidemic is minimum

(Agrawal *et al.*, 2014; Mishra *et al.*, 2004; Johnson *et al.*, 1996)

Within Year Model

The model which uses data from the current growing season only (within year model) may be beneficial in improving forecasts during a year with atypical growing conditions. These models are developed to provide forecasts of pertinent components of pests/diseases progress relying entirely on growth data collected from plant observations during the current growing season. A within year model could also be used effectively in developing objective forecast of a crop for which historical data are not available. Sometimes, past data on pests and diseases are not available but the pests and diseases status at different points of time during the crop season are available for the current season only. In such situations, within year growth model can be used for forewarning maximum disease severity/pest population, provided there are 10-12 data points between time of first appearance of pest/disease and maximum or most damaging stage. Growth models are basically non-linear in nature. A logistic model having a single dependent variable and an independent 'time' variable generally fits well to the growth process of crop yield components like dry matter accumulation, etc. The model uses repeated observations from the current year to estimate the parameters needed to forecast the dependent variable at maturity.

The form of the logistic model is

$$Y_i = \alpha / (1 + \beta\, r^{ti}) + e_i \quad i = 1,2,..,n$$

$\alpha > 0, \beta > 0, 0 < r < 1$

Y_i = Dependent growth variable

t_i = Independent time variable

e_i = Error term

The logistic growth model hypothesizes that growth of variable under study is slow during earlier stages of development, then increases at increasing rate for a period of time and then increases at a decreasing rate approaching an asymptotic maximum value (α). This asymptotic value represents the value of character at maturity. This methodology consists in fitting appropriate growth pattern to the pests and diseases data based on partial data and using this growth curve for forecasting the maximum value of variable of interest. A number of growth models such as logistic, Gompertz etc. can be used for this purpose.

Web Enabling of the Forecast System

A web based forewarning system for YSB and LF of rice was developed for the developed forecast models. The system consisted of several functional requirements such as incorporation of the statistical models, weather data entry (permitted only for administrator and authorized users), and graphic-user interface for multi users of different levels. The system was developed based on 3-tier architecture consisting of Client Side Interface Layer (CSIL), Application Logic Layer (ALL) and Database Layer (DBL). CSIL was implemented by HTML (Hyper Text Markup Language), CSS (Cascading Style Sheet) and JavaScript (for validation purpose). ALL has been implemented by the JSP (Java Server Pages) technology which provides a framework to create dynamic content on the server. Location and time specific pest forecast models have been coded in this language was saved on the server. DBL was used for storing the site and time specific weather related data (Figure 17.1). In this system, only administrators have the provision of feeding the weather information into the database. A sample template is also provided for the administrator and authorized users to upload new weather data directly to the database are given in Figure 17.2.

The system functions on a server running Windows operating system. MSSQL and Apache were used for database management server and web server, respectively. Weather data acquisition and process is site and time specific. After

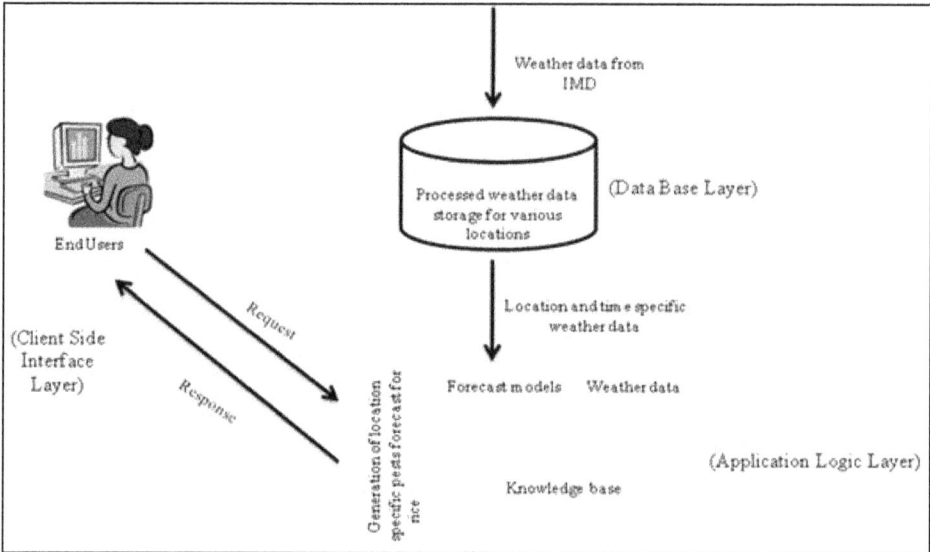

Figure 17.1: Overall Architecture of the System.

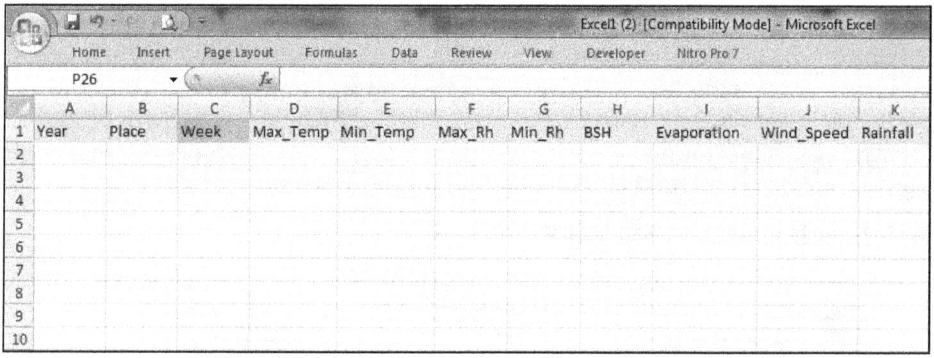

Figure 17.2: Sample Template for Administrator.

selecting the projected place and session corresponding to the crop-pest the system integrates weather data with specific forecast model to forecast the pests of rice for the particular site and session. System can be browsed over internet from any client machine having Internet Explorer, Netscape or any other web browsers.

Based on these models a *Weather based Rapeseed Mustard Aphid forewarning system* (http://www.drmr.res.in/aphidforecast/index.php) were developed. This internet-based system to forecast rapeseed-mustard aphid occurrence, has been implemented by embedding most effective earlier developed location-specific statistical models for aphid forecast. This web-based tool developed for mustard growers to the status of aphid infestation in crops for different locations which will decide the schedule of insecticide application. The user has to input weather parameter by selecting location closest to their crop planting area and system will provide a forecast of aphid incidence along with recommendations for insecticide application. The forecast regarding occurrence of aphid (*Lipaphis erysimi*) on oilseeds *Brassica* crops in season can be available to farmers with sufficient lag period for taking necessary action. This tools enables to avoid unwarranted sprays of insecticide to prevent avoidable expenditure of the farmer and also safeguard the environment from undue pesticide load. Weather indices based regression models are used in the backend for the online aphid forewarning systems (Kumar *et al.*, 2012).

References

Agrawal Ranjana, Mehta S.C., Bhar L.M. and Kumar Amrender (2004). Development of weather based forewarning system for crop pests and diseases - Mission mode project under NATP.

Agrawal Ranjana, Kumar Amrender and Singh S.K. (2014). Forecasting podfly (*Melanogromyza obtusa*) in late pigeonpea (*Cajanus cajan*). *Indian Journal of Agricultural Sciences*, 84 (2), pp. 214–217.

Bahuguna G.N. and Chandrahas (1992). Models for forecasting aphid pest of mustard crop. (IASRI Publication).

Chattopadhyay C., Agrawal R., Kumar A, Bhar L.M., Meena P.D., Meena R.L., Khan S.A., Chattopadhyay A.K., Awasthi R.P., Singh S.N., Chakravarthy N.V.K., Kumar A., Singh R.B. and Bhunia C.K. (2005-a). Epidemiology and forecasting of Alternaria blight of oilseed Brassica in India – a case study. *Zeitschrift für Pflanzenkrankheiten und Pflanzenschutz (Journal of Plant Diseases and Protection)*, 112(4), 351-365.

Chattopadhyay C., Agrawal R., Kumar Amrender, Singh Y.P., Roy S.K., Khan S.A., Bhar L.M., Chakravarthy N.V.K., Srivastava A., Patel B.S., Srivastava B., Singh C.P. and Mehta S.C. (2005-b). Forecasting of *Lipaphis erysimi* on oilseed Brassicas in India – a case study. *Crop Protection*, 24, 1042-1053.

Coakley S.M., Mcdaniel L.R. and Shaner G. (1985). Models for predicting severity of septoria tritici blotch on winter wheat. *Phytopathalogy*, 75(11): 1245-51.

Desai A.G., Chattopadhyay C., Agrawal Ranjana, Kumar A., Meena R.L., Meena P.D., Sharma K.C., Srinivasa Rao M., Prasad Y.G. and Ramakrishna Y.S. (2004). *Brassica juncea* powdery mildew epidemiology and weather- based forecasting models for India – a case study. *Zeitschrift für Pflanzenkrankheiten und Pflanzenschutz (Journal of Plant Diseases and Protection)* 111(5), 429-438.

Dewolf E.D. and Francl L.J. (1997). Neural network that distinguish in period of wheat tan spot in an outdoor environment. *Phytopathalogy*, 87(1): 83-7.

Dewolf E.D. and Francl L.J. (2000). Neural network classification of tan spot and stagonespore blotch infection period in wheat field environment. *Phytopathalogy*, 20(2):108-13.

Dhar Vishwa, Singh S.K., Kumar M., Agrawal R. and Kumar Amrender (2007). 'Prediction of pod borer (*Helicoverpa armigera*) infestation in short duration pigeonpea (*Cajanus cajan*) in central Uttar Pradesh', *Indian Journal of Agricultural Sciences*, 77(10), 701-04.

Han J. and Kamber M. (2001). *Data Mining Concepts and Techniques.* Morgan Kaufmann Publisher.

Johnson D.A., Alldredge J.R. and Vakoch D.L. (1996). Potato late blight forecasting models for the semi-arid environment of South-Central Washington. *Phytopathalogy*, 86(5): 480-84.

Komorowski J., Pawlak Z., Polkowki L. and Skowron A. (1999). Rough Sets: A Tutorial. In: *Rough Fuzzy Hybridization, Pal S.K. and Skowron, A.(eds.),* Springer, 3-99.

Kumar A., Srinivas P.S., Mishra A.K. and Chandrasekhran H. (2014). Fuzzy regression interval models for forewarning onion thrips. *IEEE - International Conference on Computing for Sustainable Global Development (INDIACom)*, pp.197-201.

Kumar Amrender, Ramasubramianian V. and Agrawal Ranjana (2010). Neural Network Based Forecast Modelling in Crops. IASRI Publication.

Kumar Amrender (2013). Forewarning Models for Alternaria blight in mustard crop. *Indian Journal of Agricultural Sciences*. 83 (1), pp. 116–8

Kumar Amrender, Agrawal Ranjana and Chattopadhyay C (2013). Weather based forecast models for diseases in mustard crop. *Mausam*, 64(4), pp. 663-670

Kumar Vinod, Kumar Amrender, Chattopadhyay Chirantan (2012). Design and implementation of web-based aphid (*Lipaphis erysimi*) forecast system for oilseed Brassicas. *The Indian Journal of Agricultural Sciences*, 82 (7), 608–14.

Laxmi R.R. and Kumar Amrender (2011a). Weather based forecasting model for crops yield using neural network approaches. Statistics and Applications, 9 (1 and 2 New Series), pp. 55-69.

Laxmi R.R. and Kumar Amrender (2011b). Forecasting of powdery mildew in mustard (*Brassica juncea*) crop using artificial neural networks approach. *Indian Journal of Agricultural Sciences*, 81(9), pp. 855–60.

Mishra A.K., Prakash O. and Ramasubramanian V. (2004). Forewarning powdery mildew caused by *Oidinm mangiferae* in mango (*Mangifera indica*) using logistic regression models. *Indian Journal of Agricultural Sciences*, 74(2): 84-7.

Pujari A.K. (2000). Data Mining Techniques. Universities Press.

Quinlan JR (1993). *C4.5:* Programs for Machine Learning. Morgan Kauffman.

Trivedi T.P., Paul Khurana S.M., Jain R.C., Mehta S.C. and Bhar L.M. (1999). Development of Forewarning system for aphids (*Myzus persicae*) on potato, Annual Report NCIPM, New Delhi.

Witten I.H. and Frank E. (1999). Data Mining: Practical Machine Learning Tools and Techniques with Java Implementations. Morgan Kaufmann Publishers.

Chapter 18

ICT Initiatives for Human Resource Development in Agricultural Education e-KrishiShiksha: An e-Learning Portal on Agricultural Education

R.C. Goyal, Sudeep Marwaha,
Rajni Bala Grover, Rama Dahiya

ICAR-IASRI, New Delhi-110 012

SUMMARY

For Agricultural Education, the Indian Council of Agricultural Research (ICAR) under financial support of National Agricultural Innovation Project (NAIP) has taken an initiative to develop UG level interactive and multimedia e-Course contents in seven major discipline viz. Agricultural Science; Fisheries Science; Dairy Science; Veterinary and Animal Husbandry; Horticultural Science; Home Science and Agricultural Engineering. The e-Course Contents are developed by Subject Matter Specialist of respective disciplines at State Agricultural Universities (SAUs) and Deemed to be Universities (DUs) in India. The course material is strictly prepared as per ICAR approved syllabus for the benefit of under-graduate students already enrolled in Indian Agricultural Universities.

To provide free online access of the interactive and multimedia UG level e-Course contents a centralized e-learning portal that provides 24/7 services to all the teachers and students learners in the field of agricultural education has been designed and developed and hosted on the web accessible at http://ecourses.iasri.res.in for the users' community. The online access of e-Course contents is made available as guest users.

Moreover, for offline usage of the e-course contents, facility has been provided to free download the desired e-course material. The downloaded file content folder could be independently executed offline on the local computers and courseware contents can be read and utilised exactly in the same manner as the contents made available on CDs/DVDs created for offline e-learning are used. This may act as a tool to aid, improve and complement the conventional learning-skills.

Keywords: *ICT, Education, Initiatives, Challenges, Teacher, Students, Infrastructure.*

Review of ICT in Education

Broadly, ICT in education can be defined as "diverse set of technological tools and resources used to communicate, and to create, disseminate, store, and manage information."[i] These technologies include computers, the Internet, broadcasting technologies (radio and television), and telephone communication. It should be understood that information and communication or ICT singularly does not generate learning.

Various Information and Communication Technology (ICT) tools such as radio, television, mobile phone and internet are effectively utilised to enhance, improve and complement the conventional learning-skills for human resource development in education [ii]. Many Indian universities are contemplating Technology enabled free access of education resources and an increased trend is being observed towards creation of a digital repository of books to create a digital learning environment for students. However, as Jaminson and McAnany (1978)[ii] stated, the three main strengths of radio are a) improving education quality and relevance, b) lowering educational costs, and c) improving access to educational inputs, particularly to disadvantaged groups. The University Broadcast Project started in 1965 and the Language Learning Project started in 1979-80 were worthy precursors of the next chain of radio-programmes that were adopted by IGNOU as part of their distance learning, the IGNOU-AIR Broadcast and the IGNOU-AIR Interactive Radio Counselling. In November, 2001, Gyan Vani, an FM Radio channel started functioning as media operatives, with day-to-day programmes contributed by various ministries, educational institutions and NGOs. EDUSAT, the first Indian satellite designed and developed exclusively for serving the educational sector was launched by the Indian Space Research Organisation (ISRO) in September, 2004. This system was primarily for school and college education, but beside the formal sector, it was also supposed to support the non-formal educational sector. Meanwhile, the Information Technology Act 2000 emphasized technical higher education, so that students would get better placement opportunities in the emerging IT sector in India. This also was bolstered by the Science and Technology Policy 2001 that called for the teaching of science at school and college levels.

Most recently, the National Mission on Education through Information and Communication Technology (NME-ICT) seeks to holistically change the educational environment of the country by an aggressive campaign to introduce ICT-enabled education in India, by assuring network access to remote corners, development of quality e-content, as well as empowering student-community by providing low-cost tablet PCs, named Akash.

In the last decade rapid changes in the education sector has been observed. During this period the higher education, in particular, has undergone a transition towards open mode with e-learning platforms. As a result the spreading of the effectiveness of education has crossed all geographical boundaries.

Incidentally, video sharing sites like YouTube came into vogue in 2006 has paved way to the surge in use and popularity for video-based content through internet, with initiatives through simple and innovative portals.

From the context of education in India, a significant initiative in the form of National Programme on Technology Enhanced Learning (NPTEL) came into being in 2003 involving seven Indian Institutes of Technology (IITs). NPTEL offered video lecture courses for wider access to learners in different engineering disciplines.

Agricultural Education in India has also received a major boost through development of e-courses, under Learning and Capacity Building program of National Agricultural Innovation Project (NAIP). In this, a total of 414 courses at Under Graduate (UG) level interactive multimedia e-Courseware contents has been developed in seven disciplines *viz.* Agricultural Science (49 courses); Fisheries Science (49 courses); Dairy Technology (49 courses); Veterinary and Animal Husbandry (64 courses); Horticulture (50 courses); Home Science (89 courses) and Agricultural Engineering (64 courses). The contents have been developed at SAUs and ICAR DUs organisations. This is a very significant move towards technology enhanced content development in agricultural education.

One of the significant aspects of these courses is the adoption of common protocol for hosting them in an open source Learning Management System Moodle and its portable version Poodle. This strategy facilitated to development of e-courses for both online and offline modes.

e-KrishiShiksha: An e-Learning Portal on Agricultural Education

From the context of agricultural education in India, ICAR under the financial support of NAIP has taken an initiative in the form of development of e-courses for the teachers and students learner at UG level in all major disciplines of agriculture and allied sciences. The e-Course Contents are developed by Subject Matter Specialist of respective disciplines at State Agricultural Universities (SAUs) and Deemed to be Universities (DUs) in India. The course material is strictly prepared as per ICAR approved syllabus for the benefit of under-graduate students already enrolled in Indian Agricultural Universities.

For Refinement, Updation, Maintenance and Sustenance of the UG level e-courses developed on different major disciplines of agricultural and allied sciences, an e-learning portal on agricultural education namely e-KrishiShiksha has been designed and developed and hosted on the web accessible at **http://ecourses.iasri.res.in**. The portal provides 24/7 services to the users' community. Home Page of e-learning Portal on Agricultural Education (e-KrishiShiksha) is presented as Figure 1. The online access to UG level e-Course contents of six disciplines namely Agriculture, Horticultural Science, Fisheries Science, Dairy Technology, Home Science, Veterinary and AH is made available. The portal is accessible to all Faculty, Teachers, Students and any one interested in the field of Agricultural Sciences.

Further for offline usage, the e-course contents of 414 courses related to seven disciplines namely Agriculture, Agriculture Engineering, Horticultural Science, Fisheries Science, Dairy Technology, Home Science, Veterinary and AH are made available as free downloadable component from the same portal. The downloaded file content folder could be independently executed offline on the local computers and courseware contents can be used for teaching/learning exactly in the same manner as any educational CDs/DVDs contents are used for offline e-learning.

Since, some of the SAUs have already created farmers level Information Systems, Expert Systems and e-Contents for short term training programmes for farmers on agriculture, horticulture, fisheries etc., and an attempt has also been made to collect e-contents, compile and made available through a sub-module created under this portal for the farmers.

Design of e-Learning Portal

The Portal is developed using Client Server web technology in .Net framework environment.

1. Client Side Interface Layer (CSIL) has been implemented using Hyper Text Markup language (HTML), JavaScript and Cascading Style Sheet (CSS). The CSIL consists of forms for accepting information from the user and validation those forms using JavaScript

2. Server Side Application Layer (SSAL) has been implemented using Java Server Pages (JSP). The JSP provides the web developers with a framework to create dynamic content on the server which is secure, fast and independent of server platform. The technology generates HTML pages according to the user's action and request.

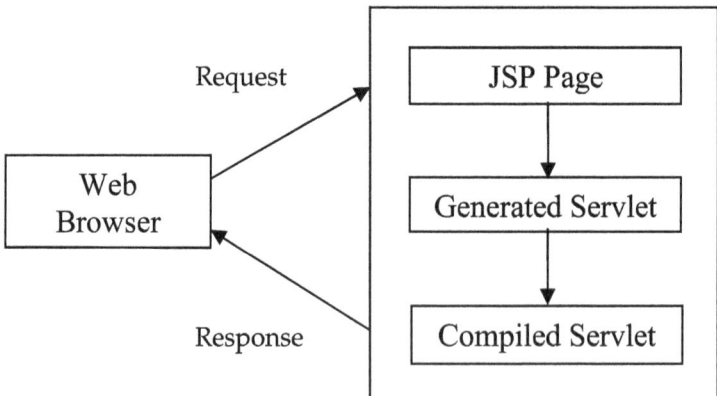

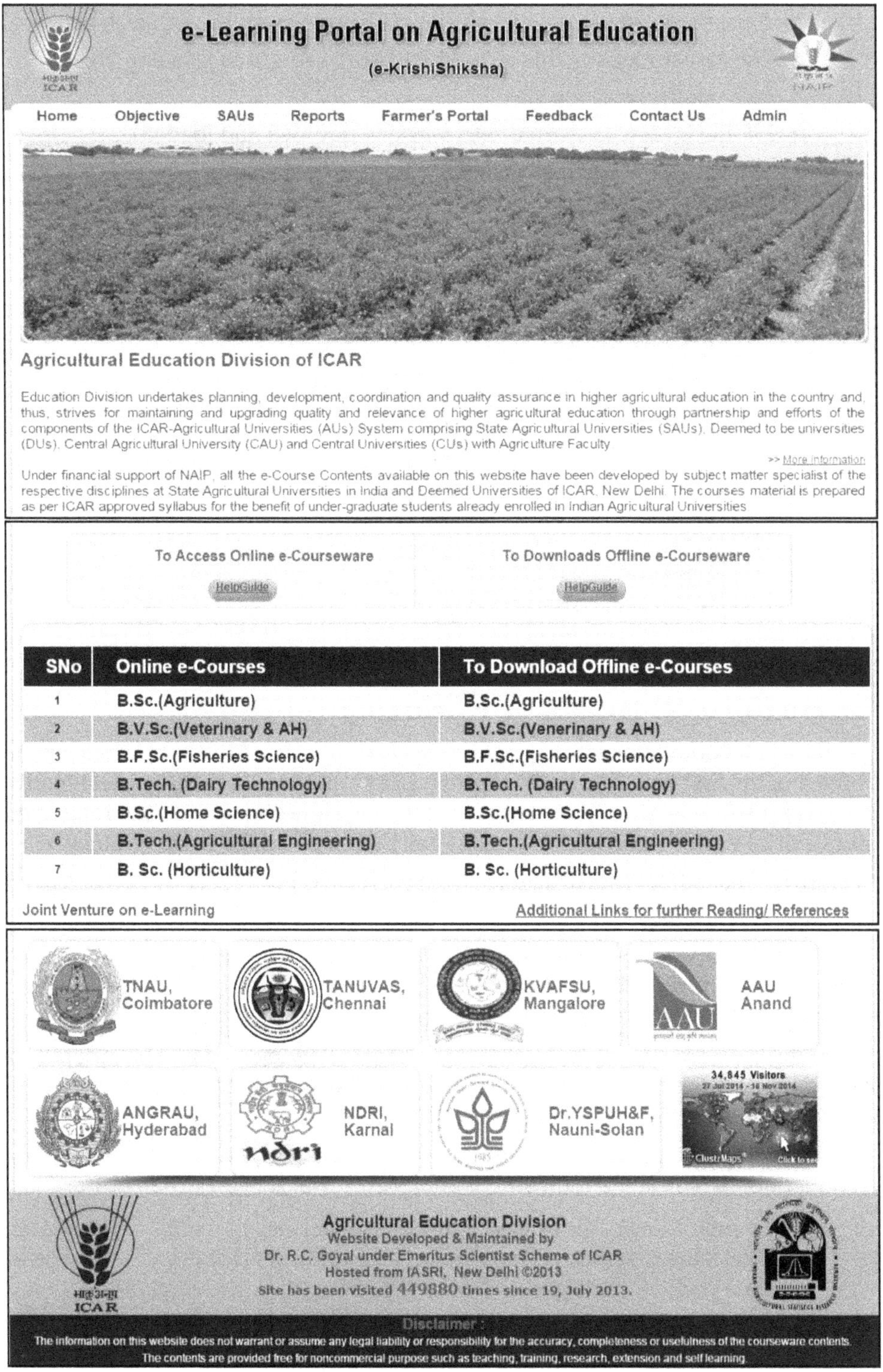

e-Learning Portal on Agricultural Education
(e-KrishiShiksha)

Home   Objective   SAUs   Reports   Farmer's Portal   Feedback   Contact Us   Admin

Agricultural Education Division of ICAR

Education Division undertakes planning, development, coordination and quality assurance in higher agricultural education in the country and, thus, strives for maintaining and upgrading quality and relevance of higher agricultural education through partnership and efforts of the components of the ICAR-Agricultural Universities (AUs) System comprising State Agricultural Universities (SAUs), Deemed to be universities (DUs), Central Agricultural University (CAU) and Central Universities (CUs) with Agriculture Faculty

>> More Information

Under financial support of NAIP, all the e-Course Contents available on this website have been developed by subject matter specialist of the respective disciplines at State Agricultural Universities in India and Deemed Universities of ICAR, New Delhi. The courses material is prepared as per ICAR approved syllabus for the benefit of under-graduate students already enrolled in Indian Agricultural Universities

To Access Online e-Courseware   To Downloads Offline e-Courseware

HelpGuide   HelpGuide

SNo	Online e-Courses	To Download Offline e-Courses
1	B.Sc.(Agriculture)	B.Sc.(Agriculture)
2	B.V.Sc.(Veterinary & AH)	B.V.Sc.(Venerinary & AH)
3	B.F.Sc.(Fisheries Science)	B.F.Sc.(Fisheries Science)
4	B.Tech. (Dairy Technology)	B.Tech. (Dairy Technology)
5	B.Sc.(Home Science)	B.Sc.(Home Science)
6	B.Tech.(Agricultural Engineering)	B.Tech.(Agricultural Engineering)
7	B. Sc. (Horticulture)	B. Sc. (Horticulture)

Joint Venture on e-Learning   Additional Links for further Reading/ References

TNAU, Coimbatore   TANUVAS, Chennai   KVAFSU, Mangalore   AAU Anand

ANGRAU, Hyderabad   NDRI, Karnal   Dr.YSPUH&F, Nauni-Solan   34,845 Visitors

Agricultural Education Division
Website Developed & Maintained by
Dr. R.C. Goyal under Emeritus Scientist Scheme of ICAR
Hosted from IASRI, New Delhi ©2013
Site has been visited 449880 times since 19, July 2013.

Disclaimer :
The information on this website does not warrant or assume any legal liability or responsibility for the accuracy, completeness or usefulness of the courseware contents. The contents are provided free for noncommercial purpose such as teaching, training, research, extension and self learning

Figure 18.1: Home page of e-Learning Portal on Agricultural Education.

☆ A user requests some information by http request through web browser.

☆ The server receives this request and send request to java engine.

☆ Java engine reads.jsp file.

☆ JSP file is then converted into servlet (compiled and loaded).

☆ The servlet then gathers the information needed to satisfy the user's request and constructs a web page in HTML containing the information.

☆ Java Engine then sends HTML to server.

☆ That web page is then displayed on the user's browser.

Modules of e-Learning Portal

The e-Learning Portal has the following 7 Modules:

1. Online e-Learning for UG courses
2. Off-line e-Learning: Free Download facility for - UG Courses
3. e-learning for Farmers
4. Contents Data Management
5. Contents Refinement Process
6. System Administration
7. Reports

Access to Portal for Online e-Learning

Reference Guide for online access has been prepared and made available on the portal. For the first time, one has to register as new user by submitting brief identity details and subsequently the email-Id is used for authentication of the registered users. Portal visitor's and User's records has been maintained in the system.

Briefly, the following instructions may be followed to have access of the desired e-course contents online.

For online access, click on the link of the desired UG level e-course discipline (B.Sc. (Horticulture) on the Home Page. The page as Figure 18.2 for the user authentication to access online will appear.

In case you are already a registered user, the following step will be ignored by the system and directly the webpage containing link of all e-courses of the desired selected discipline to have online access will appear.

For the first time, new user will have to register him/her self by submitting brief identity details in the following registration form as Figure 18.3.

☆ On submitting of the brief identification details, a page containing message "Welcome to online e-Learning on Agricultural Education" will appear. Then click on Continue.

☆ The desired page Link will open

☆ Use "login as a guest" to read the desired course contents.

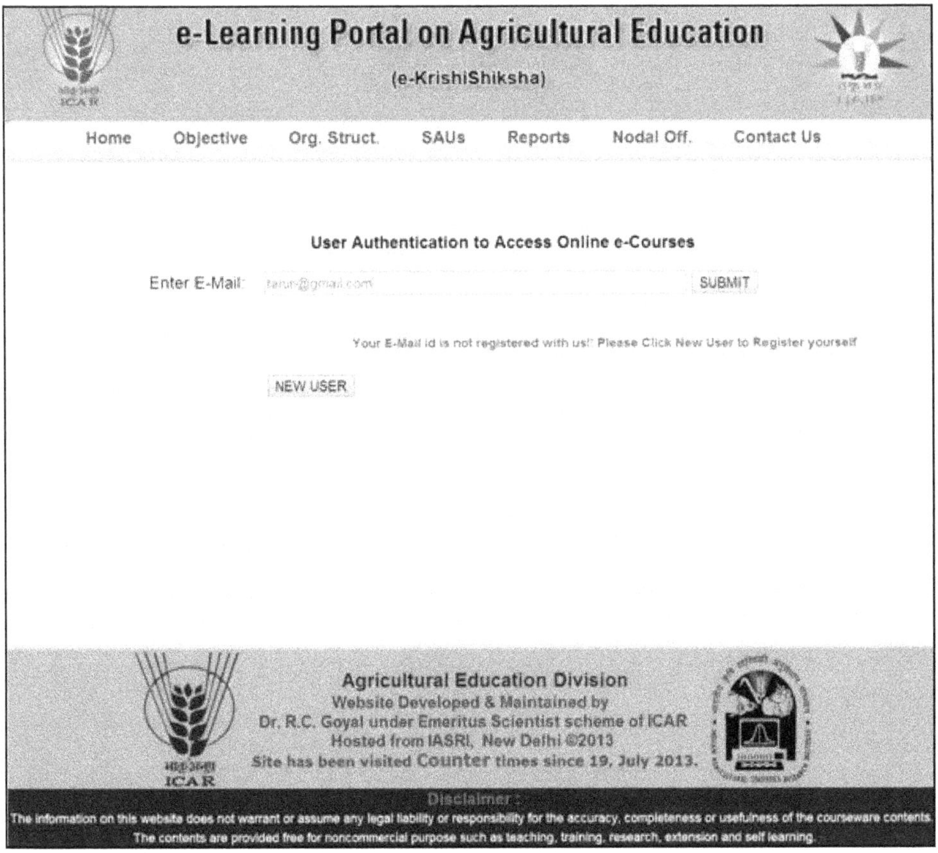

Figure 18.2: User Authentication.

Access to Portal for Free Download facility for Off-line e-Learning

For remote area institutions/faculty/students, free download facility is provided for using the e-Courseware contents offline. The downloaded file content folder could be independently executed from desktop and used for teaching/learning exactly in the same manner as any CD/DVD contents are used for offline e-learning.

Reference Guide for Free Download facility for Off-line e-Learning has been prepared and made available on the portal. To free download, for the first time, one has to register as new user by submitting brief identity details and subsequently the email-Id is used for authentication of the registered users.

Briefly, the following instructions may be followed to download of the desired e-course contents. The downloaded file is zipped in Winrar format. A link to download Winrar software is also made available on the portal and subsequently may be used to unzip the downloaded e-course file.

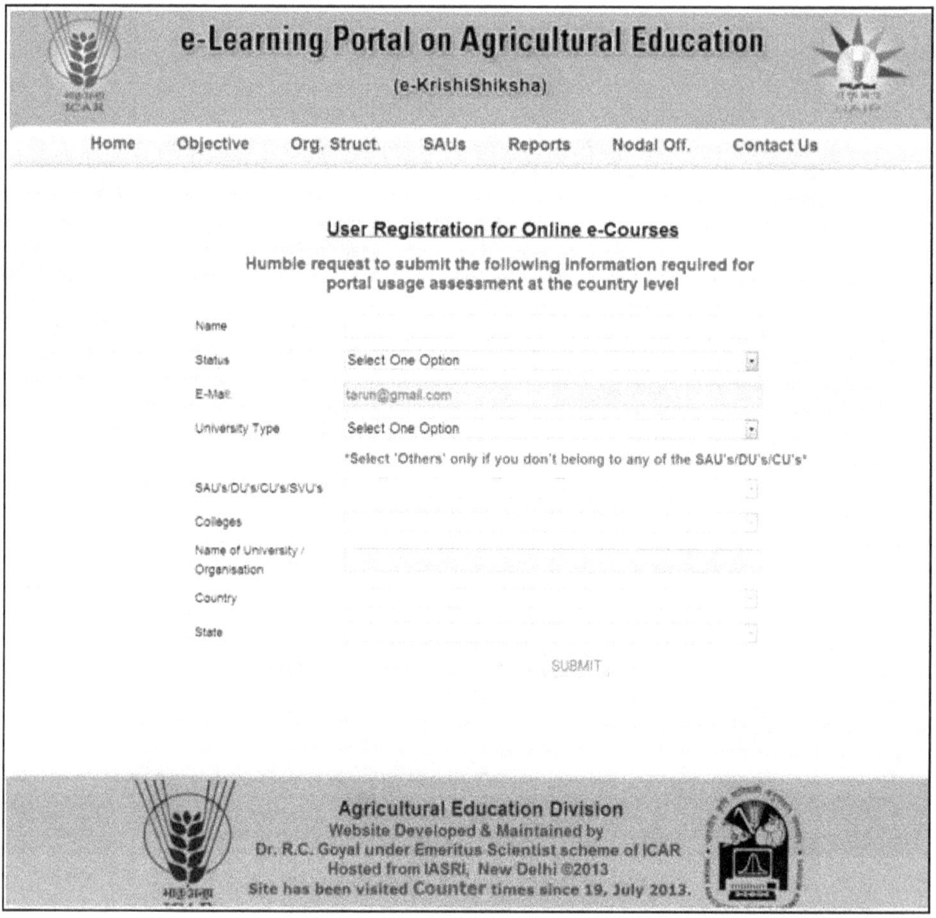

Figure 18.3: User Registration.

For offline usage, e-course contents of 414 e-courses of following disciplines are made available as free downloadable component from the portal.

☆ B.Sc (Agriculture)	49 courses
☆ B.Sc (Horticulture)	50 courses
☆ B.Sc (Home Science)	89 courses
☆ BFSc (Fisheries)	49 courses
☆ BVSc (Veterinary and A.H.)	64 courses
☆ B.Tech. (Dairy Technology)	49 courses
☆ B.Tech. (Agri. Engineering)	64 courses

Briefly, the following instructions may be followed for download of the desired e-course contents for offline usage.

For download, click on the link of the desired UG level e-course discipline (B.Sc. (Horticulture) on the Home Page. The page as Figure 18.2 for the user authentication will appear. For the first time, new user will have to register by submitting his/her brief identity details on submitting of the brief details, a new page will appear containing links of different e-courses of the desired selected discipline. Through this option, the linkage of different disciplines leading to the respective discipline e-courses available in the system is made available to the user. The user is able to download and save the desired e-course contents on desktop. The downloaded file can be independently executed and run and used for learning from the desktop.

The following instructions may be followed to download e-course content files and its offline usage from the computer.

1. Download the desired e-course contents and save it on your desktop. The downloaded file is in Winrar format.
2. Close your mozilla firefox browser.
3. Extract the downloaded e-course content file using Winrar software on the desktop.
4. Incase, Winrar software does not exist on your system, first download Winrar software.
5. Download the flash plugins or flash player to open the flash visuals. Ignore if Flash Software is already installed in the system.
6. Look for extracted file folder and double-click the same.
7. Double-click the "Startportableapps" application file.
8. You will find a new window popping up.
9. Click "Moodle start".
10. You will find "http://localhost:8101/moodle/" and various courses being listed.
11. Click a particular lecture you want to browse and enjoy offline e-learning.
12. In some cases it may ask for Username and Password. You need to enter Username as "admin" and password as " admin" (please mind the lowercase as the login is case sensitive) and enjoy reading the course

e-learning for Farmers

Since, some of the SAUs have already created farmers level Information Systems, Expert Systems and e-Contents for short term training programmes for farmers on agriculture, horticulture, fisheries etc. An Attempt is being made to collect e-contents, compile and provide access through this portal. On the home page of the portal an option e-learning for farmers/women (Figure 18.4) level short e-training material under different disciplines has been made available. The material is also available in different regional languages.

Portal Utilization Trend

At present more than 14,075 users for online access and 20,738 users for offline free downloads have been registered from SAUs in India. In addition to this a large number of users other than NARS from India and abroad have registered

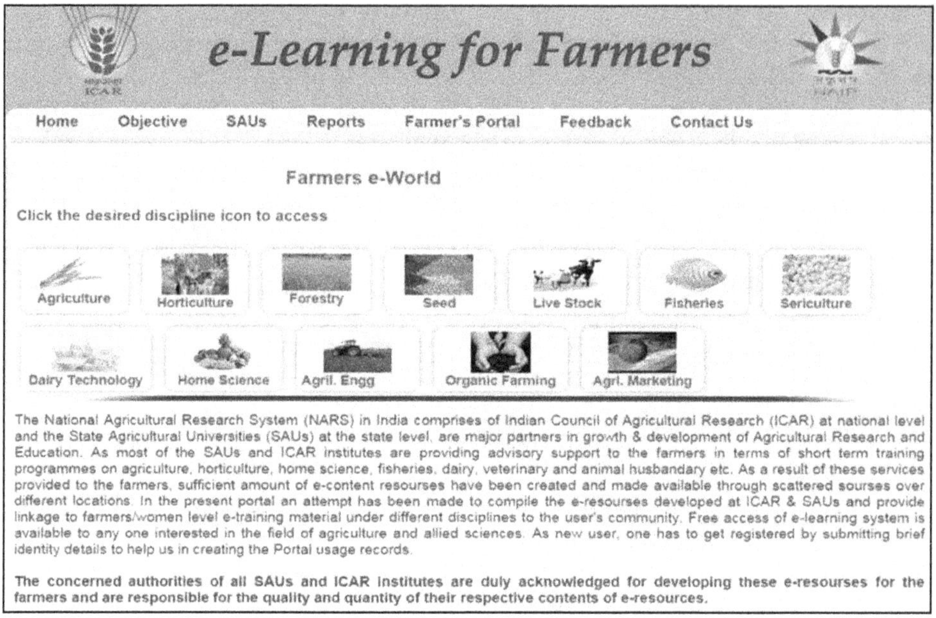

Figure 18.4: e-Learning for Farmers.

and visited the portal. Although there are some notable exceptions, women are generally underrepresented among faculty as well as students in agriculture programs, particularly at higher education levels. From the data it is observed that against seven men only one women faculty memeber/students has registered for downloading the e-courseware from the portal. More than 1,11,401 e-course content files of different disciplines have been downloaded by the registered users from NARS. Total hits on the portal are more than 6,65,067.

In view of the above efforts need to be made for wide publicity of these developments among faculty, teachers and students at SAUs. Although, the portal link has been provided on the ICAR as well as SAUs web sites. Sensitization cum awareness workshops in collaboration with the SAUs for different disciplines have been organized.

e-Courses Offline Usage

More than 20,738 users have been registered from NARS for e-courses offline usage. The monthwise status of e-Courses downloaded by Administrators, Faculty, Teachers, UG, PG and PhD students from different SAUs during June 2013 to June 2015 is presented in Figure 18.5. From the monthly trend it has been observed that the maximum number of users were registered during September 2014 and that may be due to the awareness meetings organised at some of the SAUs and the trend clearly envisaged that awareness workshops need to be organised to increase the usage of the e-learning portal.

Friday, June 26, 2015
Time 4:02:41 PM

Monthwise Registered Users for Offline Usage at SAUs

Print

Sno	Month	Year	Administrator	Faculty	Teacher	UG-Student	PG-Student	Ph.D-Student	Others	Total
1	June	2013	9	107	76	115	48	28	25	408
2	July	2013	6	141	101	146	67	38	31	530
3	August	2013	9	125	90	255	114	59	58	710
4	September	2013	11	117	80	311	124	60	62	765
5	October	2013	8	135	67	247	119	79	53	708
6	November	2013	5	169	66	379	117	50	66	852
7	December	2013	9	95	48	267	95	45	62	621
8	January	2014	14	125	59	314	78	48	66	704
9	February	2014	10	95	73	332	74	28	80	692
10	March	2014	13	154	99	379	129	60	71	905
11	April	2014	10	69	39	279	107	42	51	597
12	May	2014	2	26	18	145	59	23	27	300
13	June	2014	9	92	84	1015	34	23	36	1293
14	July	2014	9	137	135	1430	52	19	37	1819
15	August	2014	7	93	83	871	141	42	50	1287
16	September	2014	4	113	86	1734	154	45	42	2178
17	October	2014	3	40	34	423	145	16	39	700
18	November	2014	8	60	40	510	151	37	62	868
19	December	2014	5	26	27	282	73	20	28	461
20	January	2015	7	92	54	534	127	28	50	892
21	February	2015	9	65	64	678	129	49	63	1057
22	March	2015	7	30	16	250	30	13	30	376
23	April	2015	3	44	30	484	76	25	48	710
24	May	2015	7	43	43	348	84	34	50	609
25	June	2015	4	67	44	422	86	35	38	696
	TOTAL		**188**	**2260**	**1556**	**12150**	**2413**	**946**	**1225**	**20738**

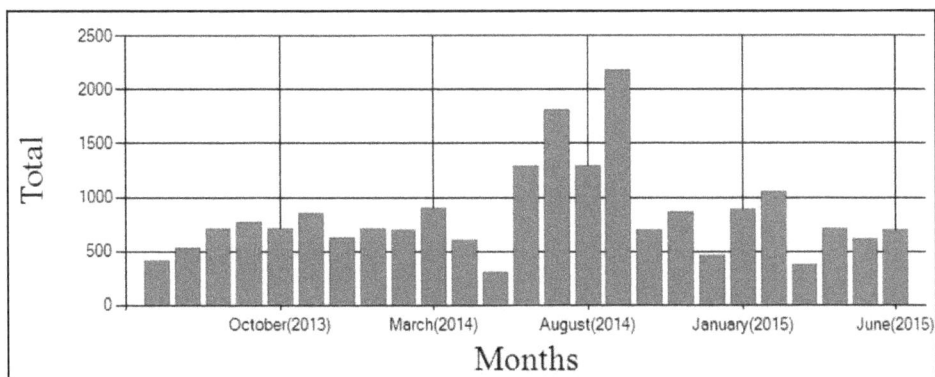

Figure 18.5: Users Registered from SAUs for Offline Usage.

e-Courses Monthwise Download Status at SAUs

About 87,646 e-course contents have been downloaded by faculty and students from NARS. The monthwise status of e-Courses downloaded by Administrators, Faculty, Teachers, UG, PG and PhD students from different SAUs during June 2013 to June 2015 is presented in Figure 18.6. From the monthly trend it has been observed that the maximum total number of downloads during August2014, September 2014 and February 2015and that may be due to the awareness meetings organised at

Friday, June 26, 2015
Time 4:08:39 PM

Monthwise Downloads Status at SAUs

Print

Sno	Month	Year	Administrator	Faculty	Teacher	UG-Student	PG-Student	Ph.D-Student	Others	Total
1	June	2013	3	237	167	199	196	142	29	973
2	July	2013	22	592	376	587	453	275	256	2561
3	August	2013	33	381	328	940	476	153	307	2618
4	September	2013	38	373	369	1055	654	224	326	3039
5	October	2013	37	391	375	1383	590	418	249	3443
6	November	2013	21	601	239	1508	671	218	304	3562
7	December	2013	16	370	214	1374	660	381	326	3341
8	January	2014	44	534	375	1695	461	252	292	3653
9	February	2014	9	453	362	1819	450	159	282	3534
10	March	2014	49	679	366	1824	650	441	308	4317
11	April	2014	94	507	202	1448	682	348	442	3723
12	May	2014	13	332	87	967	474	211	147	2231
13	June	2014	25	301	210	1111	266	114	89	2116
14	July	2014	12	383	202	1530	308	78	102	2615
15	August	2014	20	605	375	2703	641	279	629	5252
16	September	2014	73	436	280	2953	872	246	334	5194
17	October	2014	22	271	182	1822	335	118	209	2959
18	November	2014	32	385	238	2646	629	192	364	4486
19	December	2014	60	271	178	1427	425	161	128	2650
20	January	2015	26	432	281	3174	613	225	235	4986
21	February	2015	30	463	413	4240	979	348	502	6975
22	March	2015	7	162	107	1160	158	75	213	1882
23	April	2015	10	274	123	2236	619	200	114	3576
24	May	2015	33	246	260	2261	472	250	362	3884
25	June	2015	15	387	261	2608	509	189	107	4076
		TOTAL	744	10066	6570	44670	13243	5697	6656	87646

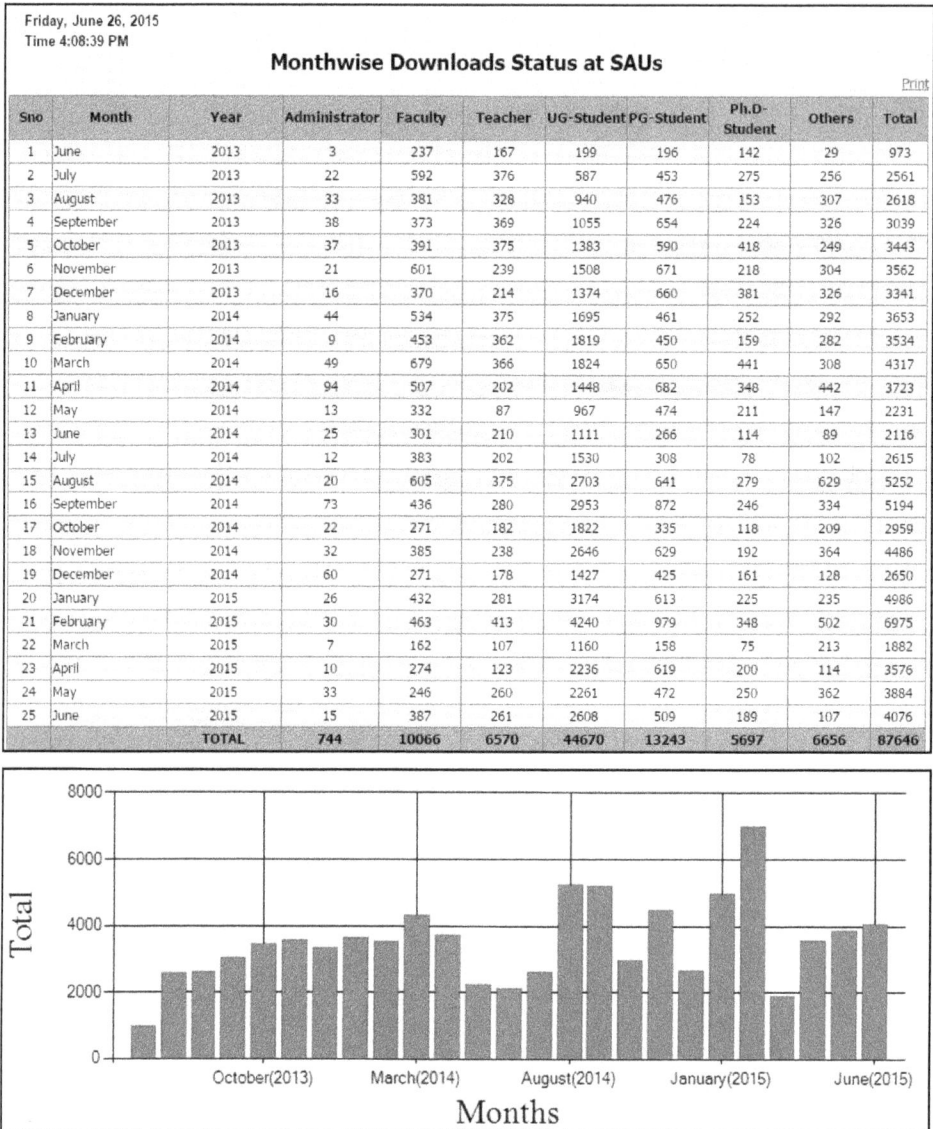

Figure 18.6: Monthwise Download Status at SAUs.

some of the SAUs and the trend clearly envisaged that awareness workshops need to be organised to increase the usage of the e-learning portal.

Conclusion

The centralized e-learning portal on agricultural education that provides 24/7 services to all the teachers and students learners in the field of agricultural education has been made accessible to the faculty, teachers, students and all others interested in learning about agricultural and allied sciences. For offline usage, the e-courseware contents are made available as downloadable component from the same portal for remote area institutions/faculty/students. This may eliminate the process of physical supply of e-course contents on (CDs/DVDs) by post/courier services. For wide publicity of these developments among faculty, teachers and students community e-KrishiShiksha (http://ecourses.iasri.res.in) link has been provided on most of the SAUs web site.

The establishment of this e-learning portal will also act as an effective tool and solution for Refinement, Updation, Maintenance and Sustenance of the e-learning courseware contents developed under Learning and Capacity Building program of NAIP. It is becoming a useful and powerful tool for the agricultural education e-courses data management related to all disciplines of Agriculture Sciences including Veterinary, Animal Science, Fisheries, Dairy, Horticulture and Home science etc.

Finally, it may act as a tool for institutional reforms as the availability of e-courses helps in introducing the advanced technology and culture in the education system.

References

http://siteresources.worldbank.org/Resources/Guidelines.pdf

Radio for education and development, www.getcited.org/pub/101781064

B.G.Sudha A, S.Ramesh. "Integration of ICT in Education – Need for Competency Enhancement" in Patil, S.S. *et al.* (Eds). *ICT in Education: Recent Trends*. Jaipur, Prateeksha Publications, 2012, p.58.

http://aview.in/allevents/Join-NME-ICT-mission-and-reap-benefits.

http://en.wikipedia.org/wiki/List_of_countries_by_English-speaking_population

http://www.dise.in

Integrating ICT in Teaching Learning Framework in India: Initiatives and Challenges, Rumpa Das, Mahestala College, West Bengal, India, 2012.

Technology Enhanced Learning in Agricultural Education: Need of the Hour; G.R.K. Murthy, D. Thammi Raju, K.M. Reddy and P. Ramesh; National Academy of Agricultural Research Management, Rajendranagar, Hyderabad.

Chapter 19

Introduction to Geographic Information System

Prachi Misra Sahoo

ICAR-IASRI, New Delhi – 110 012

Introduction

Geographic Information System (GIS) is a computer based information system used to digitally represent and analyse the geographic features present on the Earth surface and the events that take place on it. The meaning to represent digitally is to convert analog into a digital form. "Every object present on the Earth can be geo-referenced", is the fundamental key of associating any database to GIS. Here, term 'database' is a collection of information about things and their relationship to each other, and 'geo-referencing' refers to the location of a layer or coverage in space defined by the co-ordinate referencing system. Evolution of GIS has transformed and revolutionized the ways in which planners, engineers, managers etc. conduct the database management and analysis.

Defining GIS

A GIS is an information system designed to work with data referenced by spatial/geographical coordinates. In other words, GIS is both a database system with specific capabilities for spatially referenced data as well as a set of operations for working with the data. It may also be considered as a higher order map. A Geographic Information System is a computer based system which is used to digitally reproduce and analyse the feature present on earth surface and the events that take place on it. In the light of the fact that almost 70 per cent of the data has geographical reference as it's denominator, it becomes imperative to underline the importance of a system which can represent the given data geographically.

Three Perspectives on GIS

1. GIS as a toolbox -> if so then what kind of tools?

   ☆ Classification based on functional tasks of GIS.

   ☆ Tools for automating *spatial data* (data capture via digitizing, scanning, remote sensing, satellite geo-position system)

   ☆ For storing spatial data (data bases and data structures)

   ☆ For spatial data management/retrieval

   ☆ For analysis (overlay, buffering, proximity, network functions, spatial statistics)

   ☆ For display of spatial data and analysis of results

2. GIS as an Information System

   ☆ Definition of GIS as a specialized information system stresses "spatially distributed features (points, lines, areas), activities (physical and human-invoked), and events (time)

   ☆ Definition of GIS: A system of hardware, software, data, people, organizations, and institutional arrangements for collecting, storing, analyzing and disseminating information about areas of the earth.

3. GIS as an approach to Geographic Information Science

   ☆ Research on GIS (algorithms, analytical methods, visualization tools, user interfaces, human-computer-human interaction)

   ☆ Research with GIS: GIS as a tool used by many substantive disciplines in their own ways (anthropology, archeology, forestry, geology, engineering, business and management sciences)

History of GIS

Work on GIS began in 1950s, but first GIS software came only in late 1970s from the lab of the ESRI. Canada was the pioneer in the development of GIS as a result of innovations dating back to early 1960s. Much of the credit for the early development of GIS goes to Roger Tomilson. The events which took place in the development of GIS in chronological order are:

☆ Early 1950s: thematic map overlay (superimposition of maps drafted at the same scale)

☆ 1959: use of transparent blacked-out overlays to find suitable locations (overhead)

☆ 1960s: early computer mapping packages SURFACE II, SYMAP; early spatial data banks (CIA's World Data Bank)

☆ 1960s: first GIS (Canada Geographic Information System, Minnesota Land Management System)

☆ 1970s: advances in algorithms and data structures to handle spatial data, Harvard Lab for Computer Graphics (first modern GIS software)

☆ 1980s: introduction of PC, advances in hardware, mature mainframe GIS software

☆ 1990s: desktop GIS, Internet-based GIS services, proliferation of GIS applications

☆ 2000 and beyond ??? omnipresent GIS, wireless, networked, every-day applications everywhere.

Components of GIS

GIS constitutes of five key components:

☆ Hardware
☆ Software
☆ Data
☆ People
☆ Method

Hardware

It consists of the computer system on which the GIS software will run. The choice of hardware system range from 300MHz Personal Computers to Super Computers having capability in Tera FLOPS. The computer forms the backbone of the GIS hardware, which gets it's input through the Scanner or a digitizer board. Scanner converts a picture into a digital image for further processing. The output of scanner can be stored in many formats *e.g.* TIFF, BMP, JPG etc. A digitizer board is flat board used for vectorisation of a given map objects. Printers and plotters are the most common output devices for a GIS hardware setup.

Software

GIS software provides the functions and tools needed to store, analyze, and display geographic information. GIS softwares in use are MapInfo, ARC/Info, AutoCAD Map, etc. The software available can be said to be application specific. When the low cost GIS work is to be carried out desktop MapInfo is the suitable option. It is easy to use and supports many GIS feature. If the user intends to carry out extensive analysis on GIS, ARC/Info is the preferred option. For the people using AutoCAD and willing to step into GIS, AutoCAD Map is a good option. The software for a geographical information system may be split into five functional groups as mentioned below:

(a) Data input and verification
(b) Data storage and database management
(c) Data transformation
(d) Data output and presentation
(e) Interaction with the user

Data

Geographic data and related tabular data can be collected in-house or purchased from a commercial data provider. The digital map forms the basic data input for GIS. Tabular data related to the map objects can also be attached to the digital data. A GIS will integrate spatial data with other data resources and can even use a DBMS, used by most organization to maintain their data, to manage spatial data.

People

GIS users range from technical specialists who design and maintain the system to those who use it to help them perform their everyday work. The people who use GIS can be broadly classified into two classes. The CAD/GIS operator, whose work is to vectorise the map objects. The use of this vectorised data to perform query, analysis or any other work is the responsibility of a GIS engineer/user.

Method

And above all a successful GIS operates according to a well-designed plan and business rules, which are the models and operating practices unique to each organization. There are various techniques used for map creation and further usage for any project. The map creation can either be automated raster to vector creator or it can be manually vectorised using the scanned images. The source of these digital maps can be either map prepared by any survey agency or satellite imagery.

Data in GIS

A GIS stores information about the world as a collection of themed layers that can be used together. A layer can be anything that contains similar features such as customers, buildings, streets, lakes, or postal codes. This data contains either an explicit geographic reference, such as a latitude and longitude coordinate, or an implicit reference such as an address, postal code, census tract name, forest stand identifier, or road name. There are two components: spatial data that show where the feature is; and attribute data that provide information about the feature. These are linked by the software. The fact that there are both spatial and attribute data allows the database to be exploited in more ways than a conventional database allows, as GIS provides all the functionality of the DBMS and adds spatial functionality.

Spatial data Spatial data is spatially referenced data that act as a model of reality. Spatial data represent the geographical location of features for example points, lines, area etc. Spatial data typically include various kinds of maps, ground survey data and remotely sensed imagery and can be represented by points, lines or polygons.

Attribute Data: Attribute data refers to various types of administrative records, census, field sample records and collection of historical records. Attributes are either the qualitative characteristics of the spatial data or are descriptive information about the geographical location. Attributes are stored in the form of tables, where each column of the table describes one attribute and each row of the table corresponds to a feature.

The Nature of Geographical Data

☆ **Geographical position** (spatial location) of a **spatial object** is presented by 2-, 3- or 4-dimensional coordinates in a geographical reference system (*e.g.* Latitude and Longitude).

☆ **Attributes** are descriptive information about specified spatial objects. They often have no direct information about the spatial location but can be linked to spatial objects they describe. Therefore it is often to call attributes *"non-spatial"* or *"aspatial"* information.

☆ **Spatial relationship** specifies inter-relationship between spatial objects (*e.g.* direction of object B in relation to object A, distance between object A and B, whether object A is enclosed by object B, etc.).

☆ **Time** records the time stamp of data acquisition, specifies life of the data, and identifies the locational and attribute change of spatial objects.

Representation of Spatial Data (Data Representation Models)

In GIS, two types of data models represent spatial data.

1. Vector model
2. Raster model

Vector Model

In vector models, objects are created by connecting points with straight line (or arcs) and area is defined by sets of lines. Information about points, lines and polygons is encoded and stored as a collection of x, y coordinate. Location of a point feature such as tubewell can be described by a single x, y coordinate. Linear feature such as river can be stored as a collection of point coordinates. Polygon feature, such as river catchment can be stored as a closed loop of coordinates. Vector models are very useful for describing discrete features like data represented by an area. Vector model is not much useful for describing continuously varying features such as soil type (Figure 19.1).

Raster Model

In raster model, study area is divided into a regular grid of cells in which each cell contain single value. Continuous data type, such as elevation, vegetation etc. are represented using raster model (Figure 19.2).

Methods of Data Input in GIS

Conversion of Existing Data

After receiving existing spatial data from government or private sources, GIS users often need to convert the data to a format compatible with the GIS package. Existing data cannot be easily converted because of a large variety of GIS packages and data formats in use. The choice of a conversion method basically depends upon the specificity of the data format. Some data formats are proprietary and require

Spatial Data: Vector format

Vector data are defined spatially:

Point - a pair of x and y coordinates

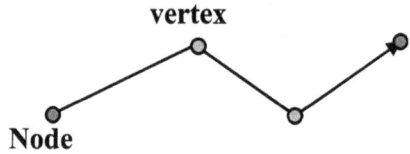

Line - a sequence of points

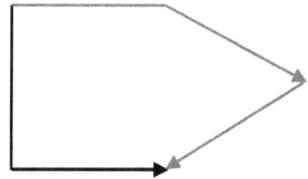

Polygon - a closed set of lines

Figure 19.1

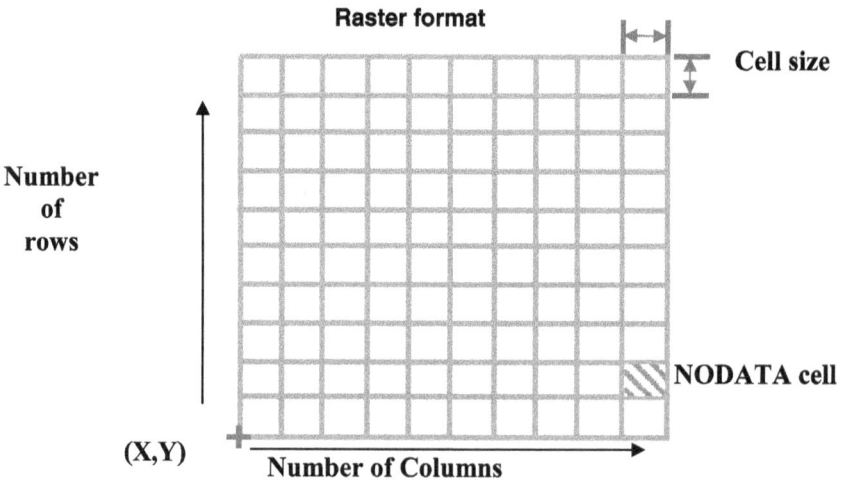

Figure 19.2

special translators for conversion of data from one GIS package to another. Such a conversion method can be described as direct translation. On the other hand, some data formats are neutral or public. In that case a GIS package needs to have translators that can work with the neutral format for importing and exporting data.

Creating New Data

You can create new data by using primary data sources, such as satellite or GPS (Global Positioning System) data, or secondary data sources, such as paper maps. The process of converting paper maps to digital data is called digitizing, and it can be done using digitizer or scanner technology.

Digitizing

Digitizing using a digitizing tablet is also called manual digitizing. The digitizing tablet has a built-in electronic mesh and can sense the position of the cursor and transmit it to the computer. The units of measurement on digitized coverages are in inches. Digitizing begins with a set of tics, which are used later for converting the coverage to real-world coordinates. Two considerations for manual digitizing are: point versus stream mode, and resolution and accuracy.

Scanning

A scanner converts a paper map to a scanned file, which contains raster data with values of 1 and 0. Pixels with the value 0 represent lines scanned from the paper map, and pixels with the value 1 represent non-inked areas. The scanned file is then converted to a coverage through tracing. GIS packages such as ARC/INFO have algorithms that enable users to perform semi-automatic tracing or manual tracing.

On-screen Digitizing

On-screen digitizing is an alternative to manual digitizing and scanning for limited digitizing work such as editing or updating an existing coverage. On-screen digitizing is manual digitizing on the computer monitor using a data source such as a DOQ as the background. This is an efficient method for digitizing, for example, new trails or roads that are not on an existing coverage but are on a new DOQ. Likewise, the method can be used for editing a vegetation coverage based on new information from a new DOQ that shows recent clear-cuts or burned areas. Obviously, the major shortcoming of this method is the resolution of the computer monitor, which is much coarser than a digitizing table or a scanner.

Basic GIS Functionality

GIS software combines computer mapping functionality that handles and displays spatial data, with database management system functionality to handle attribute data. The basic functionality of GIS is as follows:

- ✿ Querying both spatially and through attribute
- ✿ Manipulating the spatial component of the data: for example, through changing projections, rubber sheeting to join adjacent layers of data together, and calculating basic statistics such as areas and perimeters of polygons

☆ Buffering where all locations lying within a set distance of a feature or set of features are identified

☆ Data integration, either informally by simply laying one layer over another, or formally through a mathematical overlay operation

☆ Areal interpolation

Uses of GIS

There are three basic categories of use that GIS can be put to:

☆ As a spatially referenced database;

☆ As a visualisation tool; and

☆ As an analytic tool.

A spatially referenced database allows us to ask questions such as 'what is at this location?', 'where are these features found?', and 'what is near this feature?'. It also allows us to integrate data from a variety of disparate sources. For example to study the dataset on hospitals we might also want to use census data on the population of the areas surrounding each hospital. Census data are published for districts that can be represented in the GIS using polygons as spatial data. As we have the coordinates of the hospitals and the coordinates of the district boundaries we can bring this data together to find out which district each hospital lay in, and then compare the attribute data of the hospitals with the attribute data from the census. We may also want to add other sorts of data to this: for example data on rivers represented by lines; or wells represented by points to give information about water quality. In this way information from many different sources can be brought together and interrelated through the use of location. This ability to integrate is one of the key advantages of GIS.

Once a GIS database has been created, mapping the data it contains is possible almost from the outset. This allows the researcher a completely new ability to explore spatial patterns in the data right from the start of the analysis process. As the maps are on-screen they can be zoomed in on and panned around. Shading schemes and classification methods can be changed, and data added or removed at will. This means that rather than being a product of finished research, the map now becomes an integral part of the research process. New ways of mapping data are also made possible, such as animations, fly-throughs of virtual landscapes, and so on. It is also worth noting the visualization in GIS is not simply about mapping: other forms of output such as graphs and tables are equally valid ways of visualising data from GIS.

Although visualisation may answer some of the questions a researcher has about a dataset, more rigorous investigation is often required. Here again GIS can help. The combined spatial and attribute data model can be used to perform analyses that ask questions such as 'do cases of this disease cluster near each other?' in the case of a single dataset; or 'do cases of this disease cluster around sources of drinking water?' where more than one dataset is brought together. To date, this form of analysis has been well explored using social science approaches to quantitative GIS data. It has not been so well explored using humanities approaches to qualitative data, but this is one area where historians are driving forward the research agenda in GIS.

Questions GIS can answers

Till now GIS has been described in two ways:

1. Through formal definitions, and
2. Through technology's ability to carry out spatial operations, linking data sets together.

However there is another way to describe GIS by listing the type of questions the technology can (or should be able to) answer. Location, Condition, Trends, patterns, Modelling, Aspatial questions, Spatial questions. There are five type of questions that a sophisticated GIS can answer:

Location What is at.............?

The first of these questions seeks to find out what exists at a particular location. A location can be described in many ways, using, for example place name, post code, or geographic reference such as longitude/latitude or x/y.

Condition Where is it.............?

The second question is the converse of the first and requires spatial data to answer. Instead of identifying what exists at a given location, one may wish to find location(s) where certain conditions are satisfied (*e.g.*, an unforested section of at-least 2000 square meters in size, within 100 meters of road, and with soils suitable for supporting buildings)

Trends What has changed since.............?

The third question might involve both the first two and seeks to find the differences (*e.g.* in land use or elevation) over time.

Patterns What spatial patterns exists.............?

This question is more sophisticated. One might ask this question to determine whether landslides are mostly occurring near streams. It might be just as important to know how many anomalies there are that do not fit the pattern and where they are located.

Modelling What if................?

"What if…" questions are posed to determine what happens, for example, if a new road is added to a network or if a toxic substance seeps into the local ground water supply. Answering this type of question requires both geographic and other information (as well as specific models). GIS permits spatial operation.

Aspatial Questions

"What's the average number of people working with GIS in each location?" is an aspatial question - the answer to which does not require the stored value of latitude and longitude; nor does it describe where the places are in relation with each other.

Spatial Questions

" How many people work with GIS in the major centres of Delhi" OR " Which centres lie within 10 Kms. of each other? ", OR " What is the shortest route passing through all these centres". These are spatial questions that can only be answered using latitude and longitude data and other information such as the radius of earth. Geographic Information Systems can answer such questions.

GIS as an Integrating Technology

In the context of these innovations, geographic information systems have served an important role as an integrating technology. Rather than being completely new, GIS have evolved by linking a number of discrete technologies into a whole that is greater than the sum of its parts. GIS have emerged as very powerful technologies because they allow geographers to integrate their data and methods in ways that support traditional forms of geographical analysis, such as map overlay analysis as well as new types of analysis and modeling that are beyond the capability of manual methods. With GIS it is possible to map, model, query, and analyze large quantities of data all held together within a single database.

The importance of GIS as an integrating technology is also evident in its pedigree. The development of GIS has relied on innovations made in many different disciplines: Geography, Cartography, Photogrammetry, Remote Sensing, Surveying, Geodesy, Civil Engineering, Statistics, Computer Science, Operations Research, Artificial Intelligence, Demography, and many other branches of the social sciences, natural sciences, and engineering have all contributed. Indeed, some of the most interesting applications of GIS technology discussed below draw upon this interdisciplinary character and heritage.

Application Areas

GIS are now used extensively in government, business, and research for a wide range of applications including environmental resource analysis, landuse planning, locational analysis, tax appraisal, utility and infrastructure planning, real estate analysis, marketing and demographic analysis, habitat studies, and archaeological analysis.

One of the first major areas of application was in **natural resources management**, including management of

- ☆ Wildlife habitat,
- ☆ Wild and scenic rivers,
- ☆ Recreation resources,
- ☆ Floodplains,
- ☆ Wetlands,
- ☆ Agricultural lands,
- ☆ Aquifers,
- ☆ Forests.

One of the largest areas of application has been in **facilities management**. Uses for GIS in this area have included

- ☆ Locating underground pipes and cables,
- ☆ Balancing loads in electrical networks,
- ☆ Planning facility maintenance,
- ☆ Tracking energy use.

Local, state, and federal governments have found GIS particularly useful in **land management**. GIS has been commonly applied in areas like

- ☆ Zoning and subdivision planning,
- ☆ Land acquisition,
- ☆ Environmental impact policy,
- ☆ Water quality management,
- ☆ Maintenance of ownership.

More recent and innovative uses of GIS have used information based on **street-networks**. GIS has been found to be particularly useful in

- ☆ Address matching,
- ☆ Location analysis or site selection,
- ☆ Development of evacuation plans.

The range of applications for GIS is growing as systems become more efficient, more common, and less expensive. Some of the newest applications have taken GIS to unexpected areas. The USGS and the city of Boulder, Colorado have come up with some innovative uses for GIS:

- ☆ Global Change and Climate History Project
- ☆ Emergency Response Planning
- ☆ Site Selection of Water Wells
- ☆ Boulder, Colorado, has used GIS to develop a Wildfire Hazard Identification and Mitigation System

References

Antenucci, John C.; Brown, Kay; Croswell, Peter L.; Kevany, Michael J.; and Archer, Hugh N. 1991. "Introduction," "Evolution of the Technology," and "Applications." Chaps. 1-3 in Geographic Information Systems: A Guide to the Technology. New York: Van Nostrand Reinhold.

Burrough, P.A. 1986. "Geographic Information Systems." Chap. 1 in Principles of Geographic Information Systems for Land Resources Assessment. Oxford: Oxford University Press.

Huxhold, William E. 1991. "Information in the Organization" and "Applications of Urban Geographic Information Systems." Chaps. 1 and 3 in An Introduction to Urban Geographic Information Systems. New York: Oxford University Press.

Star, Jeffrey and John Estes. 1990. "Introduction" and "Background and History." Chaps. 1 and 2 in Geographic Information Systems: An Introduction. Englewood Cliffs, NJ: Prentice- Hall.

Tobler, W.R. 1959. "Automation and Cartography." Geographical Review 49: 526-534.

Chapter 20

AGRIdaksh: A Tool for Development of Online Expert Systems for Crops

Sudeep Marwaha

Division of Computer Applications,
ICAR-IASRI, New Delhi-110 012

A knowledge based system has knowledge and inference procedures that are difficult enough to be solved require human expertise for their solution. The knowledge necessary to perform at such a level plus the inference procedures used can be thought of as a model of the expertise of the best practitioners in the field. Expert system is designed to simulate the problem-solving behaviour of a human who is an expert in a domain or discipline. An expert system is normally composed of a knowledge base (information, heuristics, *etc.*), inference engine (analyzes the knowledge base), and the end user interface (accepting inputs, generating outputs). One of the most powerful attributes of expert systems is the ability to explain reasoning. Since, the system remembers its logical chain of reasoning, a user may ask for an explanation of a recommendation and the system will display the factors it considered in providing a particular recommendation.

Developing an expert system in a specific knowledge domain is quite a difficult task as it requires team of experienced knowledge engineers, programmers as well as domain experts. Agriculture, being a very vast and varied domain of knowledge with over a hundred crops distributed in different geographic regions having varied climatic conditions, building such a team in every domain of knowledge of agriculture is itself a challenging and huge task. Knowledge engineers gather

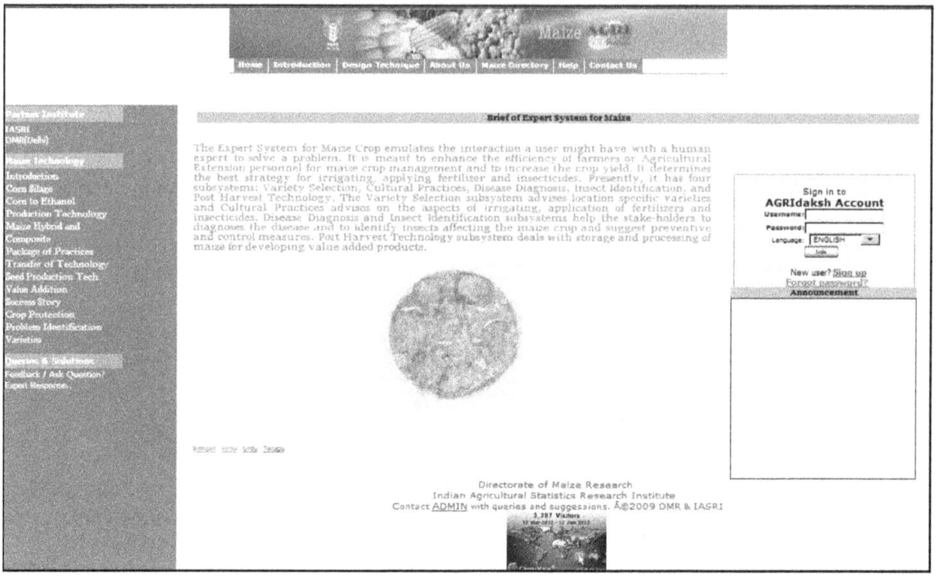

Figure 20.1: Maize AGRIdaksh Home Page.

knowledge from domain experts and put it in such a form that system can use for inferring and reasoning using some knowledge representation technique. Programmers than build an online interface so that the end users can use the system over the Internet.

AgriDaksh, a tool for building online expert system has been developed at Division of Computer Applications, IASRI to overcome these hurdles. AgriDaksh is available online through IASRI web site http://www.iasri.res.in or at its direct link http://expert.iasri.res.in/agridaskh. AgriDaksh enables domain experts to build online expert system in their crops with minimal intervention of knowledge engineers and programmers. With its use, it is possible to build online expert system for each and every crop in significantly less time and resources. Online expert systems have the capability to transfer location specific technology and advice to the farmers efficiently and effectively. This in turn can reduce losses due to diseases and pests infestation, improve productivity with proper variety selection and increase in income of the farmer. **Maize AgriDaksh** is the first system developed using AgriDaksh.

AgriDaksh Features

☆ One system for all crops with ability to create knowledge models for new crops

☆ Location specific variety information with the ability to add multiple pictures for each variety

☆ Comprehensive plant protection sub module with

   a. Diseases

   b. Insects

      c. Weeds

      d. Nematodes

      e. Physiological Disorders

☆ Ability for domain experts to define problems online and create decision trees to solve the problems

☆ Ontology based diseases and insects identification and variety selection

☆ Ability to add static web pages

☆ Powerful administrative module

☆ Full featured online help

☆ Semantic web compliant

☆ Built on robust, platform independent java technology using n-tier web architecture

System Architecture

Technology has evolved to a point where Web applications are very complex and have many parts. Figure 20.2 shown below shows the structure called the N-Tier Web. The N-Tier Web, also known as distributed systems, is where the Web is today in its evolution.

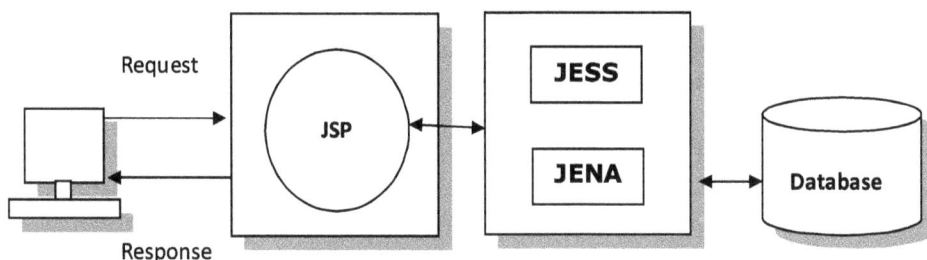

Figure 20.2: N-Tier Architecture.

The Figure can be divided into multiple sections: the client Layer, the application logic level, and the data level. Let's begin dissecting this structure starting with the client layer. Different kinds of clients can be in this structure. For example, a Web Client is accessing a Web server using TCP/IP and making requests with HTTP. Another type of client, a Java application, also can access the application server through other communication protocols such as Remote Method Invocation (RMI) and Internet Inter-Orb Protocol (IIOP).

The application logic can be spread over a Web Server and a Application Server. The Web Server can handle request from Web Clients and service simple HTML documents. If the request is for an application, it can forward the request on to the Application Server. The application Server can handle larger programs than the Web Server can. The last layer in this structure is the data level. The data level can be made up of one or more databases, and it can also include legacy systems, such as mainframes.

Thus the essence we have is that, if a Web Server concentrates on serving Web Pages, it should be able to optimize that process and serve them efficiently. If an application server focuses on serving applications, it should be able to offer services that almost all applications use, such as security. Finally, if a database is responsible for handling data, it can focus on providing services, such as caching, to access data faster. Another benefit of breaking up the facilities is that it is easier to write and maintain smaller components than large, bulky applications.

Java Server Pages (JSPs) are a technology defined by Sun Microsystems to create dynamic content on the Web. They are HTML documents that are interleaved with Java, which provides the dynamic content.JSPs are a server-side application; they accept a request and generate a response. Generally the requests are made from a Web client, and the response is generated HTML document that gets sent back to the Web client. Because JSPs are a server-side application, they have access to the resources on the server, such as Servlets, Java Beans, EJBs and databases.

JDBC is an Application Programming Interface (API) that allows Java programs to connect and interact with databases. The API set of classes and interfaces packaged under the Java packages java.sql and javax.sql. The goal of the JDBC APIT is to provide a consistent and standard way of accessing databases from a number of diverse drivers. The JDBC API strives to shield developers from having to deal with the details of which database vendor is being used. This is achieved by using drivers provided by the database vendors. JDBC Drivers are classes provide by the database vendors, Java programs, including Java Server Pages, use JDBC drivers to obtain a connection to a database and then use the connection to query and update the database.

JESS is an expert system shell and scripting language written entirely in Sun Microsystems's Java language. Jess supports the development of rule-based expert systems which can be tightly coupled to code written in the powerful, portable Java language. Jess language supports a comprehensive list of supported functions. It provides the facility of calling Java functions from Jess, of extending Jess by writing Java code, and of embedding Jess in Java applications.

In the context of computer and information sciences, the definitions of ontology can be categorized into roughly three groups:

☆ Ontology is a term in philosophy and its meaning is "theory of existence".

☆ Ontology is an explicit specification of conceptualization.

☆ Ontology is a body of knowledge describing some domain, typically common sense knowledge domain.

The first definition is the meaning in philosophy as we have discussed above, however it has many implications for the AI purposes. The second definition is generally accepted as a definition of what an ontology is for the AI community. The last third definition views an ontology as an inner body of knowledge, not as the way to describe the knowledge. The second definition of ontology mentioned above, "explicit specification of conceptualization", comes from Thomas Gruber. Explicit specification of conceptualization means that an ontology is a description (like a formal specification of a program) of the concepts and relationships that can exist for an agent or a community of agents. A conceptualization can be defined as an intensional semantic structure that encodes implicit knowledge constraining the structure of a piece of a domain. Ontology is a (partial) specification of this structure, *i.e.*, it is usually a logical theory that expresses the conceptualization explicitly in some language. Ontology is important for the purpose of enabling knowledge sharing and reuse. An ontology is in this context a specification used for making ontological commitments. Agents then commit to ontologies and ontologies are designed so that the knowledge can be shared among these agents.

The World Wide Web is possible because a set of widely established standards guarantees interoperability at various levels. Until now, the Web has been designed for direct human processing, but the next-generation Web, which Tim Berners-Lee and others call the "Semantic Web," (Lee, *et al.*, 2001) or Web 3.0 aims at machine-processible information. Semantic Web is a group of methods and technologies to allow machines to understand the meaning - or "semantics" - of information on the World Wide Web. The term was coined by World Wide Web Consortium (W3C) director Tim Berners-Lee. He defines the Semantic Web as "a web of data that can be processed directly and indirectly by machines".

Resource Description Framework (RDF) was originally created in 1999 as a standard on top of XML for encoding metadata information. The RDF is used for encoding information about Web resources as well as information about and relations between things in the real world: people, places, concepts, etc. RDFS is used to create vocabularies that describe groups of related RDF resources and the relationships between those resources. An RDFS vocabulary defines the allowable properties that can be assigned to RDF resources within a given domain. RDFS also allows creating classes of resources that share common properties.

The Web Ontology Language (OWL) is a family of knowledge representation languages for authoring ontologies. The languages are characterized by formal semantics and RDF/XML-based serializations for the Semantic Web. OWL is endorsed by the World Wide Web Consortium (W3C) and has attracted academic, medical and commercial interest. The OWL Web Ontology Language is designed for use by applications that need to process the content of information instead of just presenting information to humans. OWL facilitates greater machine interpretability of Web content than that supported by XML, RDF, and RDF Schema (RDF-S) by providing additional vocabulary along with a formal semantics. OWL has three increasingly-expressive sublanguages: OWL Lite, OWL DL, and OWL Full.

JENA is a Java framework for building Semantic Web applications. It provides a programmatic environment for RDF, RDFS and OWL, including a rule-based inference engine. The Jena Framework includes modules like RDF API, ARP, Persistence, Reasoning Subsystem, Ontology Subsystem, SPARQL query language implementation. RDF API has statement and resource centric methods for manipulating RDF model, cascading method calls for more convenient programming, built in support for RDF containers, enhanced resources, integrated parsers and writers for RDF/XML (ARP), N3 and N-TRIPLES. ARP is Jena's RDF/XML Parser. ARP Jena2 version is compliant with the RDF Core recommendations.

Protégé is a free, open-source platform that provides a growing user community with a suite of tools to construct domain models and knowledge-based applications with ontologies. At its core, Protégé implements a rich set of knowledge-modeling structures and actions that support the creation, visualization, and manipulation of ontologies in various presentation formats. Protégé can be customized to provide domain-friendly support for creating knowledge models and entering data. Ontology describes the concepts and relationships that are important in a particular domain, providing a vocabulary for that domain as well as a computerized specification of the meaning of terms used in the vocabulary. SPARQL is a recursive acronym standing for SPARQL Protocol and RDF Query Language.

AgriDaksh Modules

Keeping in mind the user friendliness, the AgriDaksh has been designed with the following modules:

☆ Knowledge Model Creation

☆ Knowledge Acquisition

☆ Problem Identification

☆ Knowledge Retrieval

☆ Ask Questions to Experts

☆ Administration

Knowledge Model Creation

First step for building an expert system of a crop through AgriDaksh is to build its knowledge model. Knowledge model can be build by selecting the desired

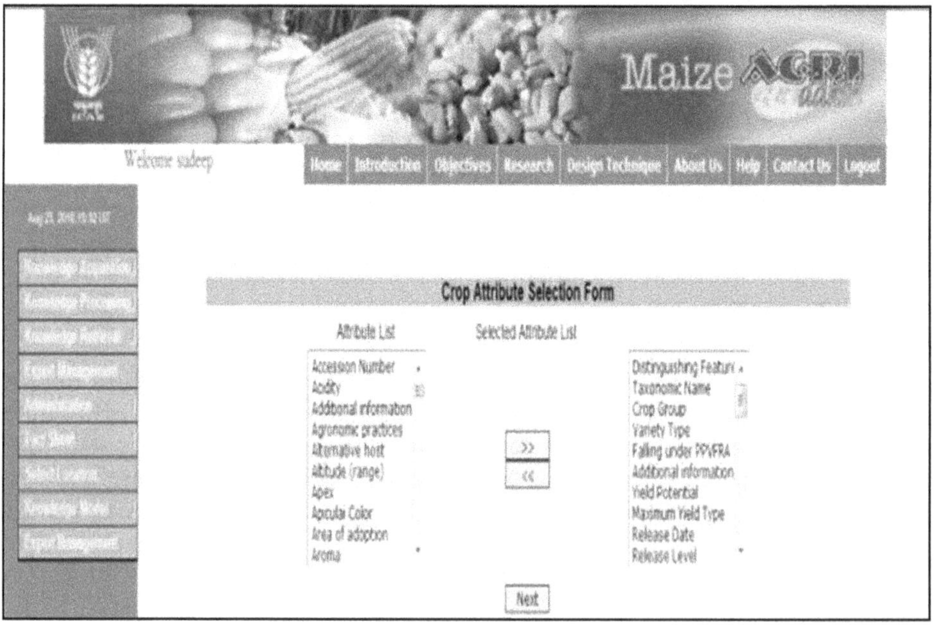

Figure 20.3: Crop Attribute Selection Form Page.

attributes from the Attributes List and moving them to Selected Attribute List. Once, the desired attributes are chosen, domain experts can enter the values of these attributes for each and every variety of the crop.

Knowledge Acquisition

Knowledge Acquisition module is used for entering knowledge about various entities such as crop varieties, diseases, insect-pests, weeds, nematodes, physiological disorders and post harvest technology.

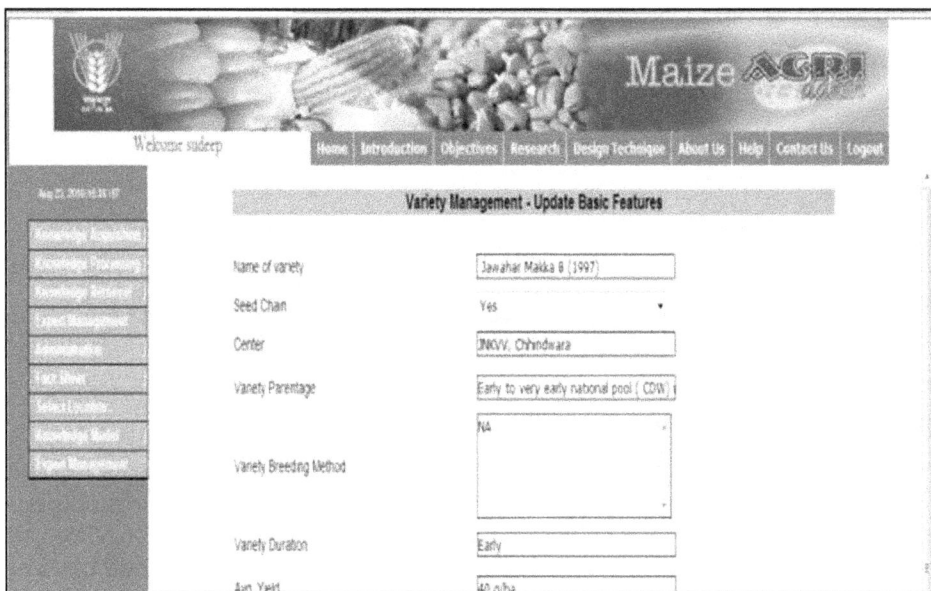

Figure 20.4: Basic Features Update Performa of Variety Management.

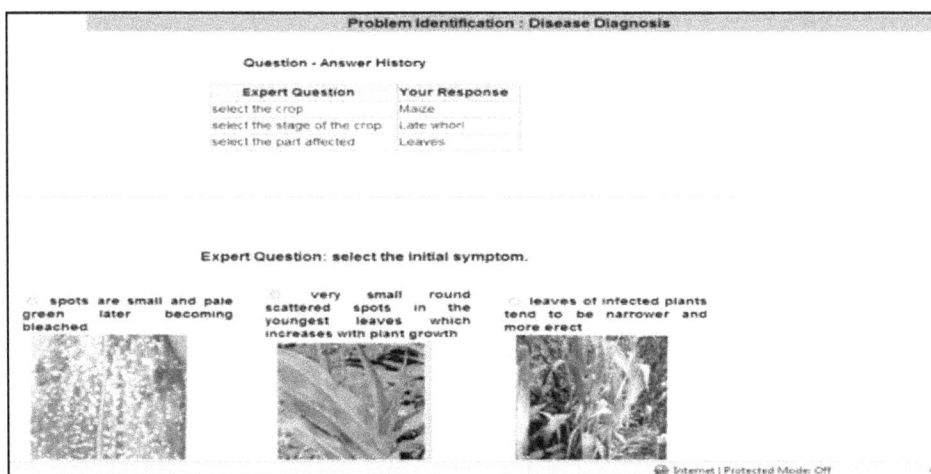

Figure 20.5: Initial Symptoms of Maize.

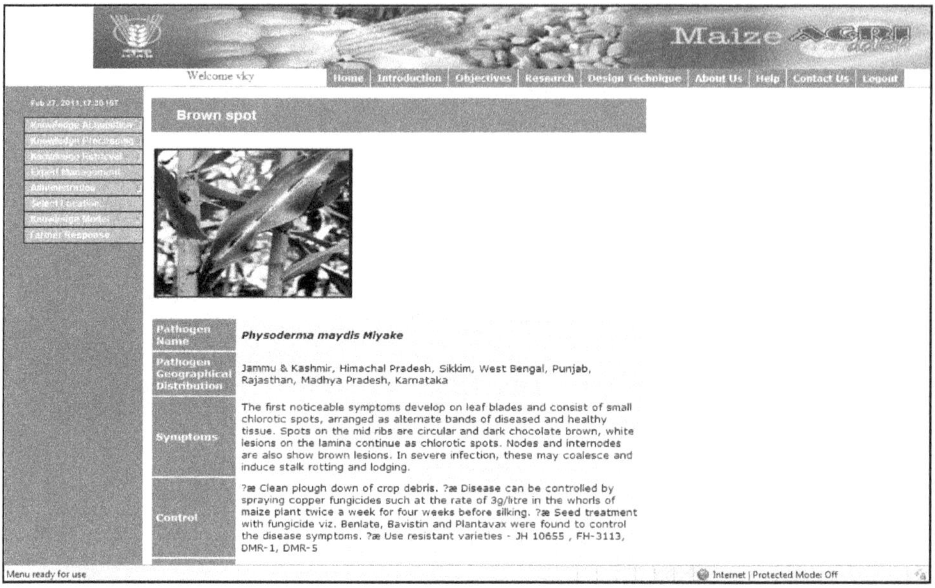

Figure 20.6: Information of a Particular Maize Disease.

Problem Identification

This module has two sub modules *viz.*, Rule based problem identification and Ontology based problem identification. First sub module allows the domain experts to define the problem and develop decision tree to solve the problem. Once the tree is developed, farmers can get the solution about the problem in their situation. The second sub module allows the farmers to identify the diseases and insects affecting their crops as well as select varieties according to their location and conditions.

Knowledge Retrieval

Knowledge Retrieval module is the most important module as far as farmers are concerned. Through this module, a farmer can get information about each and every thing that domain experts have entered *e.g.* plant protection sub module allows farmers to retrieve knowledge about diseases, insects, weeds, nematodes and physiological disorders.

Ask Questions to Experts

Using this module a farmer can ask question directly to domain experts. The system transfers the question to relevant domain experts and sends answer to the farmer thorough email. The same is displayed in the system for the benefit of other farmers.

Administration

This module is for the administrator for controlling the overall functionality of the system. Using this module administrator can create different type of users such as end users, domain experts, domain expert validators, and crop administrator. One can add a new crop and assign a crop administrator for that crop.

Chapter 21
ICT in Agriculture

U.B. Angadi and K.K. Chaturvedi

Centre for Agricultural Bioinformatics,
ICAR-IASRI, New Delhi-110 012

Introduction

Agriculture is the backbone of India's rural economy as two-third of the population lives in rural area and their source of income from farming. Low productivity of Indian agriculture is due to several factors such as inadequate updated knowledge, biotic, abiotic stress, climate change, weather parameters, problems in input supply management and availability, effective marketing strategy and poor investment in agriculture etc. Proper knowledge management and planning is required to guide or assist policy makers/extension professionals/ farmers for effective utilization of available resources to tackle the problems or issues related to biotic/abiotic stresses and market strategies.

The research and development on application of information and communication technology in agriculture (Agricultural Informatics) has a considerable influence on the agriculture production as well as better livelihood of farming community. It can play a significant role in maintaining viable information by storing and processing the diversified data, and dissemination of knowledge among stakeholders. This agricultural informatics can provide sustainable solution to increase agricultural production and helps to cope with the consequence of climate change and other management issues.

This chapter describes the priority areas, present status and challenges of research and development in agricultural informatics. At present, generally utility of information technology (IT) in agriculture is mainly restricted to researchers. This chapter focused on various approaches and opportunities for building an informatiion system for sharing agricultural and biodiversity resources in targeting all kinds of stakeholders such as farmers, extension professionals, agricultural researchers, educationists, industrialists and decision makers. Although, numbers of attempts were made to use ICT for generation and dissemination of agricultural knowledge to different stakeholders, but still country need major ICT enabled intervention for ensuring to increase production and productivity of agriculture. There are issues related to primary data collection, compilation and integration of secondary data and knowledge, sharing mechanism of data and knowledge, usage and availability of high performance computing, formulation of knowledge network, data processing and analysis, data modeling and forecasting, data storage and archival, system for automation and agriculture intelligence etc.

Primary Data Collection

Present Status and Challenges

☆ Traditional method is being continued.

☆ No standard practice of data sharing mechanism to directory of data sources and automated transaction process for request and acknowledgement.

☆ Lack of advance data collection devices.

☆ Lack of upgraded and new methodology, tools and techniques.

☆ Manual method for transformation of data into a required standard/ format.

☆ Non-availability of work flow for collection of diversified data from different sources and its integration.

☆ Standardization and development software tool for collecting/cataloguing of experimental/laboratory data.

Opportunities

☆ Exploiting opportunities using ICT enabled technologies for sensor based automated and semi-automated devices for data collection. Video and voice recorder, photos for qualitative data collection using mobile, tablet, electronic device, camera etc.

☆ Proper attribution and recognition of primary data resources, creators and curators including individuals as well as institutions. (weather, census, livestock census, land use patterns)

☆ Crowd sourcing for collecting data from different sources.

☆ Real-time data capture. (*e.g.* advance remote sensing data for grazing land/LUP, crop production)

☆ Providing advanced data collection facility and methodologies suitable for user based on ability. (web based, tale-services, mobile, tablet, handheld devices etc.)

☆ Developed precise and large volume data collection methodologies (eg. online herd management software, phenotypes data collection)

☆ Mobilize the diversified data collected from various sources, standardised and to make available promptly. (*e.g.* animal feed resources data- collecting from literature, crop production statistics, Land Use Pattern, livestock census, feed industries)

☆ Makes use of existing data resources as well as generating new data to address a specific problem.

☆ Common standards for data exchange and integration (nomenclature common portal for data exchange using XML based web services)

☆ Converting work flow into automated data collection system.

Compilation and Integration of Secondary Data and Knowledge

Present Status and Challenges

☆ Availability of wealth of data in printed forms and lying in isolated computers or incompatible digital formats or other native languages.

☆ Data and Knowledge of Indigenous technical knowledge, published materials, field surveys reports and observations (videos and audios).

☆ Valuable traditional agricultural knowledge and expertise in various local or native languages but not well documented and structured format.

☆ Workflow and automated tools for compilation, cleaning and integration.

Opportunities

☆ Data mining and semantic tools to convert the printed, unstructured and inaccessible data into digitalized and structured formats by harnessing the technology enabled Big Data.

☆ Collection of traditional indigenous technical knowledge and package of practice for commodity and location specific.

☆ Developing new methodologies and work flow on data mining to extract and document valuable knowledge.

☆ Conversion of existing knowledge from its native language to other Indian languages.

☆ Handling multiple languages for collecting data and information.

☆ Accelerating data digitalization, cleaning, compilation and integration.

☆ Data quality improvement and feedback mechanism.

Data and Knowledge Sharing

Present Status and Challenges

☆ Data and Knowledge gains more value when it is shared. No one is willing and ready to share the data generated from their studies/projects.

☆ Lack of improvement of technology and quality of knowledge without sharing and applying.

☆ Traditional paradigm of sharing scientific knowledge through publications is not sufficient to disseminate new technologies to the farming community.

☆ Cannot fill the gaps in our understanding without pooling of the data.

☆ Datasets are either built for a particular project or publication, and access is restricted; or sharing of data is neglected

☆ Inadequate infrastructure and technical support for sharing the data.

☆ Genomic research publications rely on primary data being deposited in common data storage.

☆ Open access policy/legislation for data sharing of government-funded projects.

☆ Advancement of Information and communication technologies enabled techniques for sharing of the data generated from laboratories of various organizations.

Opportunities

☆ Making awareness of data and knowledge sharing among stakeholders.

☆ Develop open access and reuse culture in research and production system of agriculture.

☆ Need to frame new policies for ensuring project data are made freely available to centralized database.

☆ Recommending and implementing a mechanism for citing data with URL.

☆ Support respecting and sharing traditional knowledge and practices by adapting the sharing culture and sustainable foundation for future research and decisions.

☆ Commitment to increase knowledge to strengthen agricultural system by making its data and information openly available.

☆ Data sharing address through permanent archives or national repositories will become part of the publication instead of just as citing or type of specimens.

☆ Share knowledge and exchange of data will create opportunities to involve more stakeholders in agricultural research and production system.

☆ Build shared expertise environment and incentives/credits and policies may be framed for sharing the data.

☆ Policies of information sharing have an impact on the sustainable use and conservation of agricultural biodiversity.

Agricultural Knowledge Network

Present Status and Challenges

☆ Agricultural research had long run and continuous culture of data collection, analysis, and annotating data, interpretation of results. The curation of knowledge base is main activity for documenting and dissemination of knowledge on new technologies and farm management activities.

☆ Although automated tools for curation of knowledge base are available but requires an experts' involvement for identifying and correcting errors. Thus, need to create an experts' network to support curation and annotation of knowledge.

☆ At present, no knowledge network exists in agricultural knowledge system for sharing and even existing weak linkages among researchers, farmers, industries policy makers, and public, private and NGO extension workers.

☆ Govt. of India initiated a project National Knowledge Network to support knowledge sharing in the country.

☆ No proper mechanism for curation of knowledge at institute level (intranet for knowledge curation), and requirement of strong functional linkages/ consortium between agricultural researchers, extension workers, farmers, industrialists and decision makers.

☆ Availability of cheap and fastcommunication technology can be used to develop knowledge network and share through social media apps.

Opportunities

☆ Framework to build agricultural knowledge network taking in all stakeholders.

☆ At institute/organization level, at least one knowledge expert may be nominated for knowledge network. Formulate his duties to collect and curate knowledge base at this level.

☆ Encourage people to contribute their expertise in improving the system and awareness about knowledge network.

☆ Need to frame mechanism for knowledge base curation (intranet) at institute level.

☆ The Network should support matrix and hierarchical mode structure, and value chain, domains and inter-domain wise.

☆ The network is state of converging and integration of information and communication technology keeps the information up-to-date and reliable

Persistent Data Storage and Archives

Present Status and Challenges

☆ There is no centralized and structured storage with the fixed function assignments

☆ Non availability of integrated data warehousing for diversified structures and data structure.

☆ Underlying data standards and its refinement.

✰ Local storage is not capable for Long-term preservation and open accessible.

✰ Useful and curated data in usable formats which are interoperable and compatible with other systems.

✰ Many of databases are already created and held in local systems or systems created for short-term projects, whose project is ended then making vulnerable or taken offline.

✰ Even when databases are still exist, data sources may disappear due to broken link or change in identifiers or protocols, or offline or unable to upgrade the system and non-availability of technical support.

✰ Handling of heterogeneous data structures, unstructured and multi-media data.

Opportunities

✰ IT Infrastructure development for long-term centralized data repositories.

✰ Centralized data repositories for all categories of data, along with consistent handling of metadata, identifiers, licences, tools and services.

✰ Significant planning, research and investment are required to deliver persistent repositories.

✰ Put in a place and ensure data are made freely and persistently available in appropriate and usable forms.

✰ Aggregating, integrating and bringing together into single database in the form distributed database structure.

✰ Standardization and ensuring the data can be understand and reused by both machines and humans across the systems and disciplines.

✰ Develop additional services to peer-review, re-annotation and to ensure that the data remain accessible.

✰ To create awareness among researchers and institutes on how best to organize their data for simple archiving.

✰ Enter data directly from field to central database and making field data should available immediately accessible in a moment it was collected.

✰ Creating architectures that can handle heterogeneous data structure and multi-media data.

High Performance Computing Facilities for Data Processing and Analysis

Present Status and Challenges

✰ Existing tools are restricted to small data sets and limited to local demand.

✰ Diversified computational tools at local system.

✰ Scientific data analysis and understanding is not proportional to what we have.

☆ Piece and duplication of demands of tools for local PC and difficult to procure and maintain. (need a tool, instead all comes with bundle)

☆ Lack of availability of all tools at single place with service support for analysis of agricultural research data.

☆ Parallel and distributed computing effort on digitisation, error detection, detecting redundancy, and correction, annotation, crowd sourcing data and analysis of data.

☆ Semantic annotations to store interpretations obtained from research (roughly, a combination of metadata labels and ontology items)

☆ Time and space complexities with Meta data.

Opportunities

☆ There is a need for centralized grid or cloud computational facilities with all required tools.

☆ Development of High Performance Computational (HPC) infrastructure for data integration, processing, fusion, analysis and mining, workflow development orchestration and execution, capture of provenance/origin, creation of lineage, knowledge extraction and its representation.

☆ Development of parallel, GPU enabled and distributed scientific analysis and processing tools.

☆ HPC broadly shares computer resources instead of using software or storage on a local PC. HPC can be utilized as new supplement, consumption and delivery model for IT services based on the public network.

☆ The centralized facility supports better resource management and effective cost control.

☆ Enabling environment to initiate and innovate IT infrastructure for agricultural models, services, and applications.

☆ Aids greater research focus on methodologies that emphasize user involvement.

☆ Leads centralized single window solution to store the data and computing facility enhances analysis capability and decipher the knowledge from the data.

☆ Promoting an interdisciplinary approach to facilitates integration of agricultural, omics data and weather parameters into complex scientific problems.

☆ Bringing together ideas, disciplines, people and organizations to provide single window solution for agricultural research and development.

☆ Development and usage of tools in collaborative mode is an opportunity to close the gap between disciplines, understanding and mobilizing available data.

☆ Developments and improvements in modelling and information processing with parallel mode to overcome time and space complexities

☆ It is possible to provide processing, analysis and presenting tools to wide range of users such as researches, farmers, students, industries and decision makers.

☆ Identity management and contribution tracking of various types of end users.

☆ Provides tools to support consistent and comprehensive results.

Projection and Estimation Models

Present Status and Challenges

☆ Existing projects and models are support only limited parameters

☆ Existing approaches have lack of advanced machine learning techniques, Big data analysis tools and methodologies

Opportunities

☆ Modelling for sustainable consumption and degrading of natural resources and habitats. The modelling will help to effectiveness of decision making and policies.

☆ Improved visualization and presentation tools to cater different needs of various categories of users.

☆ Modules to enable people and organizations to develop new projects based on current needs and offer support for particular activities.

☆ Models to assist for track projects, funding, ideas and framing project.

☆ Modules to generate thematic geographic information systems (GIS) maps on distribution of data and resources.

☆ Integrate historical data and identify the changes over time to create predictive modelling tools to support decision making, estimation and prediction the potential impact of changes.

☆ Build virtual models of KVK for knowledge sharing with collaboration with existing KVKs

☆ Phenology models to study the effect of plant and animal life cycle events which influenced by seasonal and inter-annual variations in climate.

☆ Automation of agricultural production with possible intervention factors such as input availability, resource requirements, weather etc.

☆ Optimisation model for crop production system to minimizing risk and financial investment, and maximizing profits

☆ Understanding evolutionary and ecological events to understand the present and build prediction models about future response over changing environment.

☆ Implementation of site specific prediction models.

☆ Modeling complex biological systems with the cells interaction network.

Automation and Work Flow

Present Status and Challenges

☆ Workflows are a good choice to help to automate the system

☆ Lack of semantic annotations to store and dessiminate the interpretations.

☆ Lack of knowledge on automated and semi-automated workflows, which helps to automate the system from data collection to knowledge re-presentation and visualizations.

☆ Lack of research on automation of agricultural production system (eg. Irrigation, fertilizer and pesticide application, harvesting and post harvesting process and etc.)

Opportunities

☆ Automation should be dynamic in nature and models can be customized based on external events/parameters and user interventions.

☆ Automated knowledge flow from Laboratory to field and vice-versa.

☆ Need to develop the technology wise impact analysis of tools and methodologies.

☆ Scientific workflows have emerged as a paradigm for representing and managing complex distributed scientific computations. Such workflows capture the individual data transformations and analysis steps as well as the mechanisms to carry them out in a distributed environment.

☆ Organized knowledge about individual organisms or commodities with integration of genetic data, traits, interactions, cultivation practices, ecological parameters will deliver an interconnected digital resource supporting scientific knowledge that will leads automated farming system.

Advanced Knowledge Dissemination System

Present Status and Challenges

☆ Many drawbacks in existing field extension system.

☆ Extension workers are not in adequate numbers and inadequate to update their knowledge to advice the farmers according to their needs and available resources with respect to new and improved technologies.

☆ Radio and Television: Irrelevance of knowledge delivered, does not cater to the needs of individual farm, timing and topics of broadcast clashing with farming activities. The information/knowledge is pushed to farmer in one direction and in turn receiving minimal or limited feed back.

☆ Krishi ghosti, Krishi mela, seminars, demonstration are essentially support large community of farmers and a few crops at a time.

☆ Magazines and new papers are out of reach to the majority of farmers who are illiterate or with low literacy level and inappropriate feedback

- ✩ Diversified IT based systems; available at different sources and in duplication.
- ✩ Several approaches have been made for develop and implement short-term projects but these are lying in the shelf or not updated or containing the irrelevant material.
- ✩ Developed using only inter-organizational information, does not consider inter-operatability, integration and exchange environment.

Opportunities

- ✩ User friendly knowledge presentation, visualization and dissemination system to access desire knowledge in their language from anywhere, anybody and at anytime to overcome existing extension system.
- ✩ Enabling interactive visualization tools with multi-media and multi-lingual support.
- ✩ Making all knowledge interlinked and accessible through the rich indexed system with literature, data, multimedia, graph, maps and other presentation forms.
- ✩ Need to engage specialists as game developers, graphics designer, web designers, and communications experts with the farming practice.
- ✩ Developing new interoperability standards for diversified electronic devices like mobile, computing, tablet, electronic gadget, etc. to maximize the usefulness of visualization tools and applications.
- ✩ Single window solution to provide desire knowledge to all range of users.

Benefits

- ✩ Helps to understand the status of the diversity of local crops and their farming practices which leads to a priority research task.
- ✩ Facilitate decision-making by individual, government and all stakeholders relating to the conservation and sharing of valuable genetic resources.
- ✩ Help farming communities minimize the risks associated with climate change.
- ✩ Helps to build scientific evidence for agricultural ecosystems.
- ✩ Diversification of crops due to changing markets, farming practices, environmental degradation and many other factors.
- ✩ Helps to increase value and quality of agricultural products to reduce transaction and storage costs.
- ✩ Provides improved and sophisticated media to extension workers.
- ✩ Strong linkage, single window system and consortia between farmers, researchers, students, extension workers, industries and decision and policy makers.
- ✩ Duplication of efforts of failure in technology innovation and implementation.

☆ Increasing agricultural productivity and improving livelihood in farming community

☆ Advices the farmers according to their needs with available resources in time, easy to use, cost effective to avoid knowledge distortion. (A4 - Any time, Any person, Any where and Accurate *i.e.*, the support in 24*7 manner)

☆ Provides information using multi-media technology (Text, Images, Maps, Audio, Video and Animation etc.) to increase use of smart phones.

☆ Acts as virtual extension unit and distance education to farming community

☆ Copyrights, trademarking of documents and protection of the technologies

☆ Educates the farmers to become e-literate.

☆ Establishment of strong functional linkages and consortium between agricultural researchers, extension workers, farmers, industrialists and decision makers.

Conclusion

The emergence of Information and Communication Technologies (ICT) in the last two decades has opened new avenues in research and development for application of information and communication technology in agriculture production system. This could play important roles in data collection, compilation, processing to generate knowledge, sharing, exchanging and disseminating among the researchers, farmers and policy makers. Discussed research areas will lead to a prevailing network to communicate, interact, and exchange knowledge and data, sharing computing facility, processing tools and data storage resources among stakeholders. Researches in informatics and development of IT infrastructure for agriculture have major impact on agricultural productivity. Systematic approach for knowledge generation about individual organisms or commodities with all interlinked records such as genetic data, traits, interactions with ecological parameters, the cultivable practices and market potential will deliver an interconnected digital resources supporting scientific knowledge, which will leads automated farming system.

References

A.K.Choubey (2009). ICT Initiatives in Agriculture by Government of India, Presented in FAI Workshop on 10-8-2009 at Ooty, Tamil Nadu.

Ranjeet Singh and S. Mangaraj (2006). Information Technology in Agriculture Present Scenario and Challenges, *Agricultural Engineering Today*, Vol. 30 (3).

Dhakshinamoorthy Maikandadevan (2012). Agricultural Research - Opportunities and Challenges, presented at Tamil Nadu Agricultural University on *Sep 27*.

M. A. Carravilla, J. F. Oliveira, (2013). Operations Research in Agriculture: Better Decisions for a Scarce and Uncertain World Agris on-line Papers in Economics and Informatics, Volume V, Number 2.

Richard Duncombe (2012). Mobile Phones for Agricultural and Rural Development: *A Literature Review and Future Research Directions* 2012 Published by: *Centre for Development Informatics*.

System Priorities for CGIAR Research 2005-2015 (2005). Report by CGIAR.

Zacharoula Andreopoulou *et al.*, (2011). Agricultural and Environmental Informatics, Governance and Management: Emerging Research Applications, Information Science Reference (an imprint of IGI Global).

Chapter 22
Database and Expert System on Animal Feed Resources: A Case Study

U.B. Angadi[1], S. Jash[2], Letha Devi[2] and S. Anandan[2]

[1]ICAR-IASRI, New Delhi-110 012
[2]ICAR-NIANP, Bangalore-560 030

Introduction

Sustaining the present population of livestock with the available feed resources and catering to the growing demand for livestock products triggered by the increasing income levels and changing food habits of the growing population is going to be a major challenge. In view of the multi-faceted role of livestock in promoting livelihoods, poverty alleviation, nutritional security, crop husbandry and its impact on land/water/environment, there is greater need for efficient management of resources in the livestock sector. Assessing the potential availability and requirements of feed resources is one of vital components in feed resource management. An updated feed inventory system helps in devising ways and means of optimal usage of available resources to sustain the requirements and livestock production.

The advances in Information and Communication Technologies (ICT) has provided new opportunities for ICT application in agriculture, particularly in storing and sharing data, information and knowledge about new technologies in agriculture. Unlike agriculture where many initiatives have been made, very limited attention and work has been given to the livestock sector. This chapter describes two software packages for sharing knowledge regarding livestock feed inventory and an expert system for feed formulation. 1) "FeedBase" is a Database that is user friendly providing visualization tool on district wise inventory of feed resources availability vis a vis the requirement and livestock distribution in the country. 2) "FeedAssist" is an expert system on scientific feeding of dairy animals based on production parameters from the available information on nutrient requirement and nutrient composition of feeds and fodder. These two packages were developed to cater to the needs of all stakeholder of India livestock sector represented by researches, policy/decision makers, feed industries, government departments and farmers.

'FeedBase' Availability and Requirement of Feed Resources in the Country

FEEDBASE is developed based on the premise that all the feeds are either linked to the crop production or the green biomass obtained from cultivated fodders and other categories of land. The total potential feed resources thus arrived is matched against the total feed requirements of the various categories of livestock in relation to their production potential either in quantitative terms of crop residues, greens and concentrates or qualitative terms of protein and energy. The availability of feeds is compared with the requirements of all the animals to arrive at the feed balance in terms of, adequate - where the potential availability is similar to the requirements, inadequate- where the requirements exceed the potential availability and surplus - where the potential feed availability exceeds the requirements. Using Visual BASIC as front-end tool (Figure 22.2) and MS-ACCESS as back-end tool user friendly software has been developed to access the information as per the user defined query. The approach of FEEDBASE in simple terms can be summarized in the following pictorial depiction.

Feed Resources

This module provides quantitative and qualitative availability of feeds at district, state and the country level based on crop production and land use patter statistics for period 1985 to 2012. Feed resources statistics module helps in assessing availability of animal feeds in the country and this is an essential decision support system for planning and decision making in livestock production and dairying. This has user friendly feed resources selection by tree structure, facilitating the user to choose the entire country with states as units or a state with the districts as units and for a particular period (year or series of years) (Figure 22.2). User can create a query as per his requirement and he can get the desired information in terms of class of feed resources (coarse straw, fine straw, leguminous straw, bran, chunni, cake and greens), states (all states) and districts (within each state), and the year. The information based on the customized requirement of the user is displayed in the form of table (Figure 22.3) and graphical (Figure 22.4) and GIS maps (Figure 22.5). This would be an important tool and aid for short term and long term planning for the policy makers, researchers and industries in improving the livestock productivity in the state/district.

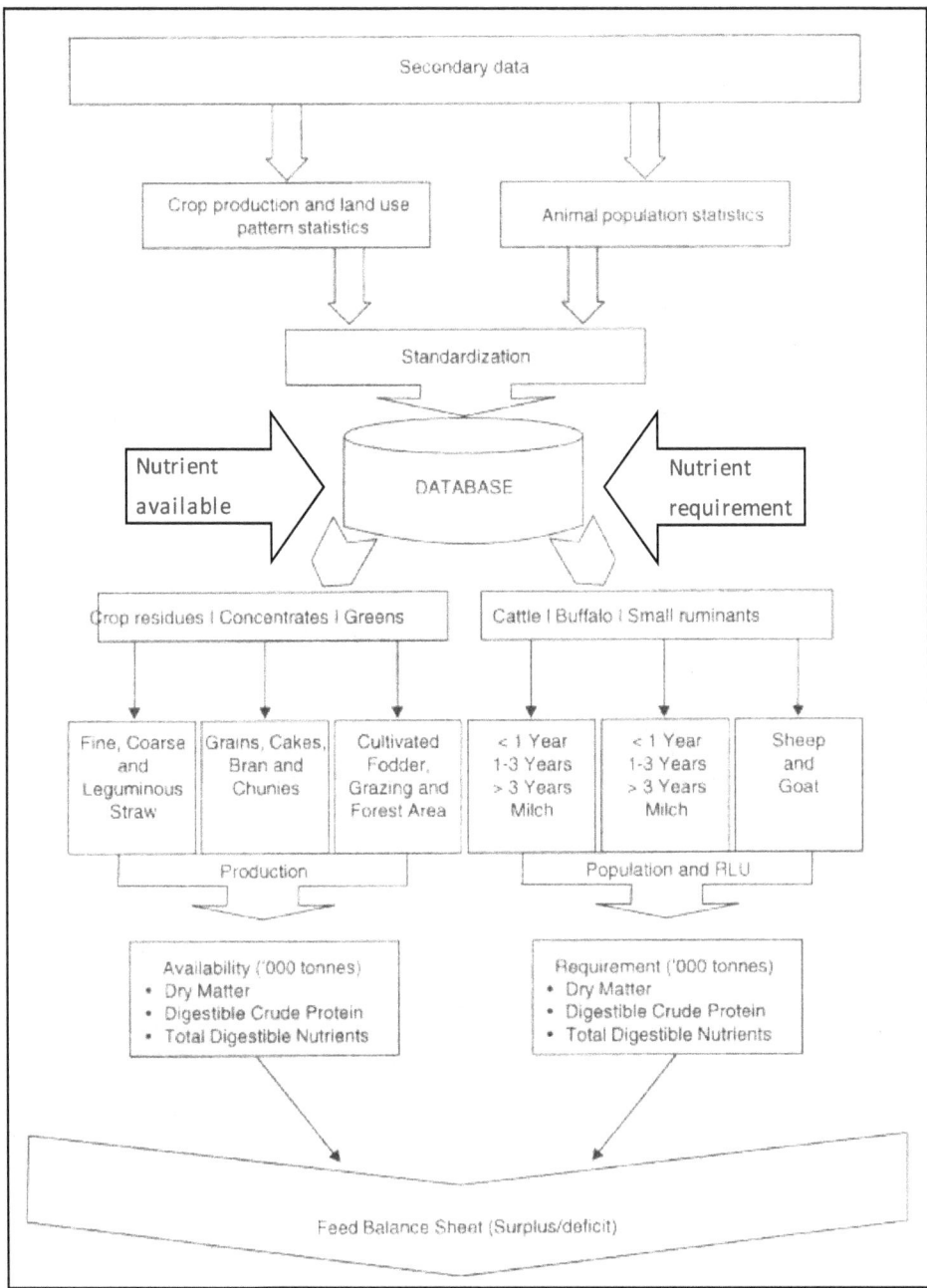

Figure 22.1: Flow Diagram.

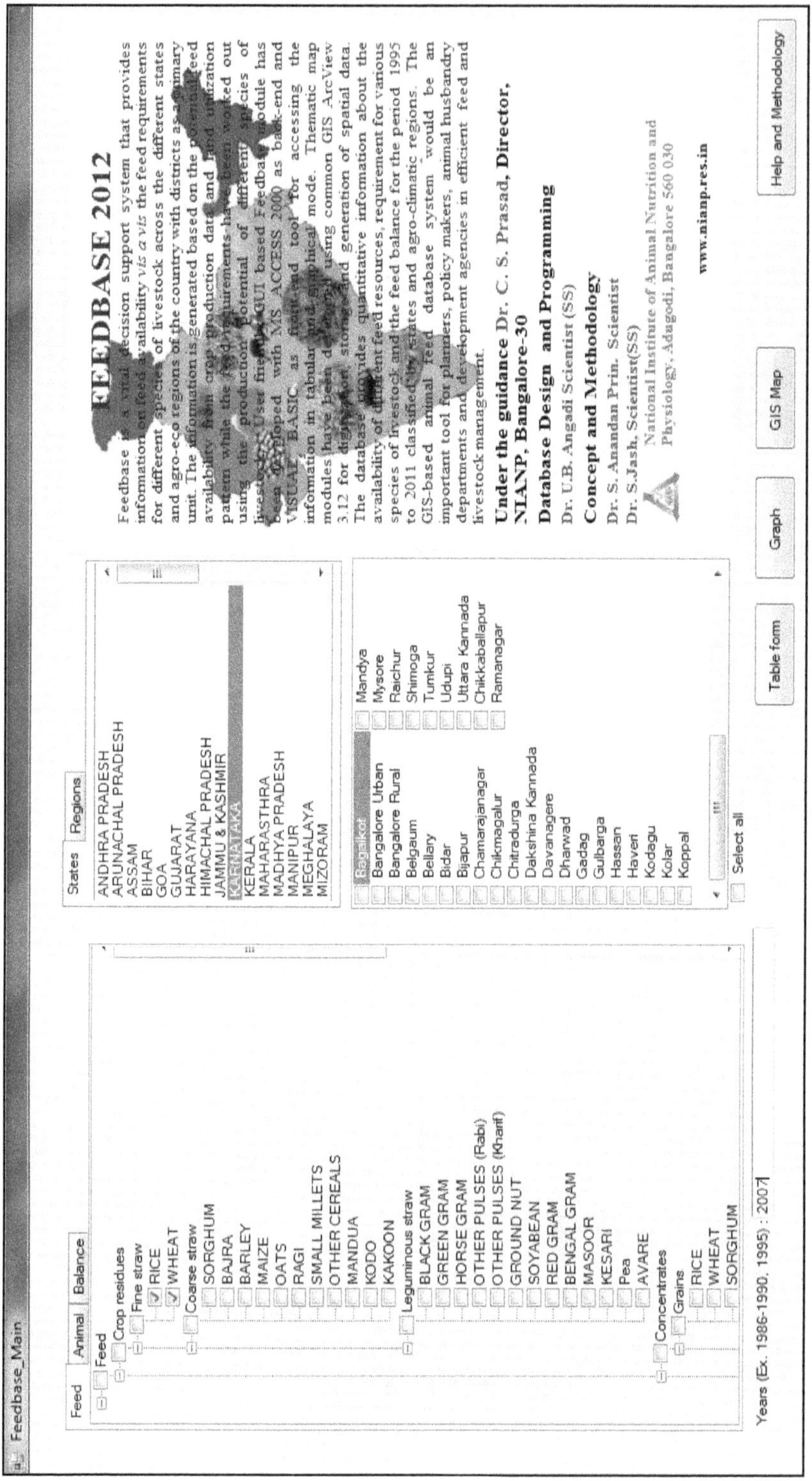

Figure 22.2: Feed Resource Main Screen.

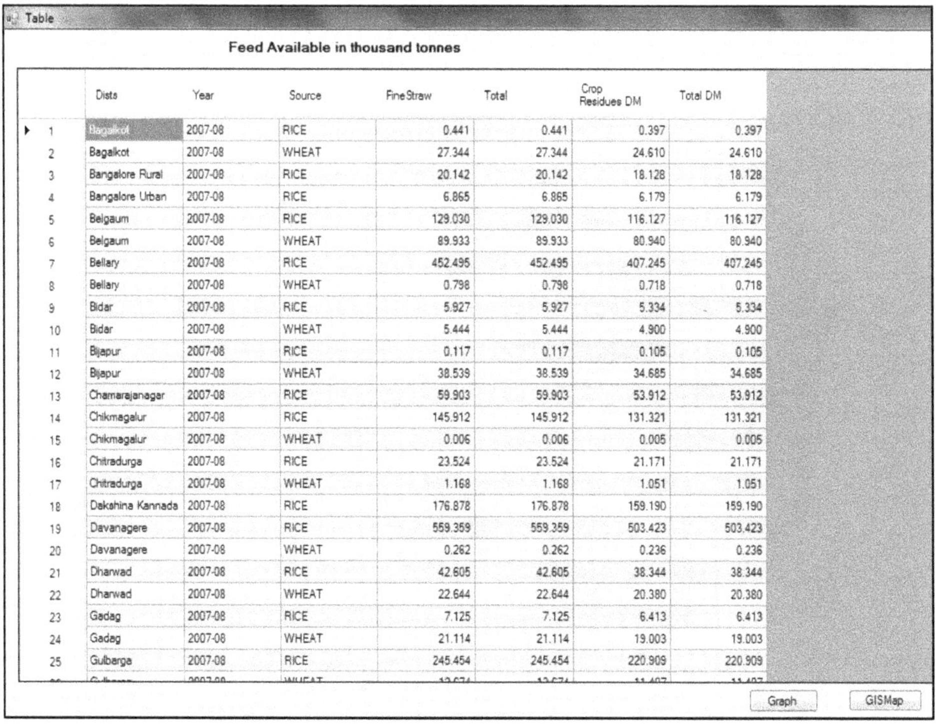

Table

Feed Available in thousand tonnes

	Dists	Year	Source	Fine Straw	Total	Crop Residues DM	Total DM
1	Bagalkot	2007-08	RICE	0.441	0.441	0.397	0.397
2	Bagalkot	2007-08	WHEAT	27.344	27.344	24.610	24.610
3	Bangalore Rural	2007-08	RICE	20.142	20.142	18.128	18.128
4	Bangalore Urban	2007-08	RICE	6.865	6.865	6.179	6.179
5	Belgaum	2007-08	RICE	129.030	129.030	116.127	116.127
6	Belgaum	2007-08	WHEAT	89.933	89.933	80.940	80.940
7	Bellary	2007-08	RICE	452.495	452.495	407.245	407.245
8	Bellary	2007-08	WHEAT	0.798	0.798	0.718	0.718
9	Bidar	2007-08	RICE	5.927	5.927	5.334	5.334
10	Bidar	2007-08	WHEAT	5.444	5.444	4.900	4.900
11	Bijapur	2007-08	RICE	0.117	0.117	0.105	0.105
12	Bijapur	2007-08	WHEAT	38.539	38.539	34.685	34.685
13	Chamarajanagar	2007-08	RICE	59.903	59.903	53.912	53.912
14	Chikmagalur	2007-08	RICE	145.912	145.912	131.321	131.321
15	Chikmagalur	2007-08	WHEAT	0.006	0.006	0.005	0.005
16	Chitradurga	2007-08	RICE	23.524	23.524	21.171	21.171
17	Chitradurga	2007-08	WHEAT	1.168	1.168	1.051	1.051
18	Dakshina Kannada	2007-08	RICE	176.878	176.878	159.190	159.190
19	Davanagere	2007-08	RICE	559.359	559.359	503.423	503.423
20	Davanagere	2007-08	WHEAT	0.262	0.262	0.236	0.236
21	Dharwad	2007-08	RICE	42.605	42.605	38.344	38.344
22	Dharwad	2007-08	WHEAT	22.644	22.644	20.380	20.380
23	Gadag	2007-08	RICE	7.125	7.125	6.413	6.413
24	Gadag	2007-08	WHEAT	21.114	21.114	19.003	19.003
25	Gulbarga	2007-08	RICE	245.454	245.454	220.909	220.909
	Gulbarga	2007-08	WHEAT	12.674	12.674	11.407	11.407

Graph   GISMap

Figure 22.3: Feed Resource Information in Table.

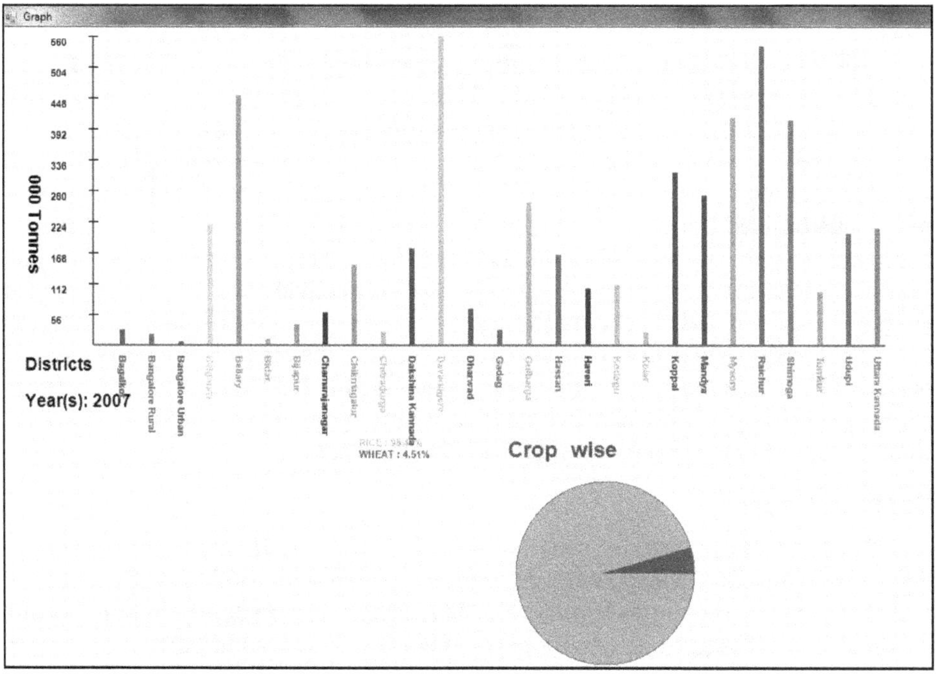

Figure 22.4: Feed Resource Information in Graph.

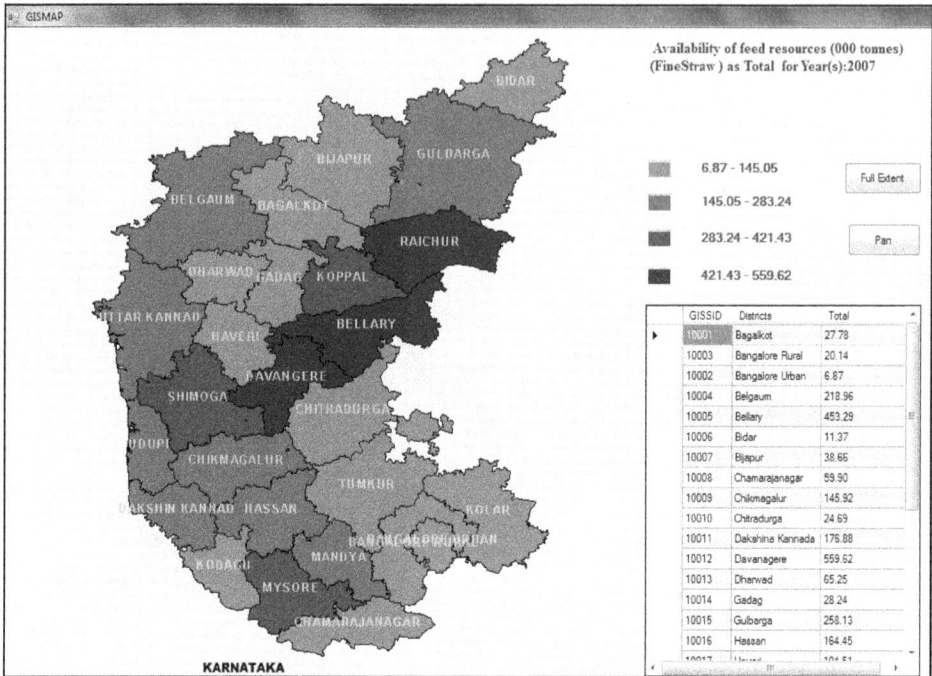

Figure 22.5: Feed Resource Information in GIS Map.

Animal Resources

This provides district wise quantitative and qualitative requirement of feeds based on the livestock census statistics for period 1985 to 2012. It contains animal census statistics that helps in assessing requirements of livestock feeds in the country and hence would be essential decision support system for planning and decision making in livestock production and dairying. The module has facility to define customized query by user using GUI tool (Figure 22.6) with tree structure based animal and category selection. Similar to feed resources statistics; list box and selection boxes for state and districts selection respectively and text entry box for years are provided. After defining the query the user can get the desired information about feed requirement for the selected category of the animals, districts and the period. The information is displayed in table (Figure 22.7) and graphical (Figure 22.8) and GIS map (Figure 22.9) forms. This would be an important tool and aid for short term and long term planning for livestock sector.

Balance Sheet

This module provides information on availability and requirement in terms of dry, green, concentrate feed resources and nutrient in terms of DM, TDN and DCP at district, state and country level for particular year (Figure 22.10). In this module user has to select region such district(s) or state(s) or country and particular year(s). It also has provision to present information in tabular (Figure 22.11), graphical

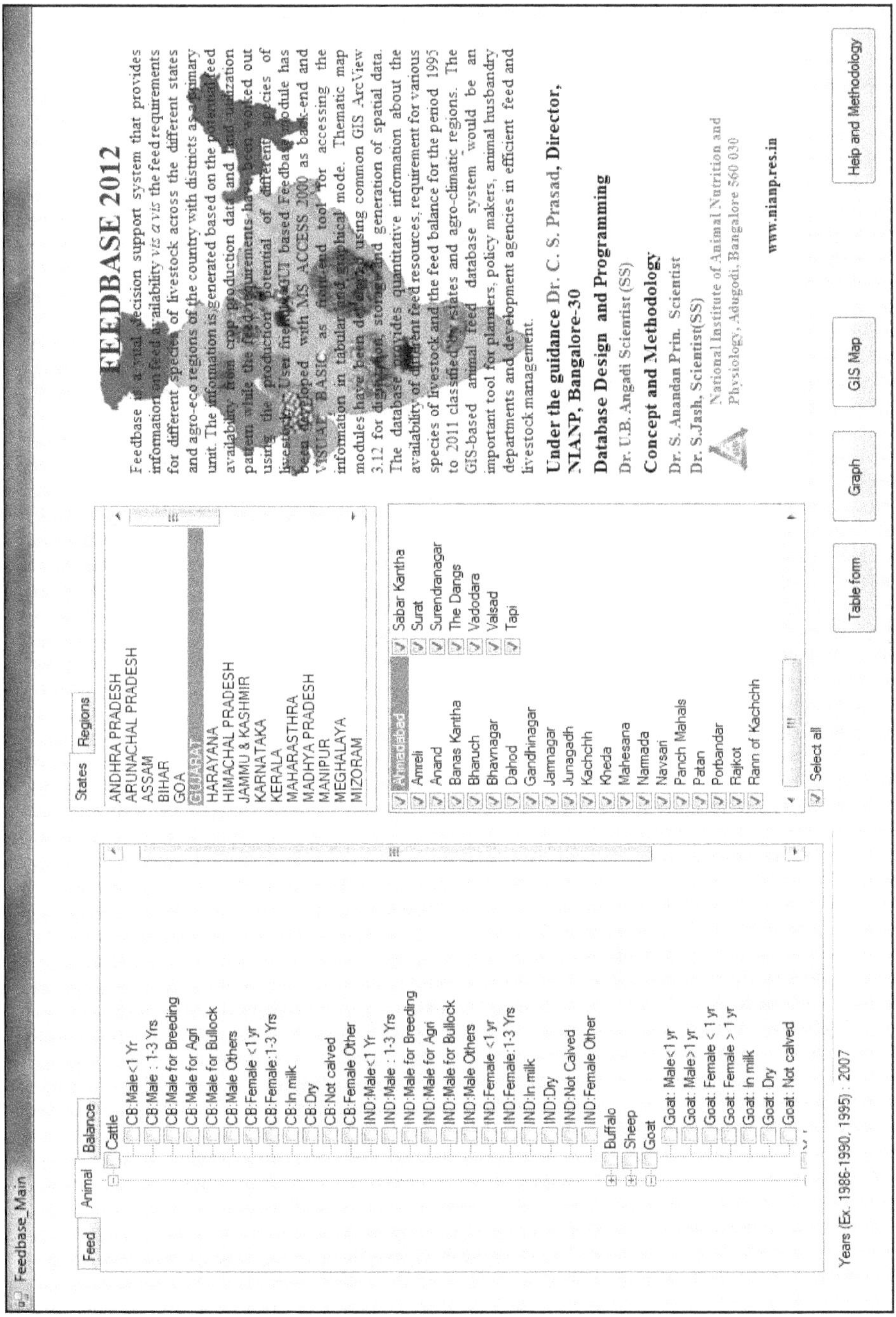

FEEDBASE 2012

Feedbase is a vital decision support system that provides information on feed availability *vis à vis* the feed requirements for different species of livestock across the different states and agro-eco regions of the country with districts as a primary unit. The information is generated based on the present feed availability, feed crop production data and feed utilization pattern while the feed requirements have been worked out using the production potential of different species of livestock. User friendly GUI based Feedbase module has been developed with MS ACCESS 2000 as back-end and VISUAL BASIC as front-end tool for accessing the information in tabular and graphical mode. Thematic map modules have been developed using common GIS ArcView 3.12 for display, storage and generation of spatial data. The database provides quantitative information about the availability of different feed resources, requirement for various species of livestock and the feed balance for the period 1995 to 2011 classified by states and agro-climatic regions. The GIS-based animal feed database system would be an important tool for planners, policy makers, animal husbandry departments and development agencies in efficient feed and livestock management.

Under the guidance Dr. C. S. Prasad, **Director, NIANP, Bangalore-30**

Database Design and Programming

Dr. U.B. Angadi Scientist (SS)

Concept and Methodology

Dr. S. Anandan Prin. Scientist
Dr. S.Jash. Scientist(SS)

National Institute of Animal Nutrition and Physiology, Adugodi, Bangalore 560 030

www.nianp.res.in

Feedbase_Main

Feed | Animal | Balance

States | Regions

States list: ANDHRA PRADESH, ARUNACHAL PRADESH, ASSAM, BIHAR, GOA, GUJARAT, HARYANA, HIMACHAL PRADESH, JAMMU & KASHMIR, KARNATAKA, KERALA, MAHARASHTRA, MADHYA PRADESH, MANIPUR, MEGHALAYA, MIZORAM

Regions: Ahmadabad, Amreli, Anand, Banas Kantha, Bharuch, Bhavnagar, Dahod, Gandhinagar, Jamnagar, Junagadh, Kachchh, Kheda, Mahesana, Namada, Navsari, Panch Mahals, Patan, Porbandar, Rajkot, Rann of Kachchh, Sabar Kantha, Surat, Surendranagar, The Dangs, Vadodara, Valsad, Tapi

Select all

Cattle: CB:Male<1 Yr, CB:Male :1-3 Yrs, CB:Male for Breeding, CB:Male for Agri, CB:Male for Bullock, CB:Male Others, CB:Female <1 yr, CB:Female:1-3 Yrs, CB:In milk, CB:Dry, CB:Not calved, CB:Female Other, IND:Male<1 Yr, IND:Male :1-3 Yrs, IND:Male for Breeding, IND:Male for Agri, IND:Male for Bullock, IND:Male Others, IND:Female <1yr, IND:Female:1-3 Yrs, IND:In milk, IND:Dry, IND:Not Calved, IND:Female Other

Buffalo

Sheep

Goat: Goat: Male<1 yr, Goat: Male>1 yr, Goat: Female < 1 yr, Goat: Female > 1 yr, Goat: In milk, Goat: Dry, Goat: Not calved

Years (Ex. 1986-1990, 1995) : 2007

Table form | Graph | GIS Map | Help and Methodology

Figure 22.6: Animal Resources Main Screen.

Population in actuals and feed requirement (Dry Matter) in tonnes

	Dists	Year	Animal	Category	Population	Crop Residues	Concentrate	Greens	Total
1	Ahmadabad	2007-08	CATTLE	CB:Male<1 Yr	1314	143.883	1007.181	287.766	1438.830
2	Ahmadabad	2007-08	CATTLE	CB:Male : 1-3 Yrs	934	613.638	511.365	920.457	2045.460
3	Ahmadabad	2007-08	CATTLE	CB:Male for Bree...	352	598.074	85.439	170.878	854.392
4	Ahmadabad	2007-08	CATTLE	CB:Male for Agri	427	725.505	103.644	207.287	1036.436
5	Ahmadabad	2007-08	CATTLE	CB:Male for Bullo...	185	314.329	44.904	89.808	449.041
6	Ahmadabad	2007-08	CATTLE	CB:Male Others	112	190.296	27.185	54.370	271.852
7	Ahmadabad	2007-08	CATTLE	CB:Female <1 yr	2633	288.314	2018.195	576.627	2883.135
8	Ahmadabad	2007-08	CATTLE	CB:Female:1-3 Yrs	2738	1798.866	1499.055	2698.299	5996.220
9	Ahmadabad	2007-08	CATTLE	CB:Dry	2111	3586.747	512.392	1024.785	5123.925
10	Ahmadabad	2007-08	CATTLE	CB:Not calved	830	1410.232	201.462	402.924	2014.618
11	Ahmadabad	2007-08	CATTLE	CB:Female Other	283	480.838	68.691	137.382	686.912
12	Ahmadabad	2007-08	CATTLE	IND:Male<1 Yr	13562	1782.047	6237.164	891.023	8910.234
13	Ahmadabad	2007-08	CATTLE	IND:Male : 1-3 Yrs	9627	3953.087	3294.239	5929.630	13176.956
14	Ahmadabad	2007-08	CATTLE	IND:Male for Bre...	2464	2922.920	449.680	1124.200	4496.800
15	Ahmadabad	2007-08	CATTLE	IND:Male for Agri	13021	15446.161	2376.333	5940.831	23763.325
16	Ahmadabad	2007-08	CATTLE	IND:Male for Bull...	4549	5396.251	830.193	2075.481	8301.925
17	Ahmadabad	2007-08	CATTLE	IND:Male Others	1195	1417.569	218.088	545.219	2180.875
18	Ahmadabad	2007-08	CATTLE	IND:Female <1 yr	28804	3784.846	13246.960	1892.423	18924.228
19	Ahmadabad	2007-08	CATTLE	IND:Female:1-3 Yrs	26587	10917.287	9097.739	16375.930	36390.956
20	Ahmadabad	2007-08	CATTLE	IND:Dry	31804	37727.495	5804.230	14510.575	58042.300
21	Ahmadabad	2007-08	CATTLE	IND:Not Calved	7127	8454.404	1300.678	3251.694	13006.775
22	Ahmadabad	2007-08	CATTLE	IND:Female Other	2769	3284.726	505.343	1263.356	5053.425
23	Ahmadabad	2007-08	Cattle	CB:In milk	5513	9121.810	6071.467	6511.404	21704.681
24	Ahmadabad	2007-08	Cattle	IND:In milk	58000	59264.400	26152.200	54044.400	139461.000
25	Amreli	2007-08	CATTLE	CB:Male<1 Yr	299	32.741	229.184	65.481	327.405

Graph   GISMap

Figure 22.7: Animal Resource Information in Table.

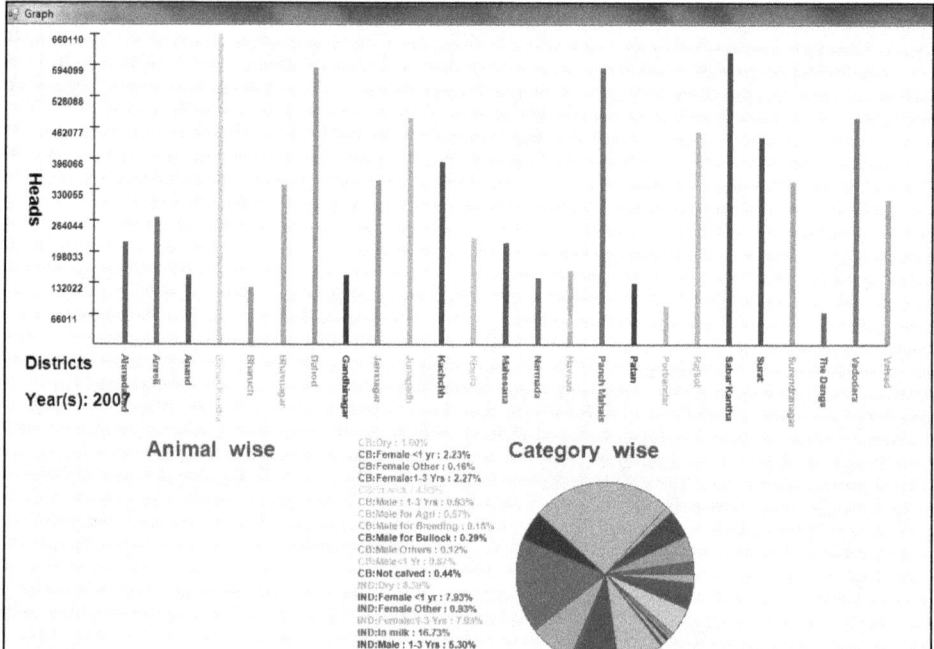

Figure 22.8: Information in Graphical Form.

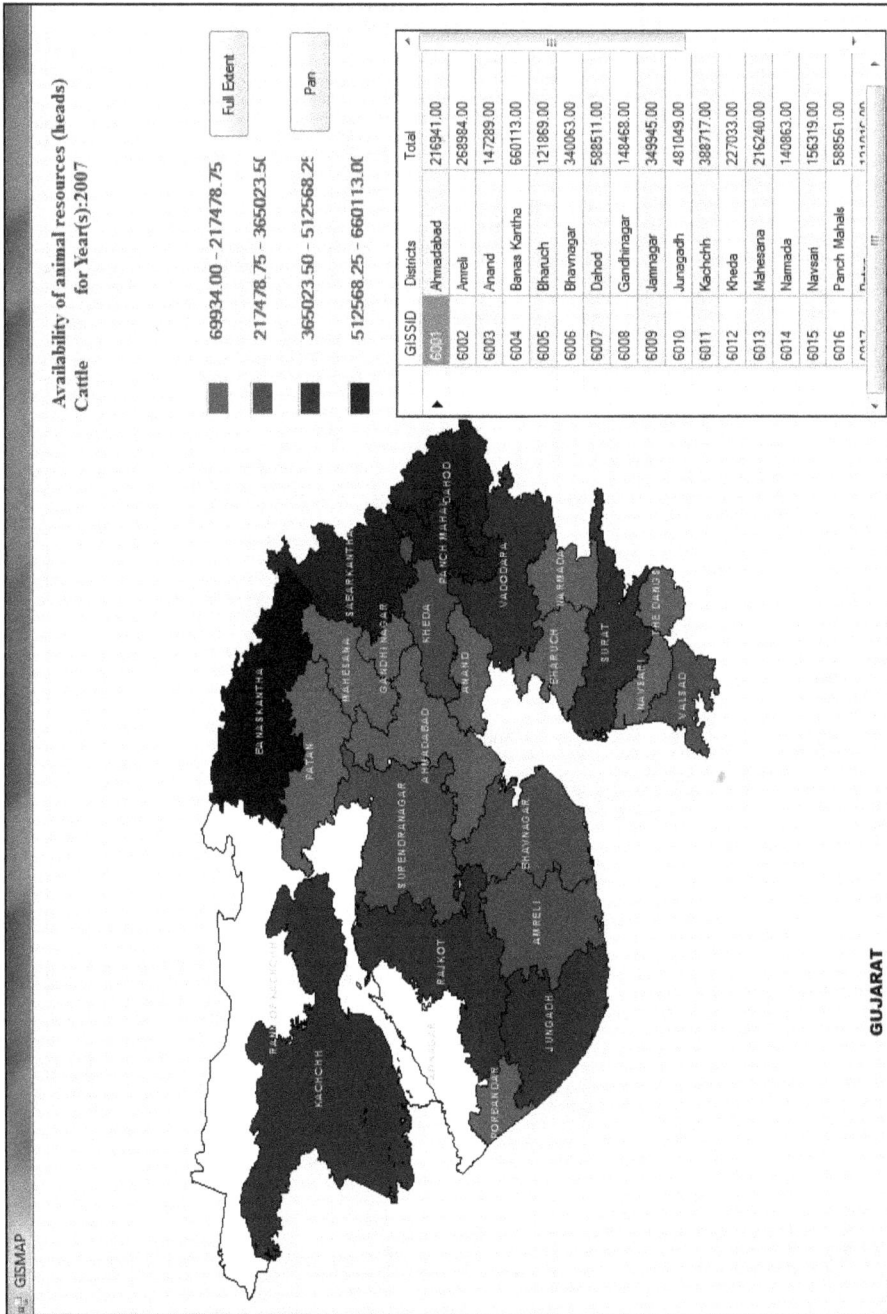

Figure 22.9: Animal Resource Information in GIS.

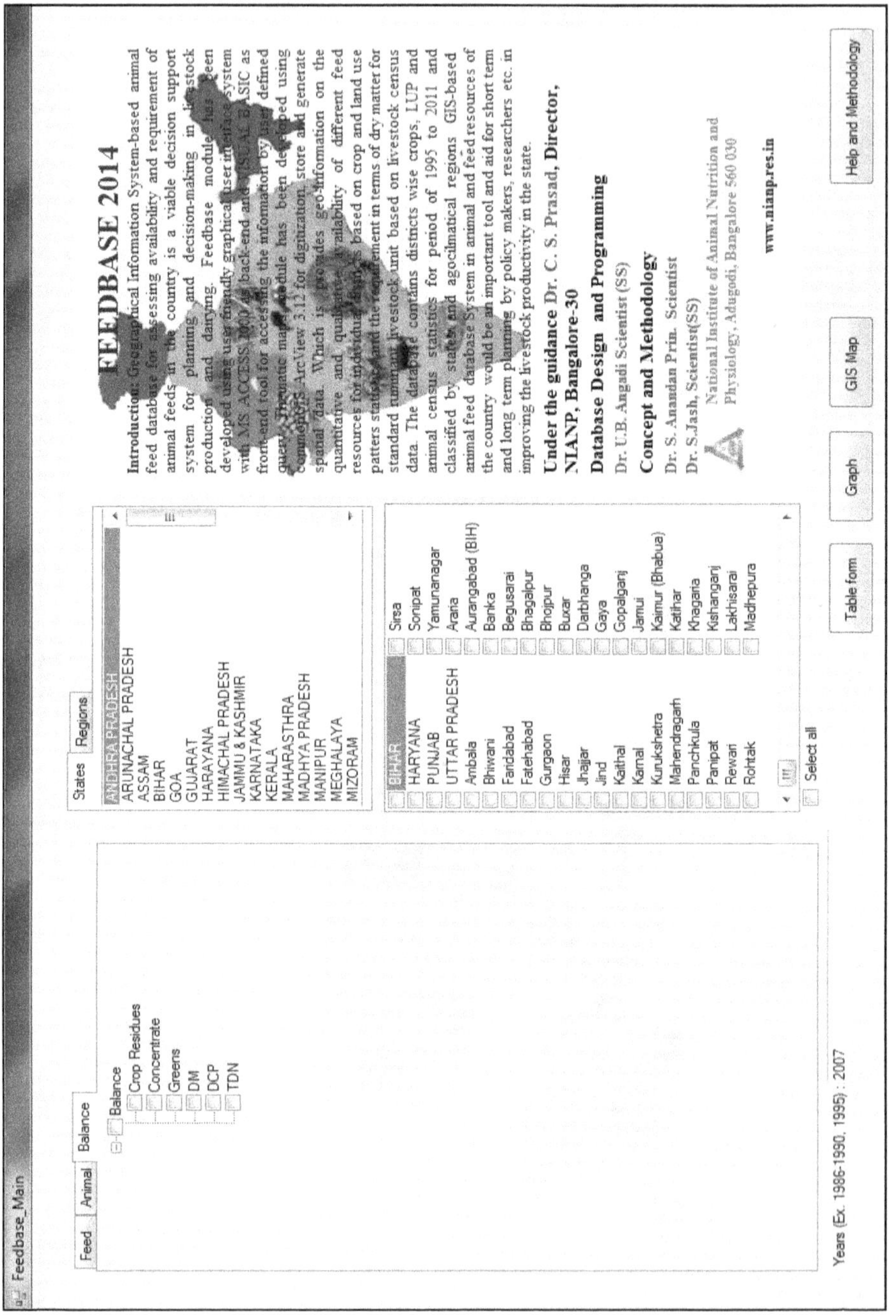

FEEDBASE 2014

Introduction: Geographical Information System-based animal feed database for assessing availability and requirement of animal feeds in the country is a viable decision support system for planning and decision-making in livestock production and dairying. Feedbase module has been developed using user friendly graphical user interface system with MS ACCESS 2007 back end and VBA & BASIC as frontend tool for accessing the information by user defined query. Thematic map module has been developed using ESRI's ArcView 3.13 for digitization, store & generate spatial data. Which provides geo-information on the quantitative and qualitative availability of different feed resources for individual taluka based on crop and land use patters statewise around the requirement in terms of dry matter for standard ruminant livestock unit based on livestock census data. The database contains districts wise crops, LUP and animal census statistics for period of 1995 to 2011 and classified by states and agoclimatical regions GIS-based animal feed database System in animal and feed resources of the country would be an important tool and aid for short term and long term planning by policy makers, researchers etc. in improving the livestock productivity in the state.

Under the guidance Dr. C. S. Prasad, Director, NIANP, Bangalore-30

Database Design and Programming

Dr. U.B. Angadi Scientist (SS)

Concept and Methodology

Dr. S. Anandan Prin. Scientist

Dr. S.Jash, Scientist(SS)

National Institute of Animal Nutrition and Physiology, Adugodi, Bangalore 560 030

www.nianp.res.in

States | Regions

ANDHRA PRADESH
ARUNACHAL PRADESH
ASSAM
BIHAR
GOA
GUJARAT
HARYANA
HIMACHAL PRADESH
JAMMU & KASHMIR
KARNATAKA
KERALA
MAHARASTHRA
MADHYA PRADESH
MANIPUR
MEGHALAYA
MIZORAM

BIHAR
HARYANA
PUNJAB
UTTAR PRADESH
Ambala
Bhiwani
Faridabad
Fatehabad
Gurgaon
Hisar
Jhajjar
Jind
Kaithal
Karnal
Kurukshetra
Mahendragarh
Panchkula
Panipat
Rewari
Rohtak

Sirsa
Sonipat
Yamunanagar
Araria
Aurangabad (BIH)
Banka
Begusarai
Bhagalpur
Bhojpur
Buxar
Darbhanga
Gaya
Gopalganj
Jamui
Kaimur (Bhabua)
Katihar
Khagaria
Kishanganj
Lakhisarai
Madhepura

Select all

Feedbase_Main

Feed | Animal | Balance

Balance
Crop Residues
Concentrate
Greens
DM
DCP
TDN

Years (Ex. 1986-1990, 1995) : 2007

Table form | Graph | GIS Map | Help and Methodology

Figure 22.10: Balance Sheet Main Screen.

Balance Sheet   Units in tonnes

	Dists Dists	YCODE	Crop Residues DM Available	Crop Residues DM Required	Crop Residues DM Balance	Concentrate DM Available	Concentrate DM Required	Concentrate DM Balance	Green DM Available	Greens DM Required	Greens DM Balance	To Av
1	Ambala	2007	604521.00	426545.93	177975.07	57645.90	217590.19	-159944.29	161107.82	382216.08	-221108.26	
2	Bhiwani	2007	1176480.00	795064.98	381415.02	214956.09	365024.02	-150067.93	389471.86	712441.50	-322963.54	
3	Faridabad	2007	502992.00	643801.34	-140809.34	47791.80	306540.16	-258748.36	132075.75	589168.26	-457092.52	
4	Fatehabad	2007	1201761.00	535375.30	666385.70	212662.89	234185.06	-21522.17	218030.07	455927.38	-237897.31	
5	Gurgaon	2007	338461.00	243565.58	94915.42	36954.90	147655.13	-110700.23	61531.44	232371.17	-170839.73	
6	Hisar	2007	1329570.00	894855.72	434714.28	253707.48	426340.55	-172633.07	335261.65	756069.05	-420807.40	
7	Jhajjar	2007	501120.00	391931.99	109188.01	73600.65	189759.66	-116159.01	137298.89	361184.89	-223886.00	
8	Jind	2007	1348263.00	849953.43	498309.57	146953.71	452284.33	-305330.62	266108.86	705210.58	-439101.72	
9	Kaithal	2007	1291419.00	662713.69	628705.31	114267.24	297480.01	-183212.77	202253.73	560257.12	-358003.39	
	Karnal	2007	1327599.00	746400.58	581198.42	117188.10	493740.68	-376552.58	264198.32	646169.60	-381971.29	
	Kurukshetra	2007	978930.00	494886.36	484043.64	90207.00	273568.66	-183361.66	204715.06	437870.31	-233155.25	
	Mahendragarh	2007	531126.00	378804.99	152321.01	107562.24	179102.34	-71540.10	140953.33	358652.57	-217699.24	
	Panchkula	2007	116055.00	144850.58	-28795.58	15034.50	289771.69	-274737.19	29887.72	126082.57	-97174.85	
	Panipat	2007	562698.00	428731.00	133967.00	51199.20	232714.47	-181515.27	141714.57	376614.48	-234899.92	
	Rewari	2007	385596.00	292351.79	93244.21	82659.78	144405.45	-61745.67	102106.69	273123.05	-171016.36	
	Rohtak	2007	500517.00	461906.95	38610.05	61452.36	223267.08	-161814.72	171828.94	410197.48	-238368.54	
	Sirsa	2007	1330893.00	732007.65	598885.35	366076.35	332266.09	33810.26	362879.52	635468.87	-272589.36	2
	Sonipat	2007	849600.00	616586.19	233013.81	80594.46	324252.96	-243658.50	215658.57	547178.18	-331519.62	
	Yamunanagar	2007	533394.00	461692.85	71701.15	50691.60	264983.69	-214292.09	292722.92	406692.69	-113969.77	
	Mewat	2007	372366.00	500680.68	-128314.68	50738.40	236598.09	-185859.69	120886.57	467494.34	-346607.77	
*	Tot		15783381.00	10702707.59	5080673.41	2231944.65	5631530.30	-3399585.65	3949692.22	9440370.16	-5490677.94	21

Figure 22.11: Balance Sheet.

(Figure 22.12) and GIS Maps (Figure 22.13) form. It depicts information in very comprehensive manner with gradient color graphs and maps to characterize surplus, deficient and sufficient areas.

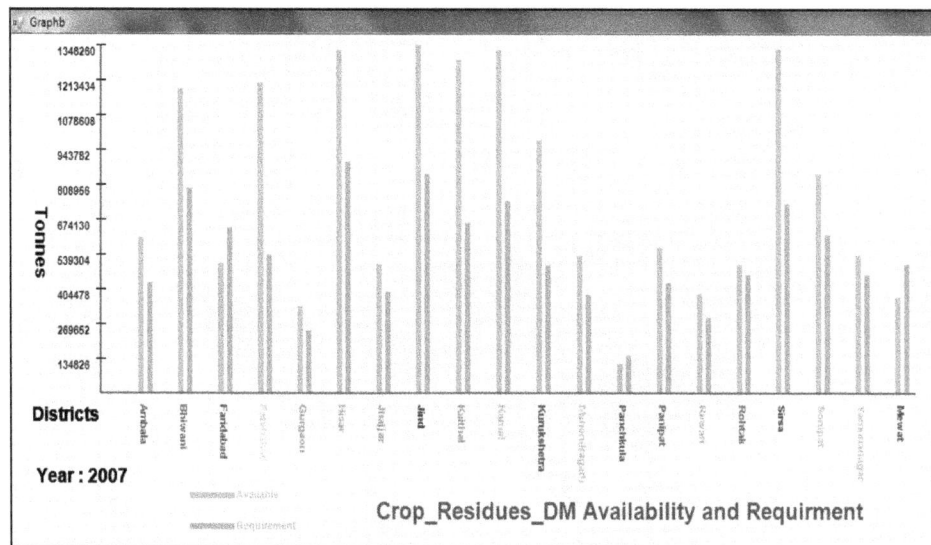

Figure 22.12: Feed Balance in Graphical Form.

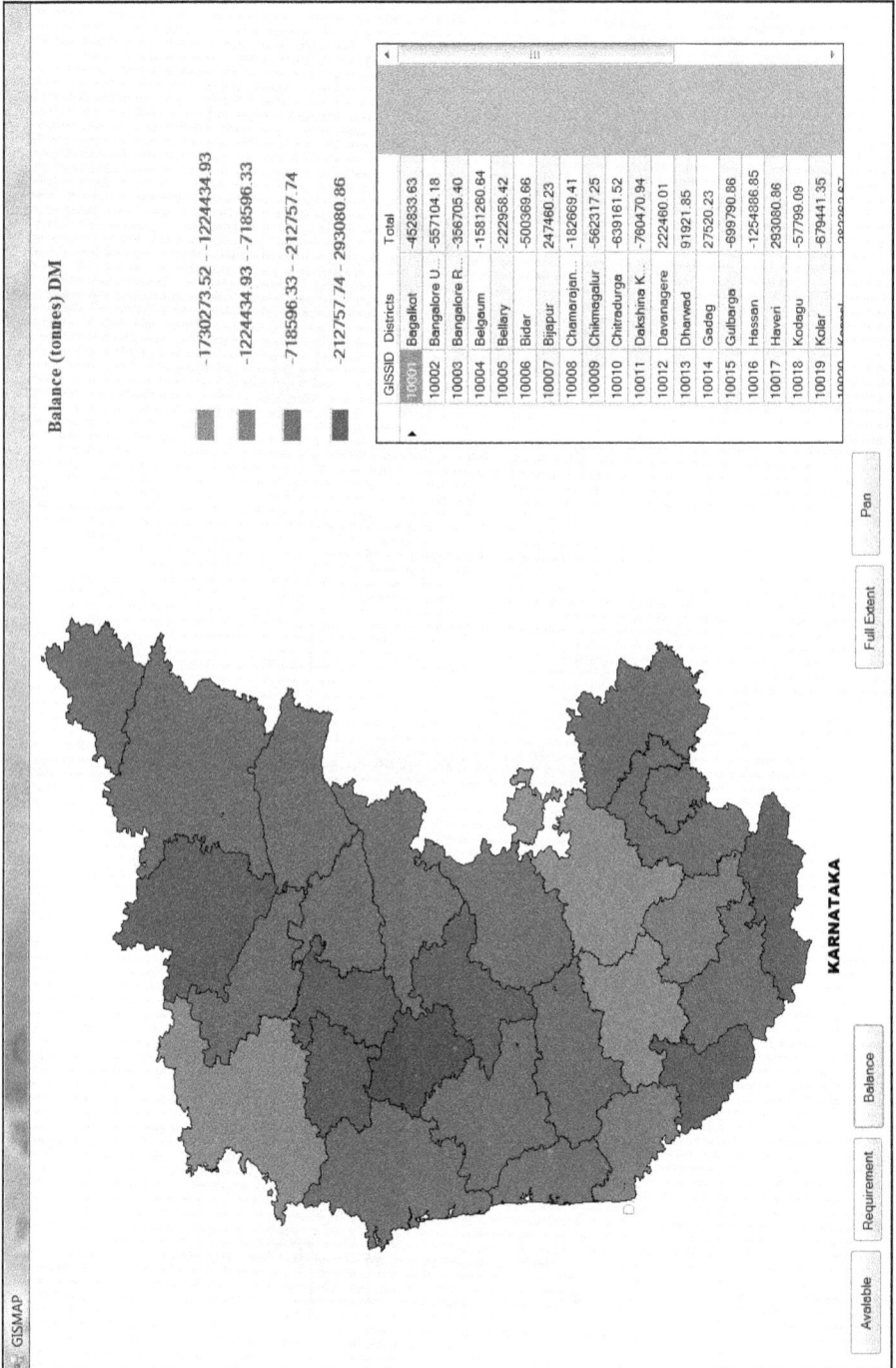

GISSID	Districts	Total
10001	Bagalkot	452833.63
10002	Bangalore U.	-557104.18
10003	Bangalore R...	-356705.40
10004	Belgaum	-1581260.64
10005	Bellary	-222958.42
10006	Bidar	-500369.66
10007	Bijapur	247460.23
10008	Chamrajan.	-182669.41
10009	Chikmagalur	-562317.25
10010	Chitradurga	-639161.52
10011	Dakshina K..	-760470.94
10012	Davanagere	222460.01
10013	Dharwad	91921.85
10014	Gadag	27520.23
10015	Gulbarga	-699790.86
10016	Hassan	-1254886.85
10017	Haveri	293080.86
10018	Kodagu	-57799.09
10019	Kolar	-679441.35

Balance (tonnes) DM

-1730273.52 – -1224434.93

-1224434.93 – -718596.33

-718596.33 – -212757.74

-212757.74 – 293080.86

KARNATAKA

Figure 22.13: Feed Resource Balance in GIS Map.

'FeedAssist': An Expert System for Balance Feeding Dairy Animals

In India, a major factor responsible for low productivity in livestock is usually attributed to animals with low genetic potential and feed shortage/poor feeding practices. With regard to the feeding practices more often the level of awareness among the end users – farmers, regarding the information on the nutrient contents of feeds (quality), their proportions to be fed for various production levels and other issues in feeding management of livestock is low and generally is overlooked or neglected. "Feed Assist": an expert system on balanced feeding for cattle and buffaloes uses linear programming for optimizing feed formulation at least cost. This enables the farmers to formulate least cost rations as per the nutrient requirements for his animal using a choice of the feed resources available with him. The categories of animals include calf, growing animals, pregnant, lactating, dry and working animals. By choosing the feed ingredients and providing the details of the animal with respect to the parameters like milk yield, body weight and growth rate the farmer can obtain a balanced diet that gives the details of different ingredients and their proportions to be fed.

Method

The least cost optimization program is developed based on Linear Programming Problem (LPP) for optimizing feed diet/ration at least cost. This is a mathematical algorithm to find the least-cost feeds that satisfy the nutritional requirements.

Database

Feed resources data with compositions and nutrient requirements in terms of DM, TDN and CP for cattle and buffalo have been collected from literature on different categories of animals(calf, growing animals, pregnant, lactating dry and working) and other parameters such as body weight, average growth rate and milk yield. Collected data was standardized, compiled to non-redundant data set and elicited standard formula to calculate feed requirements as per end-user defined animal parameters A database has been developed with various tables in MS-Access and integrated those based on RDBMS concept. The data has been uploaded into the database

Software

A VISUAL BASIC program has been written to compute balance ration for dairy animals in least cost ration as per the nutrient requirements of selected animal with nutrient profile of selected feed ingredients.A multi-lingual user and farmer friendly graphical user interface (GUI) module (Figure 22.14) has been developed to provide the details of the animal with respect to the categories and to the parameters like body weight, average daily growth rate and milk yield by user, and choose the feed resourcesb from the master list of commonly used feed resources. Based on selection of animal category and other parameters, it provides information of nutrient requirement in terms of DM, CP and TDN for maintenance, growth and production. This front end module has provision to change price of feeds stuffs and

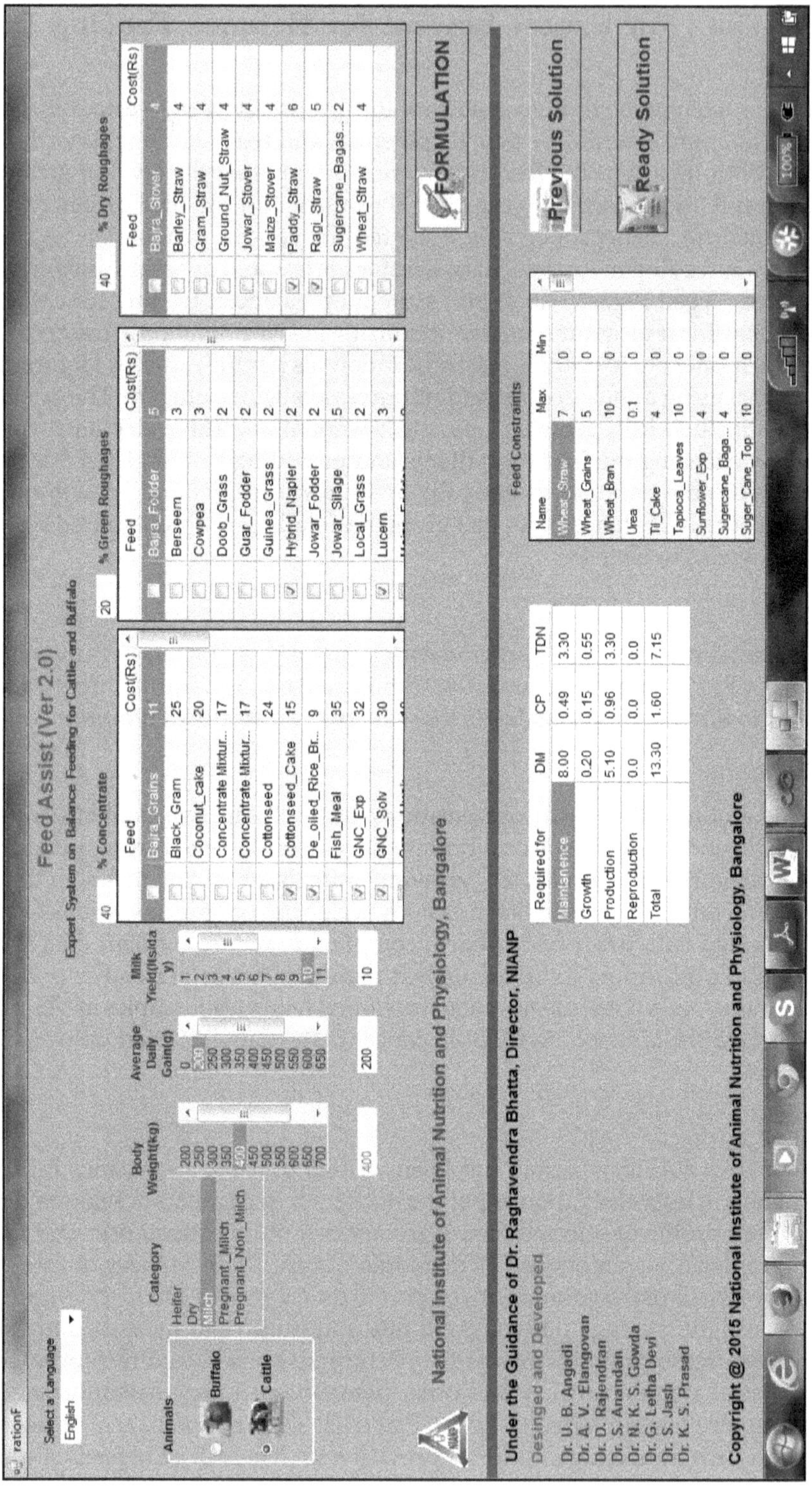

Figure 22.14: Feed Assist Main Screen.

also has facility to add, delete and modify feeds master database with local available feeds and fodders. The provision has been made for end-user to change ratio of feed components on availability as per seasonal deviation such as concentrate, greens and dry roughages. User can set constraints for fitting maximum and minimum quantity to a particular category of animal and feed ingredient. After providing animal details and selecting feed ingredients user can find solution by clicking on formulation icon that gives details of ingredients with proportion and cost of diet.

Features of Software and Steps for Formulation

a) Selection of animal category as per body weight and production status like growth or milk yield.

b) Selection of feed recourses available

c) Click on Formulation

Farmer can obtain solution by clicking FORMULATION icon and the solution will be displayed on Final Result form. The Final Result form (Figure 22.15) will represent information on selected and required feeds as balance ration with total cost of diet, nutrient requirements as per details of selected animal and nutrient available from diet. This information is presented in tabular and graphical form for easy analysis of nutrients available against requirements. Cost and feed quantity sharing in diet is depicted by pie diagram with provision to store the solution for feature use and retrieval.

The main features of the expert system which has been made user friendly are;

☆ Date maintenance – provides addition, deletion and modification of feed ingredients in the feed master table with nutrient compositions and price of feeds. Very easy system to manage ingredient composition database and editing of cost. A simple double click on feeds list box would open Feed Master Form and user can incorporate desired changes in the feeds master table.

☆ Easy to use – no need of special training and assistant to operate the system. Enhanced with touch screen user interface like ATM operation. A very easy and friendly interface to calculate nutrient requirements for various categories of animals

☆ Multi-lingual - has provision with multi-lingual, presently it is in three languages (Kannada, Hindi and English) and can be extended to other languages.

☆ Storing and retrieval – user can save the solution and retrieve the saved solutions.

☆ Display and printing - Provides results in tabular, graphical formbar chart and pie charts, which gives an instant overview of the solution and the diet. Facility for printing and downloading has been done.

☆ Available in two versions- One is professional for researchers, feed industries and commercial dairy farms, and another one customized

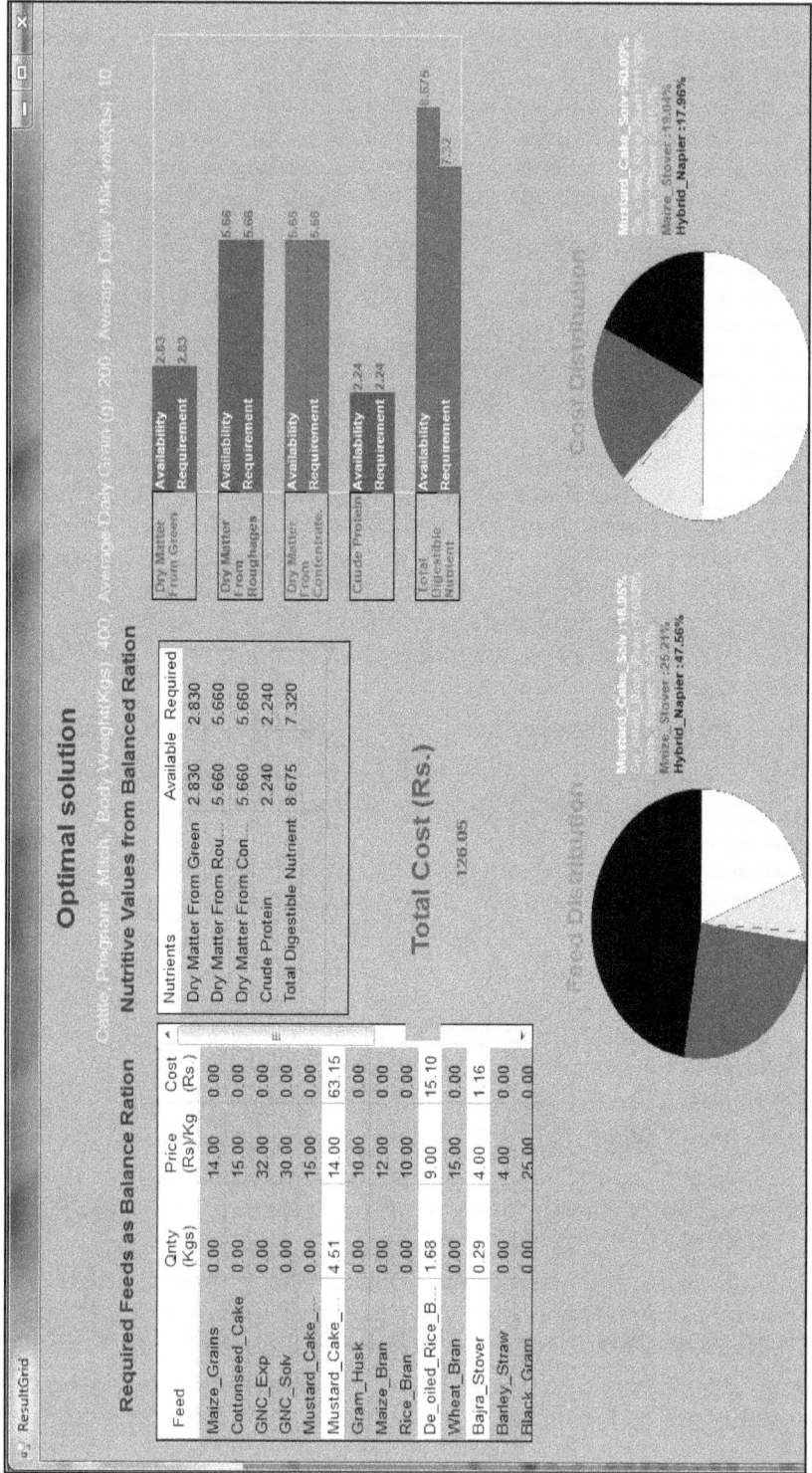

Figure 22.15. Feed Assist Optimal Solution.

version suitable for farming community. In farmer version a provision has made to calculate body weight based on girth and length of the animal.

☆ Computer configurations requirement: Hardware; Pentium Dual Core and Above with 1GB RAM, OS; windows XP and above with.net 2.3 and above.

Conclusion

The advent of Information and Communication Technologies (ICT) in the last two decades has opened new avenues in research and development for application of information and communication technology in agriculture production system. This could play a major role for sharing, exchanging and disseminating the knowledge. The packages- FEEDBASE and FEED ASSIST implementation of ICT in livestock sector will have major impact on livestock research, development and productivity.

☆ Helps to understand the status of the feed and animal resources at district and block level, which leads to a priority research task and decision making.

☆ Facilitate decision-making by individual, government and all stakeholders relating to the conservation and sharing of valuable feed resources and their management.

☆ Helps for farming communities to minimize cost associated with feed, feeding and nutrient management.

☆ Advices the farmers according to their needs with available resources in time, easily, cost effectively.

References

Angadi U.B., Anandan, S. and Ramachandra, K.S. (2009). Visual Data mining tool and Data base for assessing district wise animal and feed resources in India, *Indian Journal of Animal Sciences*. 79 (1): 89-92.

Angadi U.B., A.V.Elongovan, D. Rajendran, S. Anandan, N.K.S Gowda, Letha Devi, K.S.Prasad, Prakash Khandekar and A P Kolte (2013). "Mobile application of 'Feed Assist': Expert System on Balance Feeding of Dairy Animals"

Angadi, U.B., Raju, S.S., Anandan, S. and Ramachandra, K.S. (2005). Database on availability and requirement of animal feed resources in the Country, *Indian Journal of Animal Sciences*. 75 (9): 1083-1086.

Angadi U. B., S. Anandan and S. Jash (2012). "FeedBase-2012 District wise Feed Resource Availability and Requirements".

K. S. Ramachandra, V. K. Taneja, K.T.Sampath, S. Anandan, U.B.Angadi. (2007). "Livestock Feed Resources in Different Agro Ecosystems of India: Availability, Requirement and their Management, The Director, National Institute of Animal Nutrition and Physiology, Bangalore.

Chapter 23

Extraction of NSSO Data Using SPSS

Rajni Jain

Principal Scientist,
ICAR-NIAP, New Delhi-110 012

Introduction

In 1972-73 the National Sample Survey Organisation (NSSO) began a quinquennial series of all-India surveys on Consumer Expenditure, Employment and Unemployment at household level. NSSO provides these data in text files using binary formats. Along with the data in binary format, many associate files like documents, multiplier files, work files etc. are also provided by NSSO. All necessary instructions to generate estimates are available in Readme file. Layout. xls file provide details of field names and the position of the corresponding data in the binary file. Beside instructions which were given to field investigators, files containing codes for different states and districts are also available in the data CD. The data format and codes are different for different rounds of NSSO. All the data files are observed to be released for same fixed record-length for a specific round. This paper provides details about data extraction using one such round namely 59 round. However, the techniques presented in this article can be followed for extraction of data from other rounds also.

The millions of farmers of India have made significant contributions in providing food and nutrition to the entire nation and provided livelihood to millions of people of the country. During the five decades of planned economic development, India has moved from food-shortage and imports to self-sufficiency and exports. Food security and well being of the farmer appears to be major areas of concern of the planners of Indian agriculture. In order to have a snapshot picture of the farming community at the commencement of the third millennium and to analyze the impact of the transformation induced by public policy, investments and technological change on the farmers' access to resources and income as well as well-being of the farmer households at the end of five decades of planned economic development, Ministry of Agriculture have decided to collect information on Indian farmers through "Situation Assessment Survey" (SAS) on Indian farmers and entrusted the job of conducting the survey to National Sample Survey Organisation (NSSO).

The Situation Assessment Survey of Farmers is the first of its kind to be conducted by NSSO. Though information on a majority of items to be collected through SAS have been collected in some round or other of NSS, an integrated schedule, *viz.,* Schedule 33, covering some basic characteristics of farmer households and their access to basic and modern farming resources was canvassed for the first time in SAS. Moreover, information on consumption of various goods and services in an abridged form are also to be collected to have an idea about the pattern of consumption expenditure of the farmer households.

Schedule 33 is designed for collection of information on aspects relating to farming and other socio-economic characteristics of farmer households. The information was collected in two visits to the same set of sample households. The first visit was made during January to August 2003 and the second, during September to December 2003. The survey was conducted in rural areas only. The concepts and definitions adopted for the survey are provided in the data CD which is available from NSSO on payment basis. More details about the procurement of the data CD are available at the http://mospi.nic.in/. NSSO 59th round, schedule 33 is used in this article as an example for demonstrating the data extraction. There are two ways of extracting data through SPSS. The first method deals with using a syntax file, say schedule33.SPS. This file needs to be created in SPSS by opening a new syntax file. This file contains the desired syntax for extracting data of schedule 33 (Table 23.1). The user may choose any name to save the contents. It should be noted that line numbers are mentioned in the table to explain the purpose of each line.

Table 23.1: Sample Syntax Code for Extracting Level 1 Information for 59 Round Schedule 33

```
1.   GET DATA
2.   /TYPE=TXT
3.   /FILE='D:\ Nss59_33\AH133.TXT'
4.   /FIXCASE=1
5.   /ARRANGEMENT=FIXED
6.   /FIRSTCASE=1
7.   /IMPORTCASE=ALL
8.   /VARIABLES=/1
9.   Centre_code 0-2 F3.0
10.  Serial_No 3-7 F5.0
```

Contd...

Table 23.1–*Contd...*

```
11. Round 8-9 F2.0
12. Schedule 10-12 F3.0
13. Sample 13-13 F1.0
14. Sector 14-14 F1.0
15. State_Region 15-17 F3.0
16. District 18-19 F2.0
17. Stratum 20-21 F2.0
18. Sub_Round 22-22 F1.0
19. Sub_sample 23-23 F1.0
20. FOD_Sub_Region 24-27 F4.0
21. Hamlet_group 28-28 F1.0
22. SSS_no 29-29 F1.0
23. Visit_number 30-30 F1.0
24. Sample_hhld 31-32 F2.0
25. Level 33-34 A2
26. Filler 35-39 F5.0
27. Informant_No 40-41 A2
28. Response_Code 42-42 A1
29. Survey_Code 43-43 A1
30. Substitution_Code 44-44 A1
31. No_of_partitioned_hhlds 45-46 A2
32. Date_of_Survey 47-52 A6
33. Date_of_Despatch 53-58 A6
34. Time_to_canvass 59-61 A2
35. NSS 126-128 F3.0
36. NCC 129-131 F3.0
37. MLT 132-141 F10.0.
38. CACHE.
39. EXECUTE.
40. SELECT IF(level = '01').
41. EXECUTE.
42. SAVE OUTFILE='D:\NSSO_59\lev1331.sav'
43. /COMPRESSED.
```

Explanation of the Syntax Files and Associated Commands

In line 1, GET DATA is used here to read data from text files.

In Line 2, /type command specifies that file is of txt type. In line 3, /FILE command notifies the location and name of the data file which is 'D:\ Nss59_33\ AH133.TXT' in the given syntax file. Users should the complete path of their data file.

The FIXCASE subcommand applies to fixed data (ARRANGEMENT=FIXED) only. It specifies the number of lines (records) to read for each case. In line 4 in the above syntax, FIXCASE=1 means that only one line is to be read for each case.

The ARRANGEMENT subcommand specifies the data format. In line 5, ARRANGEMENT = FIXED means each variable is recorded in the same column location for every case.

FIRSTCASE specifies the first line (row) to read for the first case of data. This allows you to bypass information in the first n lines of the file that either don't contain data or contain data that you don't want to read. This subcommand applies to both fixed and delimited file formats. In line 6, FIRSTCASE=1 means that data will be read from 1st line itself and there is no need to skip any lines. The only specification for this subcommand is an integer greater than zero that indicates the number of lines to skip. The default is 1.

/IMPORTCASE subcommand allows you to specify the number of cases to read.

In line 7, /IMPORTCASE = ALL means all records need to be read from the given file. If we want to read say first 100 records only from then instead of all FIRST 100 should be written in the text file.

/VARIABLES subcommand in line 8 allows treating data under different columns in the data file as a variable. The following rules apply to variable names:

A. Each variable name must be unique; duplication is not allowed.

B. Variable names can be up to 64 bytes long, and the first character must be a letter or one of the characters @, #, or $. Subsequent characters can be any combination of letters, numbers, nonpunctuation characters, and a period (.).

C. Variable names cannot contain spaces.

D. The period, the underscore, and the characters $, #, and @ can be used within variable names. For example, A._$@#1 is a valid variable name.

E. Variable names ending with a period should be avoided, since the period may be interpreted as a command terminator. You can only create variables that end with a period in command syntax.

F. Reserved keywords cannot be used as variable names. Reserved keywords are ALL, AND, BY, EQ, GE, GT, LE, LT, NE, NOT, OR, TO, and WITH.

G. Variable names can be defined with any mixture of uppercase and lowercase characters, and case is preserved for display purposes.

H. When long variable names need to wrap onto multiple lines in output, lines are broken at underscores, periods, and points where content changes from lower case to upper case.

Line numbers 9-37 are used to define variables names, column position of the data and the datatype. All the three are available in the layout file which is provided by NSSO along with data. For example corresponding layout file for the above syntax is shown in Table 23.2. Depending on the requirement of users some of the variables may be omitted from the syntax file. Dot *i.e.* '.' at the end of the line 37 specifies the end of the GET DATA command.

Table 23.2: Text Data Layout for 59th Round:
Schedule-33 LEVEL – 01 Blocks 1 and 2 (VISIT NUMBER 1 AND 2)

Sl.No.	Item	Blk	Item	Col	Len	Byte Position		Remarks
1.	Centre code,Round,Shift				3	1	– 3	Generated
2.	LOT/FSU Serial No.	1	1		5	4	– 8	Generated
3.	Round	1	2		2	9	– 10	"59" Generated
4.	Schedule	1	3		3	11	– 13	"033" Generated
5.	Sample	1	4		1	14	– 14	
6.	Sector	1	5		1	15	– 15	
7.	State-Region	1	6		3	16	– 18	
8.	District	1	7		2	19	– 20	
9.	Stratum	1	8		2	21	– 22	
10.	Sub-Round	1	9		1	23	– 23	
11.	Sub-sample	1	10		1	24	– 24	
12.	FOD-Sub-Region	1	11		4	25	– 28	
13.	Hamlet group/Sub-block no.	1	12		1	29	– 29	
14.	Second-stage-stratum no.	1	13		1	30	– 30	
15.	Visit number	1	14		1	31	– 31	
16.	Sample hhld. No.	1	15		2	32	– 33	
17.	Level				2	34	– 35	"01" Generated
18.	Filler				5	36	– 40	"00000"Generated
19.	Informant Sl.No.	1	16		2	41	– 42	
20.	Response Code	1	17		1	43	– 43	
21.	Survey Code	1	18		1	44	– 44	
22.	Substitution Code	1	19		1	45	– 45	
23.	No. of partitioned hhlds (for visit-2)	1	20		2	46	– 47	
24.	Date of Survey	2	2(i)	3	6	48	– 53	"ddmmyy"
25.	Date of Despatch	2	2(iv)	5	6	54	– 59	"ddmmyy"
26.	Time to canvass(mins.)	2	4	3	3	60	– 62	
27.	Special characters for OK stamp			2	63	– 64		
28.	Blank				62	65	– 126	

In line 38, CACHE command at line 38 does not read the active dataset. It is stored, pending execution with the next command that reads the dataset. This command improves performance.

EXECUTE forces the data to be read and executes the transformations that precede it in the command sequence. EXECUTE in line 39 reads the data from text file into the variables while EXECUTE in line 41 selects the desired cases at level 01.

SELECT IF permanently selects cases for analysis based on logical conditions that are found in the data. These conditions are specified in a logical expression. The logical expression can contain relational operators, logical operators, arithmetic operations, and any functions that are allowed in COMPUTE transformations. For temporary case selection, specify a TEMPORARY command before SELECT IF.

SAVE OUTFILE command produces an SPSS-format data file, which contains data plus a dictionary. The dictionary contains a name for each variable in the data file plus any assigned variable and value labels, missing-value flags, and variable print and write formats. User can specify any other name that follows file naming conventions.

For running the syntax file following conditions must be satisfied on the users machine.

1. SPSS is loaded on the user machine with valid license.
2. Folder NSSO_59 is available on the D: drive. If it is not create it. User may make different name folder and replace the name in the syntax file.
3. The data file to be extracted *i.e.* AH133.TXT is available in this folder. If it is not copy the file from the available data CD.

After the Execution of the above syntax file a new SPSS file 'lev1331.sav' is created in the specified folder. This file can be used for further analysis using SPSS or even exported to EXCEL. Similarly, other levels can be extracted and used by the user.

SPSS WIZARD method for data extraction:

SPSS can also provide wizard based solution for extracting NSSO data. No syntax knowledge is required as we proceed through wizards. Syntax is generated by SPSS for all the steps processed. The syntax can be pasted also for further use in separate syntax file. Steps are as follows:

Step 1: From the menu choose: *File->Read Text Data* (Figure 23.1).

Step 2: Browse the location where text file of NSSO data has been kept (Figure 23.2).

Step 3: Click next on the dialog box that appears, following which screen shown in Figure 23.3 is shown. Select fixed width and click next twice.

Step 4: By clicking at require width create vertical lines in preview text box of dialog box. We can also use Insert Break button by filling appropriate value in column number text box to fill width of each column as given in Layout file (Figure 23.4). Click next after all the required fields are selected through the vertical lines.

Step 5: Rename each field by using Layout file for level 1. The names may be the ones given in the layout file or related synonyms which you can understand while analyzing the data. Click at a header to rename each field. Also choosing proper data type for each field from drop down list Data format. These fields represent the data item. Click next when you have renamed all the fields properly (Figure 23.5).

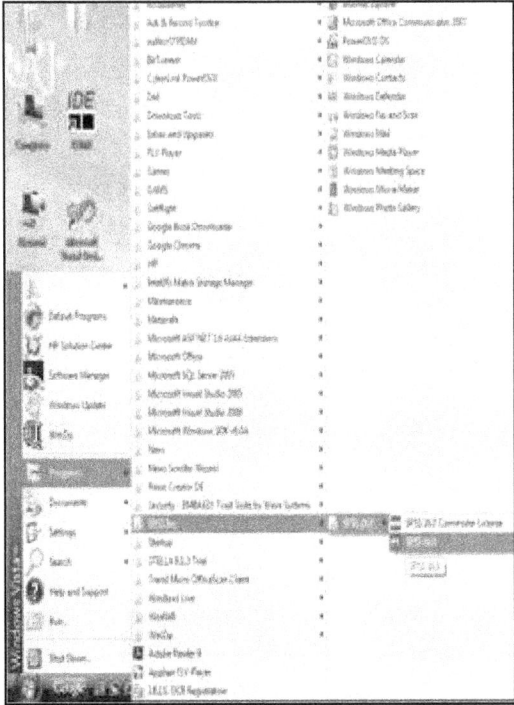

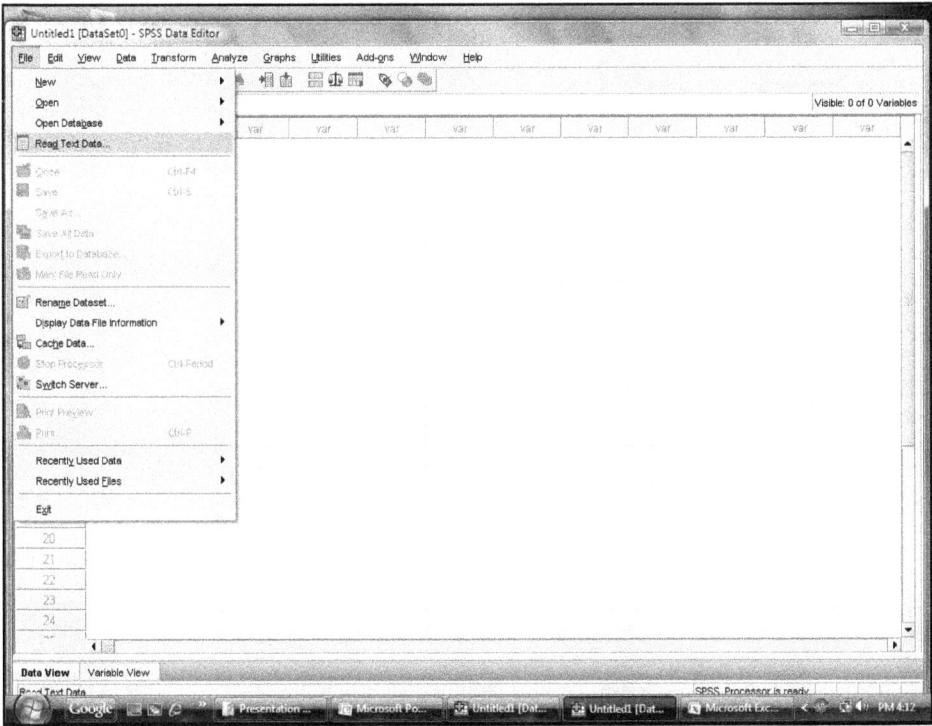

Figure 23.1: Open SPSS Blank Data File.

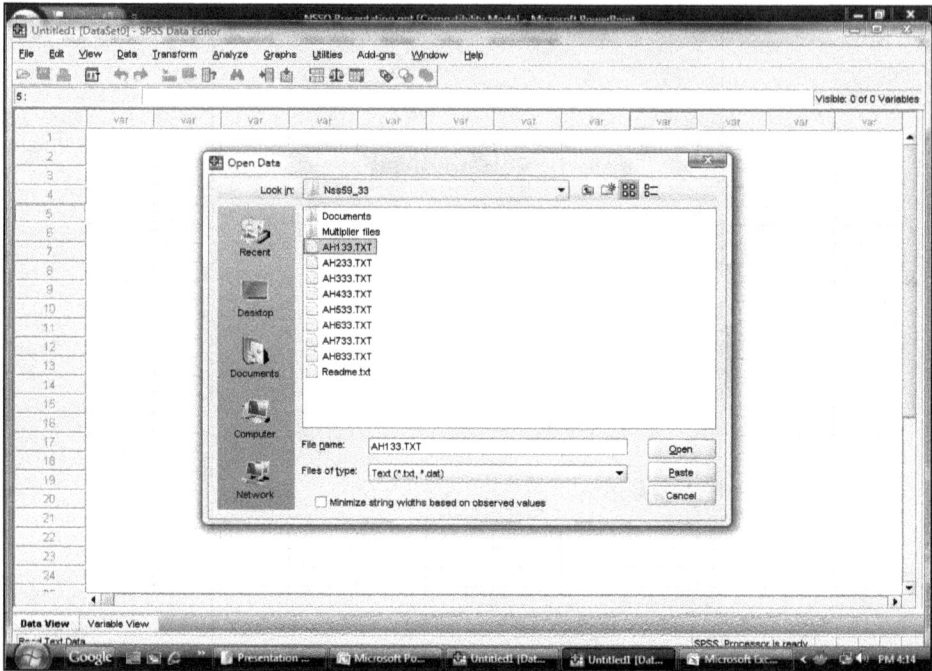

Figure 23.2: Selecting the Data File.

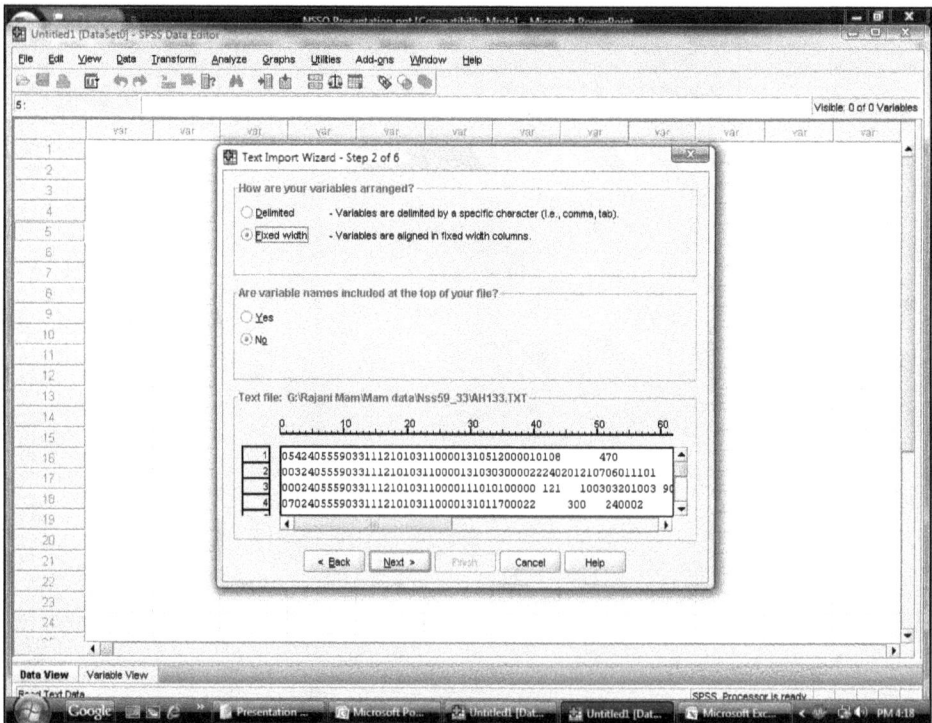

Figure 23.3: Selecting the Variable Types.

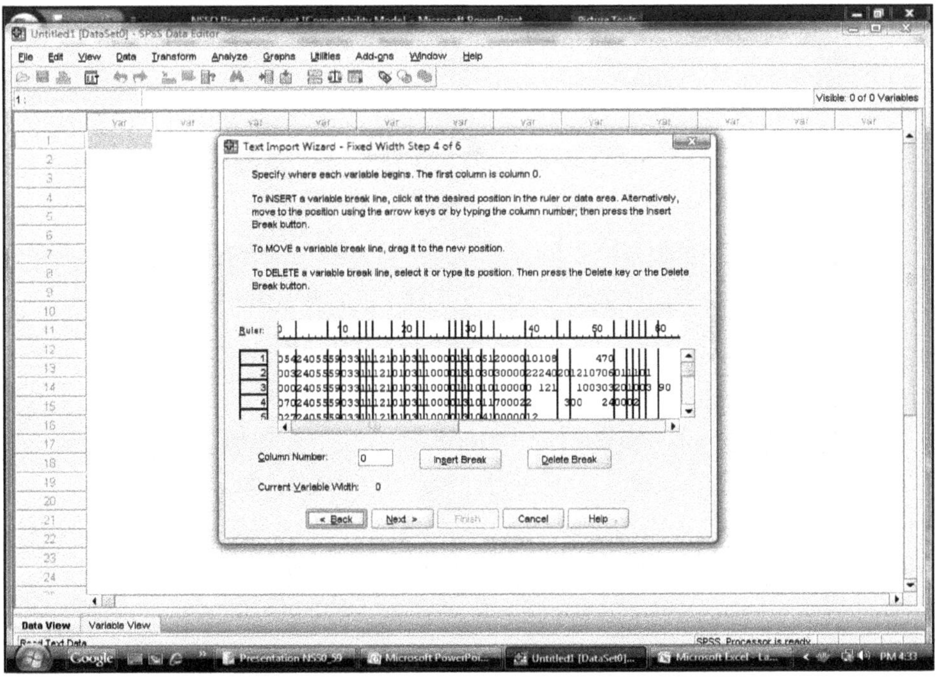

Figure 23.4: Selecting the Width of the Variables.

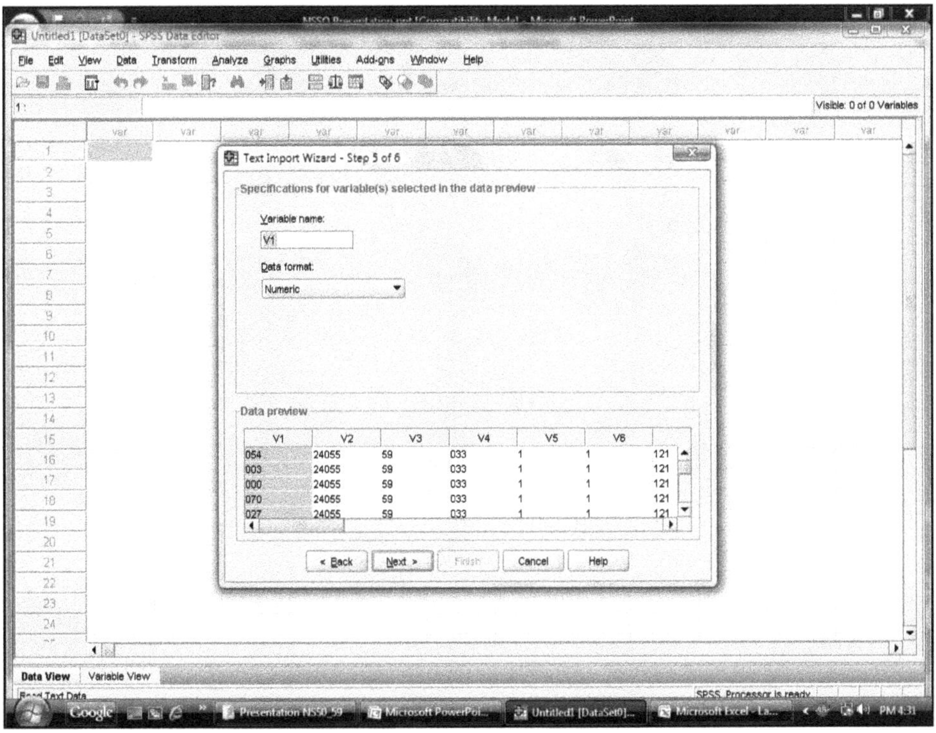

Figure 23.5: Assigning Variable Names.

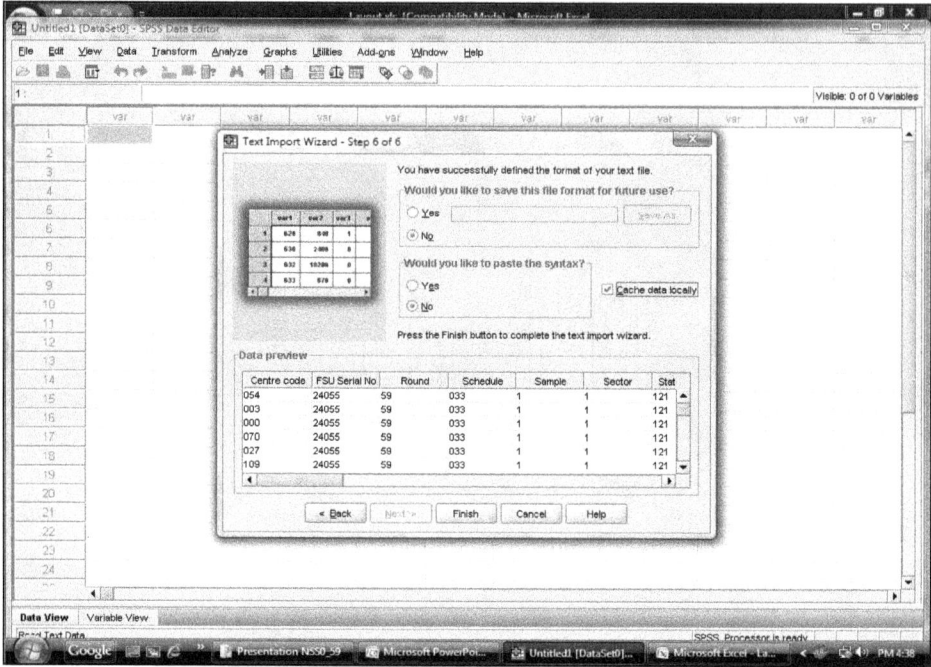

Figure 23.6: Saving the File Format.

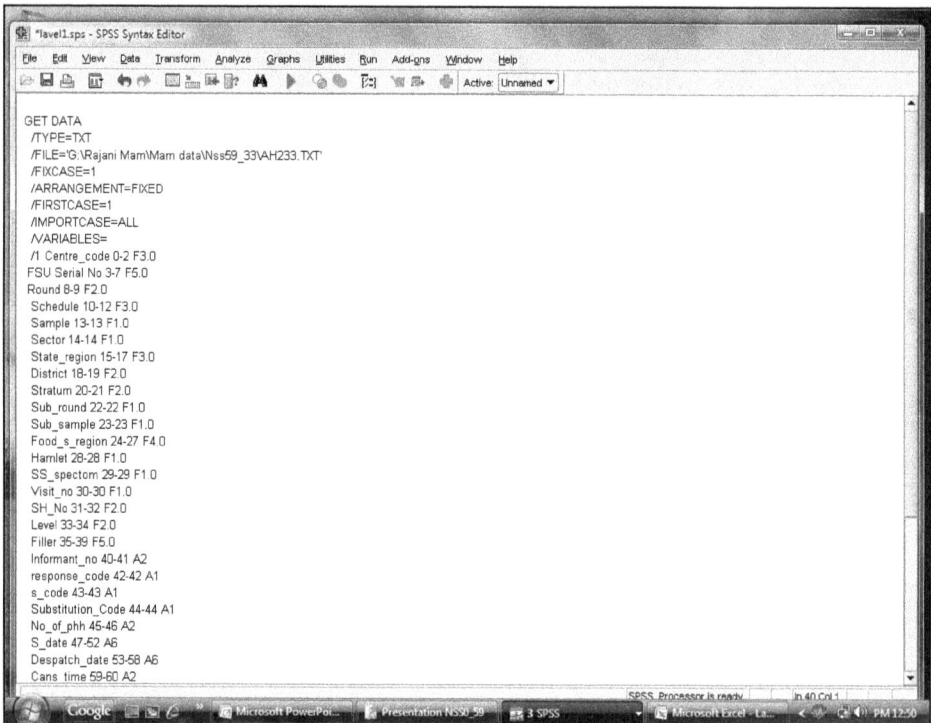

Figure 23.7: Syntax File Generated from Wizard.

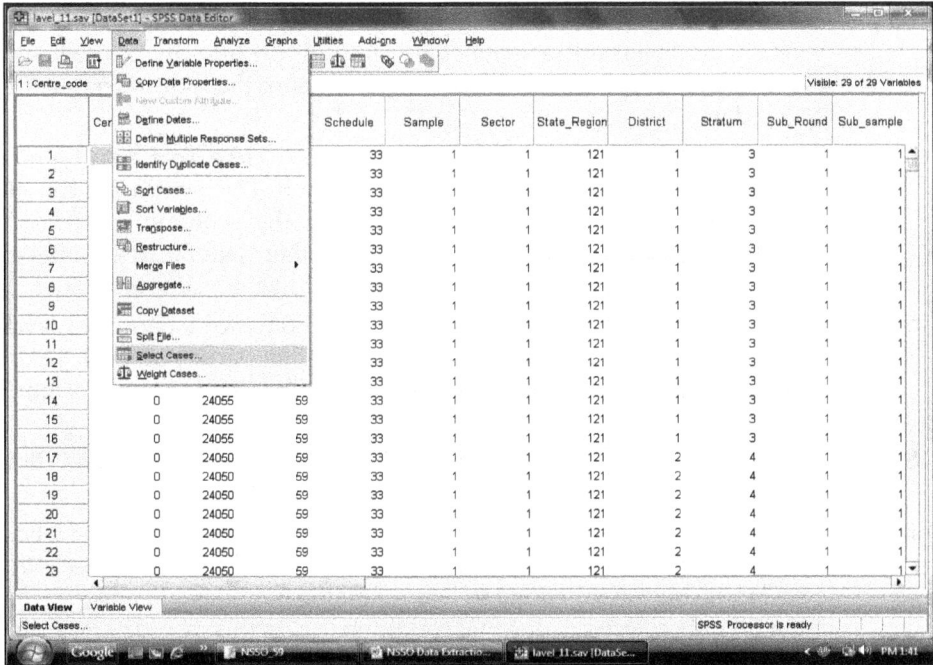

Figure 23.8: Current Status of Data File Without Selection.

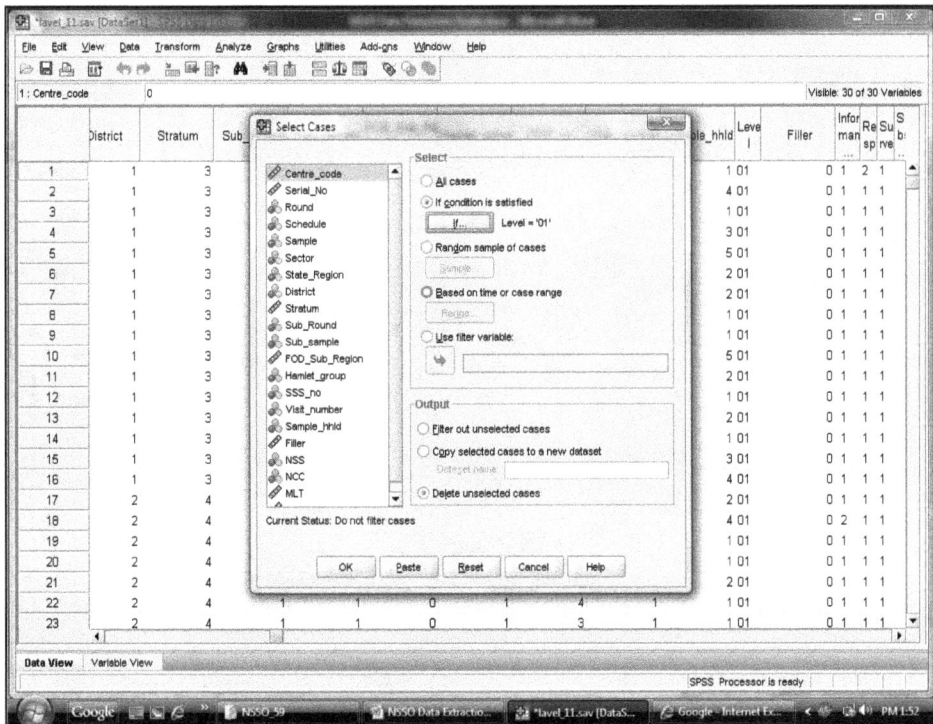

Figure 23.9: Selection of Cases.

Step 6: Select radio button Yes for the dialog *"would you like to paste syntax"* and click finish. As a result, a syntax file to import text file with desired field name and data type is generated. This file contains the code for extracting NSSO data.

Step 7: The syntax file looks as shown in Figure 23.7. Here Text data type is represented by A and Numeric data type by F. This syntax file can be manipulated by adding more data items and their column width from the layout file. Also it can be used for any other data file after suitable modifications as per the data items in the text file to be imported.

Step 8: In this case field names given by us are valid only for a particular level (*e.g.* level 2) so we have to filter only cases of that particular level. To do this in "untitled.sav" file at menu bar click Data->Select cases (Figure 23.8).

Step 9: A Dialog box opens. Select radio button *"if condition is satisfied"* and click "if "button again a sub dialog box get open (Figure 23.9).

Step 10: In the upper most text box in right panel of submenu type *"level='02' "*.Click at continue button sub dialog box get disappear. Select *"Delete unselected cases"* radio button in *"output section"* of dialog box. Now data file will be left with only selected value in if condition (*e.g.* In this case '02').From *file* menu select sub menu *"save as"* and specify the desired filename (Figure 23.10). This data can now be analyzed as per normal analytical methods.

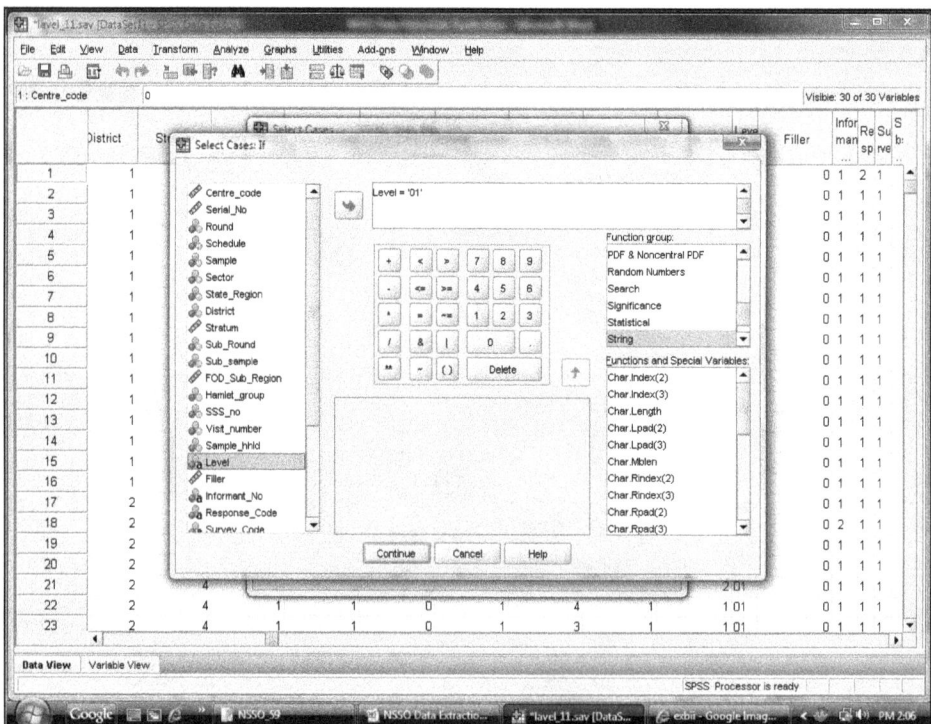

Figure 23.10: Select Case: If Dialog Box.

Merging Data Files of Different Regions

In some rounds of NSSO, data for different states is available in different text files, in such cases, user is required to merge the data of two or more states as per the need. Thus, we need to add extracted data files of same level. Step 11 explains the procedure for it.

Step 11: Open first data file of first level and select *Data->Merge file->Add Cases*. Click on *Add Cases* (Figure 23.11). A small size dialog box as shown in Figure 23.12 appears on the screen. Select "an external SPSS data file" and browse the next file of first level and click"continue". Click 'ok' without any change of next dialog box. It will add all cases (rows) of both files (Figures 23.12-23.13). This is our final data file of level 01 which can be saved for future analysis.

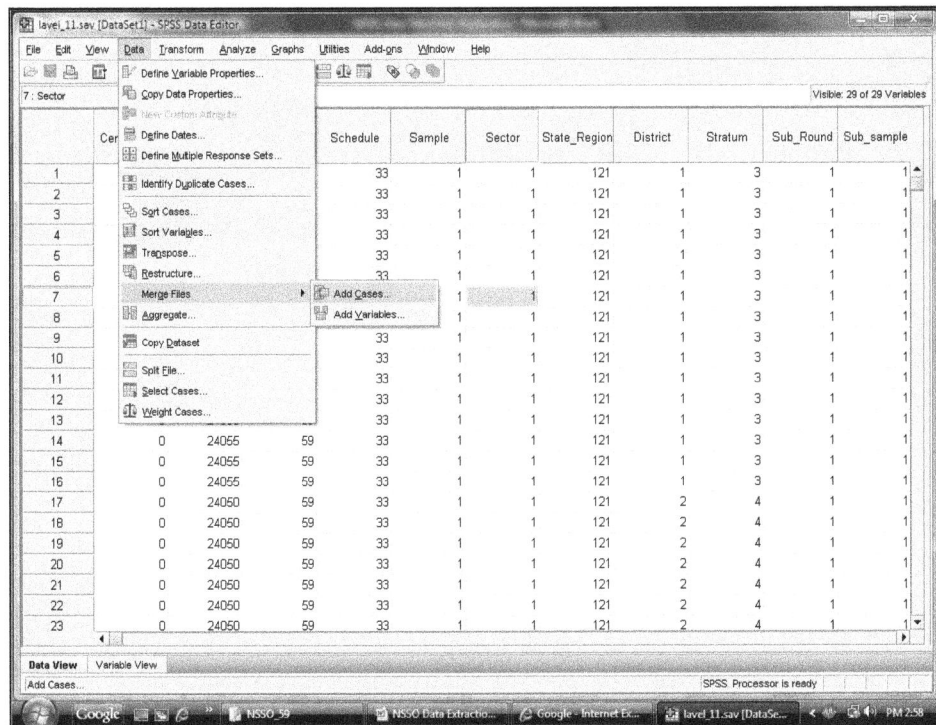

Figure 23.11: Merging of Data Files.

The extracted files which are now available in SPSS format can be easily saved in any other format like Excel or Stata using file→ save as option from the file menu.

Summary

This article has explained the extraction of data from NSSO format to SPSS or Excel files for further analysis. First method deals with using SPSS coding. The required commands for this purpose are explained in this chapter so as to allow user to use the commands judiciously. The syntax and variable names need to be

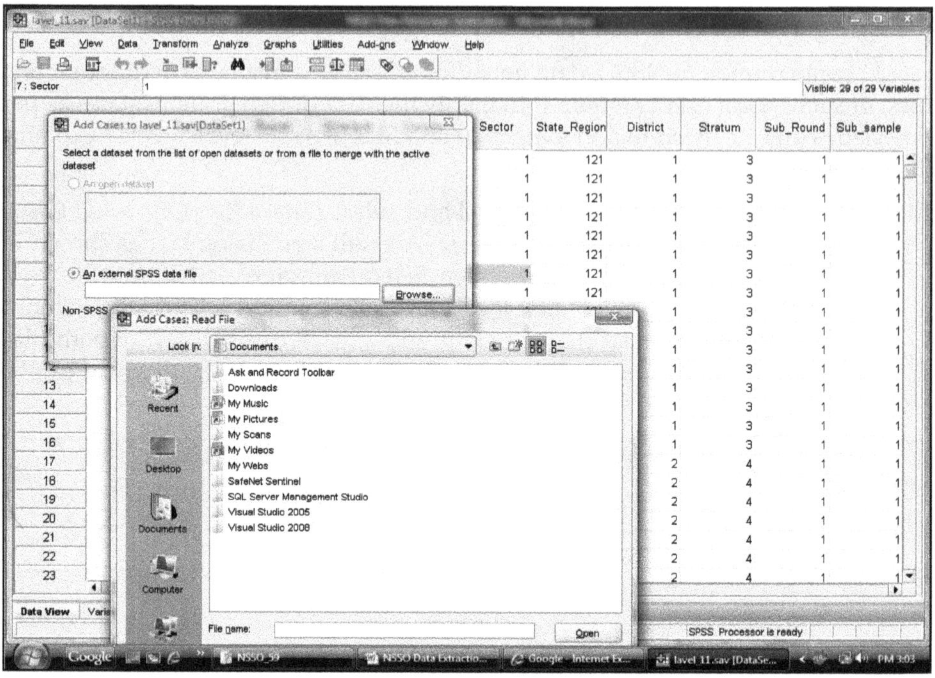

Figure 23.12: Selecting Files for Merging.

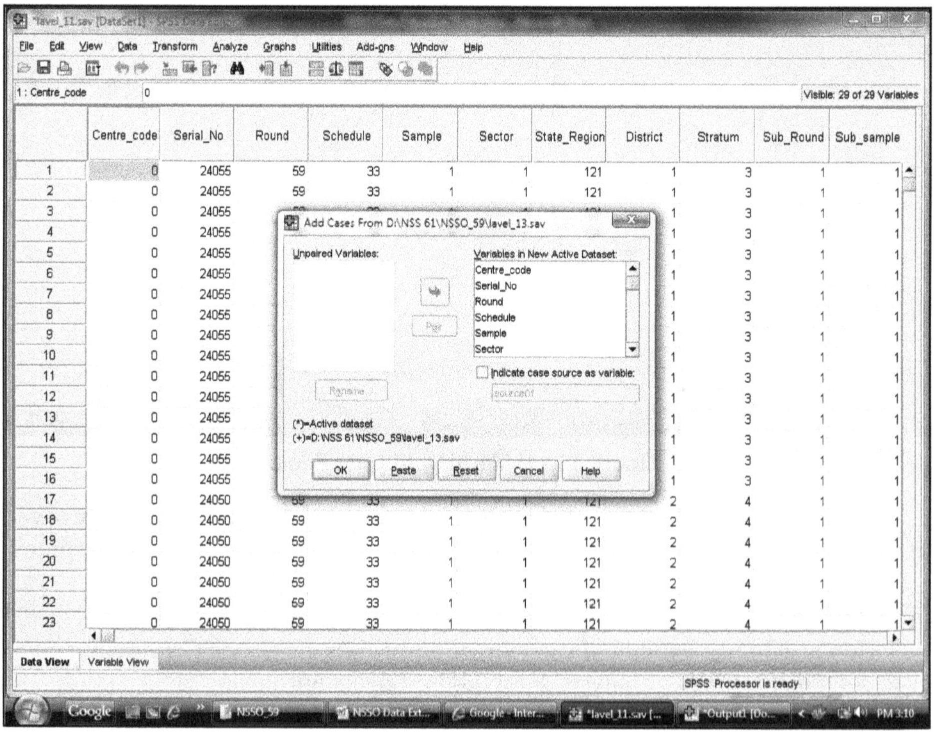

Figure 23.13: Adding Data from External File.

modified as per the layout file of the data provided. The Second method explains the extraction process using SPSS read data wizard. Many screen snapshots have been provided to help the reader in following the various steps. Finally merging of the data files for different states may be required by the user depending on the requirement which has been explained with the help of SPSS wizard.

Chapter 24

Data Center and its Services in ICAR

N. Srinivasa Rao[1], A.K. Choubey[2], Alka Arora[3],
Sudeep Marwaha[3], Mukesh Kumar[3],
Subhash Chand[4] and R.K. Saini[5]

[1]*Senior Scientist (Computer Applications),*
[2]*Head (Division of Computer Applications),*
[3]*Senior Scientist (Computer Applications),*
[4]*Senior Technical Officer &* [5]*Assistant Chief Technical Officer,*
ICAR-IASRI, New Delhi-110 012

Introduction

There was a time when our information needs were simpler. But since the dawn of the Internet, high-bandwidth broadband, smartphones and other new technologies, are constantly online and constantly demanding that data be delivered to the computers, gaming systems, TVs and phones. Electronic exchange of data is required for just about every type of business transaction, and is becoming the norm for many of our personal interactions. With this massive demand for near-instantaneous delivery of digital information came the need for concentrations of computer and networking equipment that can handle the requests and serve up the goods. Thus, the modern data center was born.

A data center is a facility that centralizes an organization's IT operations and equipment, and where it stores, manages, and disseminates its data. Data centers house a network's most critical systems and are vital to the continuity of daily operations. Consequentially, the security and reliability of data centers and their information is a top priority for organizations. It consists of servers and storage equipment that run application software, process, store data and content. The data center environment is controlled in terms of temperature and humidity, both to ensure the performance and the operational integrity of the systems within. Facilities will generally include power supplies, backup power, chillers, cabling, fire and water detection systems, security controls etc.

The main purpose of a data center is running the IT systems applications that handle the core business and operational data of the organization. It generally includes redundant or backup power supplies, redundant data communications connections, environmental controls and various security devices. Communications in data centers today are most often based on networks running the IP protocol suite. Data centers contain a set of routers and switches that transport traffic between the servers and to the outside world. Some of the servers at the data center are used for running the basic Internet and intranet services needed by internal users in the organization, *e.g.*, e-mail servers, proxy servers, and DNS servers. Network security elements such as firewalls, VPN gateways, intrusion detection systems are also usually deployed.

Data Center Goals

The benefits provided by a Data Center include traditional business-oriented goals such as the support for business operations around the clock, lowering the total cost of operation and the maintenance needed to sustain the business functions, the rapid deployment of applications and consolidation of computing resources (Mauricio and Maurizio, 2004).

These business goals generate a number of information technology initiatives, including the following:

☆ Business continuance

☆ Increased security in the Data Center

☆ Application, server, and Data Center consolidation

☆ Integration of applications whether client/server and multitier (n-tier), or web services-related applications

☆ Storage consolidation

Data Center Advantages

☆ Data centers are secure. It will typically be manned 24 hours a day 7 days a week and be physically very difficult to break in to.

☆ Server is going to be kept in a secure environment that is prepared for the eventuality of power cuts. A data center will have huge banks of batteries and generators that will keep the electricity flowing indefinitely whilst the power outage is fixed.

☆ The data center will have multiple high bandwidth and geographically diverse fiber connections to the internet.

☆ Servers doesn't overheat and the data on servers can be safely and easily backed up (Davis, 2012).

Data Center Requirements

An effective data center operation is achieved through a balanced investment in the facility and equipment housed. The elements of a data center are usable space, IT equipment which includes servers, storage hardware, cables, racks, firewalls. Also it requires support infrastructure such as uninterruptible power resources, room air conditioners, heating and exhaust systems. The operational staff is required to monitor operations and maintain IT and infrastructural equipment around the clock (Hwaiyu, 2015).

Data Center Vs Cloud Computing

The main difference between a data center and a cloud is that a cloud is an off-premise form of computing that stores data on the Internet, whereas a data center refers to on premise hardware that stores data within an organization's local network. While cloud services are outsourced to third-party cloud providers who perform all updates and ongoing maintenance, data centers are typically run by an in-house IT department.

Although both types of computing systems can store data, as a physical unit, only a data center can store servers and other equipment. As such, cloud service providers use data centers to house cloud services and cloud-based resources. For cloud-hosting purposes, vendors also often own multiple data centers in several geographic locations to safeguard data availability during outages and other data center failures (Angeles, 2013).

ICAR – Data Center and its Services

The state of art Data Center (Figure 24.1) has been created by Indian Council of Agricultural Research (ICAR) at Indian Agricultural Statistics Research Institute

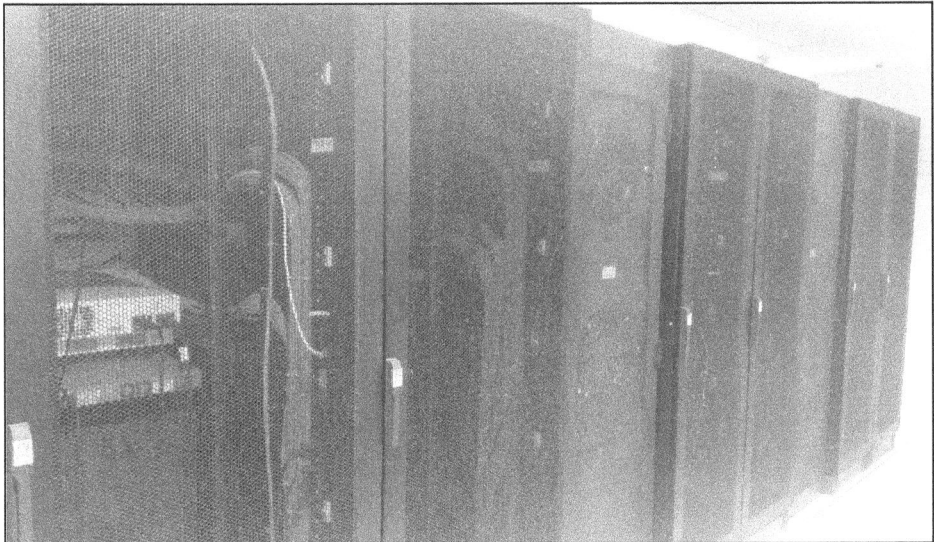

Figure 24.1: ICAR – Data Center at IASRI, New Delhi.

(ICAR- IASRI), New Delhi with the objective of providing the efficient collaboration among ICAR personnel through Unified messaging and dissemination of scientific/ research/technological/educational/extension information through hosting of web sites and applications.

It meets the international standard of Data Center Tier III specifications with adherence to ISO 27001, ITIL and TIA 942 standards. The solution is based on Structured, Scalable and Resilient Network Architecture. The data center contains servers which are connected to high performance LAN Switches, for processing millions of packets per second, depending on users and application and its contents. The computing environment consists of 448 core computing with 150TB storage space which will enable the high speed of computing/processing of data. Virtualization aids in segmentation of computing for resource allocation and making available the need based storage for different applications. In the software component Microsoft Exchange Mail server, Windows and Linux operating systems along various databases (MSAcess, MySQL, and SQL Server etc.) are available in the Data Center. The Unified messaging solution is based on Microsoft Exchange Server. The unified communication feature of the solution will help ICAR personnel to stay connected with each other via instant messaging, email, audio/video calls, persistent chat rooms, online meeting and presentations for scientific/research/ technological/educational/extension information exchange. This helps in creating Uniform Email ID of ICAR and its institutes/departments under single ICAR domain for effective communication at individual desktop (Choubey *et al.*, 2014).

Technical Architecture

This facility has IT and Non-IT parts, wherein IT part deals with hardware/ software and its integration. Installation of hardware, policy formulation, domain name registration and its configuration in the system and then loading and configuration of software as per policy requirements has been done. In the Non-IT part, Data Center environment has been created in Fire safe mode. Setup has been done for supply of water chiller based cooling and power supply. ICT infrastructure has been designed in such a way so as to provide redundancy for Power supplies, Controllers, CPUs to support 100 per cent uptime experience. The ICAR – Data center architecture is shown in Figure 24.2.

The data center has servers which are connected to high performance LAN Switches, for processing millions of packets per second, depending on users and application and its contents.

Computing Environment

The computing environment enables the high speed of computing/processing of data. Core layer switches 1G/10G/40G enabled module provides easy scalability. The following are the some major computing environment in ICAR- Data center.

- ☆ 448 Core Computing
- ☆ 150 TB storage
- ☆ Microsoft OS

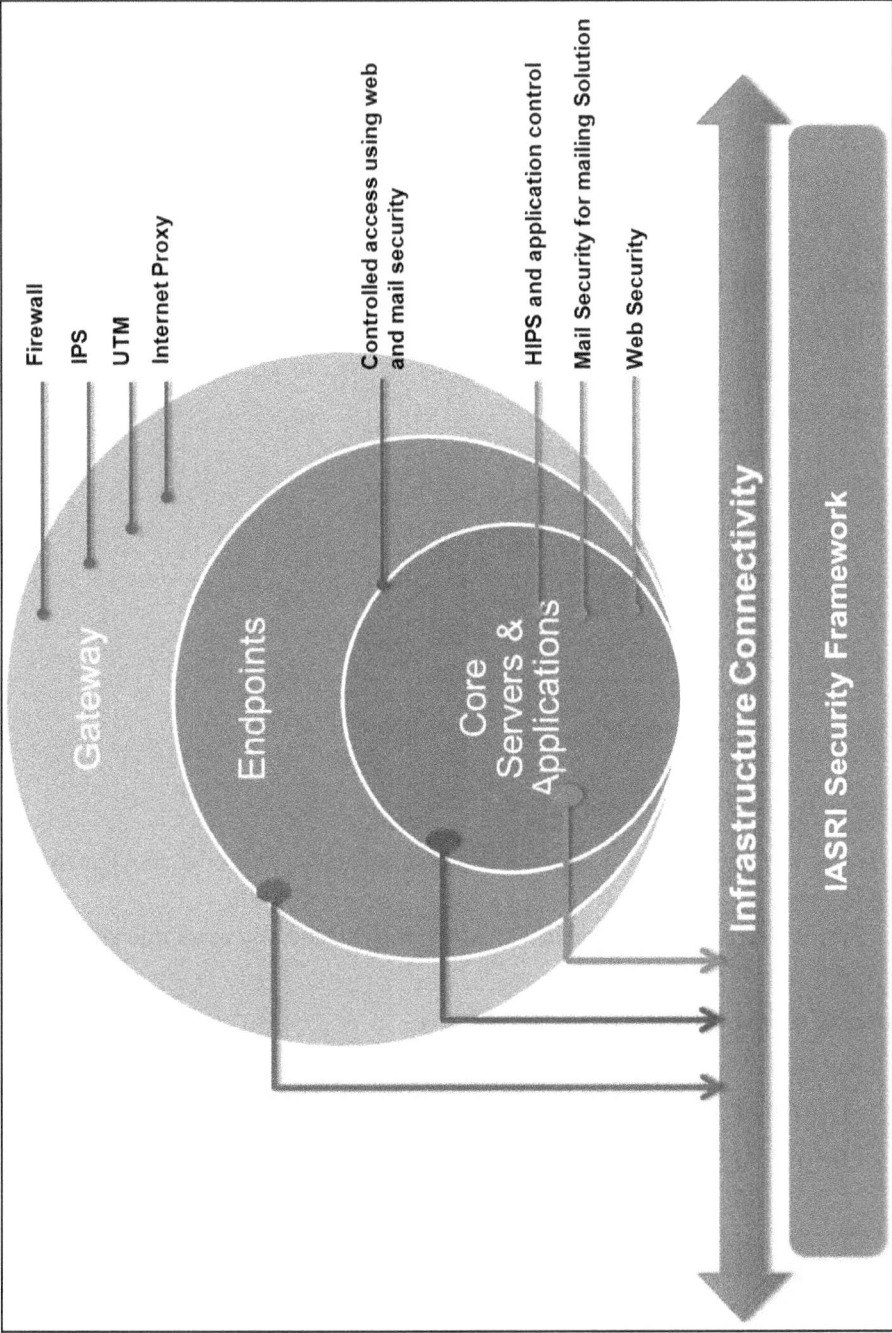

Figure 24.2: ICAR – Data Center Architecture.

- ☆ Linux OS
- ☆ Microsoft SQL DBMS
- ☆ MySQL
- ☆ Active Directory
- ☆ Microsoft Exchange 2013
- ☆ Microsoft Lync 2013
- ☆ Virtualization
- ☆ Switches

Services Offered

The following are the services offered by the ICAR – Data center.

- ☆ Virtual Machine and Data Storage
- ☆ Web hosting
- ☆ Unified Communication:
    - ☆ Messaging (Webmail and POP)
    - ☆ Phonebook
    - ☆ Calendar
    - ☆ Schedule meetings
    - ☆ Chat
    - ☆ Presence
    - ☆ Web Conferencing
    - ☆ Video Conferencing
    - ☆ Content Sharing

The concept diagram to access the unified messaging solution in ICAR is shown in Figure 24.3.

The unified communication in ICAR has been hosted and available at https://mail.icar.gov.in (Figure 24.4)

Features of the Solution

The solution has the following features:

- ☆ Scalability
- ☆ 24 x 7 availability
- ☆ Interoperability
- ☆ Security
- ☆ Manageability
- ☆ Integration
- ☆ Reliability
- ☆ Adherence to ISO 27001, ITIL, TIA 942 standards

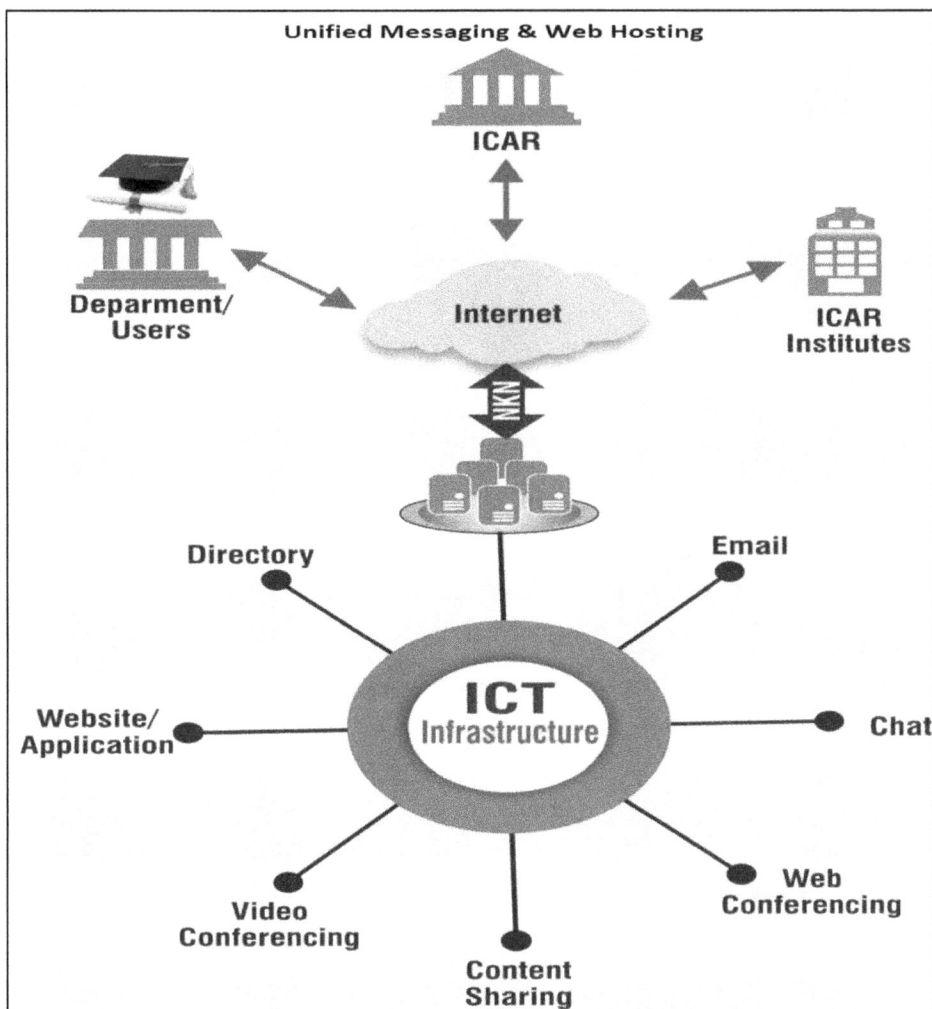

Figure 24.3: Context Diagram of Unified Messaging Solution.

Other features of the solution includes end-to-end security option with granular traffic control and monitoring smooth integration, migration, easy and centralized network management and fire protection.

Infrastructure

The following infrastructure has been established under ICAR-Data Center to provide unified mail messaging and web hosting solution in ICAR.

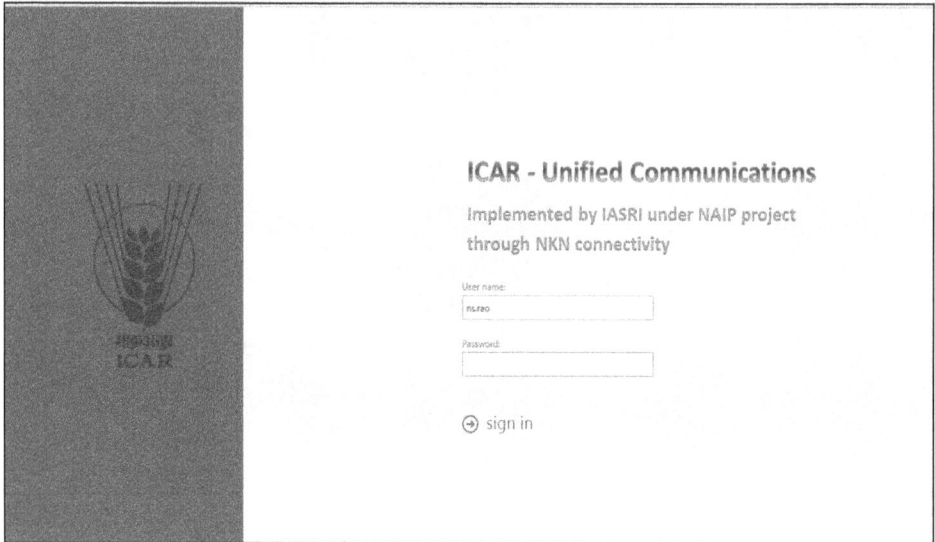

Figure 24.4: https://mail.icar.gov.in – Home Page.

Hardware

Server Devices:	CISCO UCS and CISCO Rack Servers
Storage:	EMC Networker
Network Devices:	Switches-CISCO L3 and CISCO L2 Switches, Array 2600
Security:	IPS, Firewall, IronPort, FortiGate, WebGateway
Backup and Restoration:	EMC Networker
Database:	SQL Server 2012, 2008 R2 and MY SQL
Alert Monitoring:	HPSM
Call Logging Tool:	HPSM
BMS PART:	State of the Art UPS and Air-Conditioning System, Fire Detection Control systems and Network cabling

Software

OS:	Linux 7.0, Windows Server Data center 2012 and 2008.
Application:	MS Exchange 2013, Windows AD, Lync 2013, Web Hosting, SQL

Purpose of the Infrastructure Setup

Servers

A server is a program that awaits and fulfills requests from client programs in the same or other computers. A given application in a computer may function as a client with requests for services from other programs and also as a server of requests from other programs.

Exchange Servers: Storing and accessing emails

Lync Servers: IM, Presence, audio, video chatting etc.

SQL Servers: storing application data and accessing application

Firewall

A firewall is a part of a computer system or network that is designed to block unauthorized access while permitting outward communication. It is a device or set of devices configured to permit, deny, encrypt, decrypt, or proxy all computer traffic between different security domains based upon a set of rules and other criteria.

Firewalls can be implemented in both hardware and software, or a combination of both. Firewalls are frequently used to prevent unauthorized Internet users from accessing private networks connected to the Internet, especially intranets. All messages entering or leaving the intranet pass through the firewall, which examines each message and blocks those that do not meet the specified security criteria

IronPort

The Cisco IronPort is an appliance that is deployed into an existing mail infrastructure. All emails are sent to the IronPort and the IronPort is either the last point out (most common configuration) or it can process email and then send it back to the mail server where it is sent out.

Storage

Product called **EMC VNX 5600** is used to store entire data. Total storage capacity of this data center infra comes up to approx. 140TB.

Backup

Product called **EMC Networker** is used. Data are backed up in tapes in tape library. Each tape capacity 2.5TB.

Conclusion

The information technology has revolutionized the way of living and conducting business. Organizations are experiencing a brutally competitive business environment and in order to survive, businesses have to embrace technology. It is the accelerating pace of business and the corresponding quickening of the pace of change itself that led to conceiving the idea of development of ICT infrastructure such as Data Center for ICAR. The Data Center provides the basis towards the implementation of standardized IT policy in ICAR. It also provides much secured, highly reliable, quickly scalable, efficient management and optimized utilization of resources in ICAR to deliver the Unified communications and Web Hosting services to ICAR and its institutions. It is envisioned to provide services for hosting websites and applications relating to information in the areas of education, research and extension projects of the institutes. This enables Scientist to focus on designing system for delivery of information and services and need not to spent efforts on data management and hosting of applications.

References

Angeles, S. (2013). *Cloud vs Data Center: What's the difference?* Retrieved from http://www.businessnewsdaily.com/4982-cloud-vs-data-center.html

Choubey A.K., Arora Alka, Marwaha Sudeep, Bhardwaj Anshu, Dahiya Shashi, Islam S.N., Kumar Mukesh, Rao N.S., Singh Pal and Ahuja Sangeeta (2014). *"Final Project Report on Implementation of Management Information System (MIS) including Financial Management System (FMS) in ICAR"*. IASRI, New Delhi.

Davis, T. (2012). *The advantages of using a data center.* Retrieved from http://www.timico.co.uk/blog/2012/06/21/the-advantages-of-using-a-data-centre

Hwaiyu Geng, P.E. (2015). *Data Center Handbook.* John Wiley and Sons Inc., New Jersey

Mauricio Arregoces and Maurizio Portolani (2004). *Data Center Fundamentals.* Cisco Press, Indianapolis, USA.

Chapter 25

Unit-level Cost of Cultivation Data: Extraction and Retrieving Procedure

S.K. Srivastava[1], S.S. Raju[1], Amrit Pal Kaur[1], Jaspal Singh[1], Rajni Jain[1], I. Kingly[1] and Jatinder Sachdeva[2]

[1]ICAR-NIAP, New Delhi-110 012
[2]Punjab Agricultural Universities (PAU), Ludhiana-141 004

Cost of cultivation surveys had always been an important data source for decision making on different aspects of crop production in India. The first such survey was conducted in 1954-55 under a scheme entitled "Studies in the Economics of Farm Management in India". Many useful studies were conducted using that data. However, the data lacked the consistency and uniformity in terms of concepts and definition. This led to discontinuation of the scheme. Later on, with a view to collect uniform and representative data on cost of cultivation of major crops, a scheme entitled "Comprehensive scheme for cost of cultivation of principal crops" was launched in the year 1970-71 by Directorate of Economics and Statistics, Government of India. Presently, under this scheme a representative data is collected by conducting field surveys by identified nodal agencies in 17 states using uniform schedule and survey methodology.

The data on different aspects of crop and livestock production is conducted by canvassing 40 different record types (RT). The broad theme of each RT is listed in the Table 25.1. It is to be noted that frequency of data record is different for different RT. Data on some variables are reported even on daily basis and recoded weekly/

monthly basis. The challenge therefore lies in merging RTs with different frequency levels. Further, the data is collected and reported on hard copies of schedules and afterwards recorded digitally using software "FARMAP" developed with the assistance of FAO. Once, the data is entered in FARMAP package, files containing data are encrypted into BIN format.

Table 25.1: List of RT with the Broad Theme Area

RT Number	Theme
RT110	Household members (yearly)
RT111	Household change (monthly)
RT 120	Attached farm servant (beginning of the year)
RT 121	Attached farm servant (Monthly)
RT 210	Land inventory (yearly)
RT 211	Changes in land (seasonal)
RT 230	Annual crop record (beginning and end of season)
RT 231	Perennial crop inventory (beginning and end of season)
RT 310	Animal inventory (yearly)
RT 311	Animal changes (monthly)
RT 410	Building inventory (yearly)
RT 411	Building changes (monthly)
RT 440	Irrigation structure inventory (yearly)
RT 441	Irrigation structures changes (monthly)
RT 450	Machinery and implements inventory (yearly)
RT451	Machinery and implement changes (monthly)
RT 510	Credit outstanding
RT 511	New Loan taken out (Monthly)
RT 512	Loan repayment (Monthly)
RT 610	Receipts and disposal of important crop production (yearly)
RT 710	Crop operation hours (Daily/monthly)
RT 711	Crop operation labour payments (daily/monthly)
RT 712	Crop physical inputs and other payments (monthly)
RT713	Crop outputs (monthly)
RT 714	Crop transport and marketing operations (monthly)
RT 715	Crop transport and marketing operations payments (monthly)
RT 716	Crop marketing cost incurred (monthly)
RT 720	Animal upkeep operation hours (monthly)
RT 721	Animal upkeep operation causal labour payments (monthly)
RT 722	Animal upkeep physical inputs and other payments (monthly)
RT 723	Animal non-milk outputs (monthly)
RT 724	Animal and milk products (monthly)

Contd...

Table 25.1–*Contd...*

RT Number	Theme
RT 730	Special activity operations hours (monthly)
RT 731	Special activity operations payments (monthly)
RT 732	Special activity physical inputs and payments (monthly)
RT 733	Special activity outputs (monthly)
RT 740	Machine upkeep operation hours (monthly)
RT 741	Machine upkeep physical inputs and payments (monthly)
RT 742	Machine upkeep physical inputs and payments (monthly)
RT 743	Machin power provided output farm (monthly)

The procedure of data extraction and retrieving includes following broader steps.

1. The BIN file containing raw data on 40 RTs are accessed using MS-DOS (command prompt) and converted into any usable format (DAT, PRN, etc) recognizable by any data analysis software. For conversion of file format from BIN to PRN, a software "DATAMAN (FARMAP)" is used.

2. PRN files are imported in data analysis software (SAS in our case) and different RTs are extracted individually.

3. Individual RTs are merged together on the basis of requirement of research objectives. We have developed a SAS programme for extracting and merging different RT file and estimating coefficients for different aspects of farm enterprises.

Snapshot 1a and 1b: MS-DOS for merging RT files (BIN format) if they are given separately.

A glimpse of the data extraction and retrieving procedure is shown below by different snapshots.

Note: Due to space limitation full SAS code could not be given and can be requested from shivendraiari@gmail.com if needed.

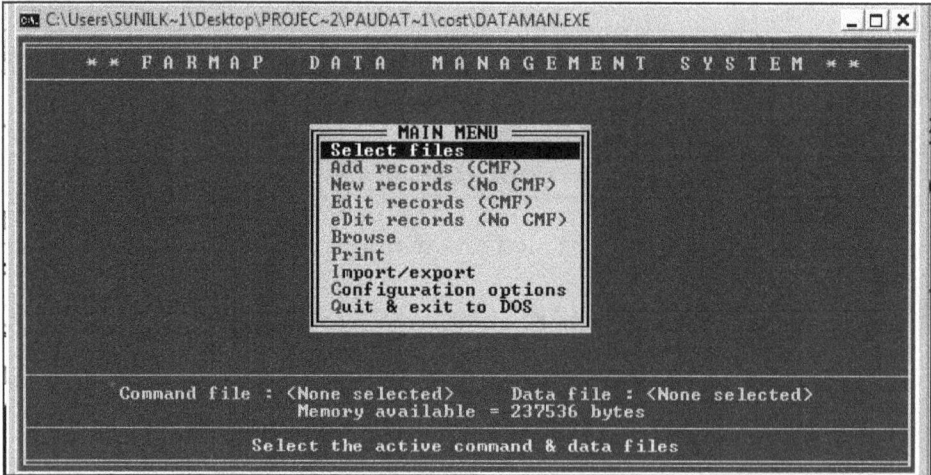

Snapshot 2. Open DATAMNAN and select appropriate option for accessing BIN file.

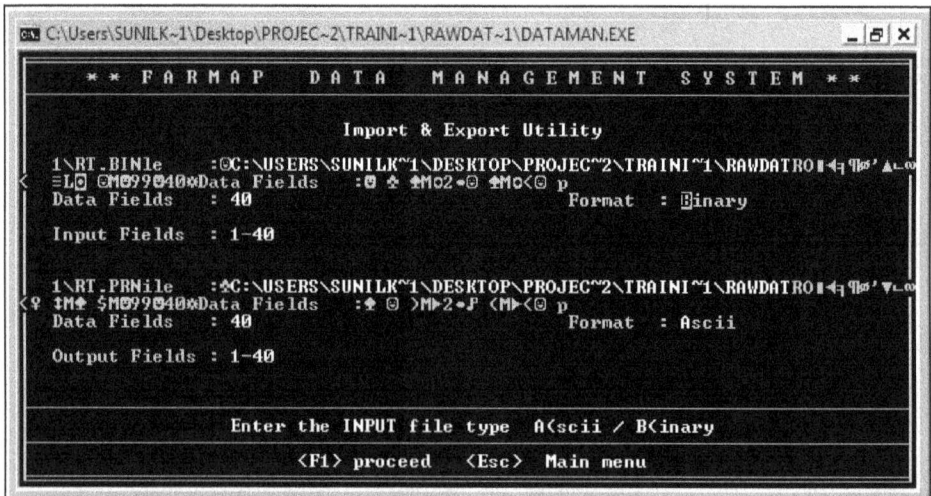

Snapshot 3: Specify input files path, output file path and data field (1-40 if wish to extract all RTs). Check format and input file (Binary) and opt for output file format (Ascii for PRN format).

C:\Users\SUNILK~1\Desktop\PROJEC~2\TRAINI~1\RAWDAT~1\DATAMAN.EXE _ □ ×

R	Data Field	Lower Value 1	Upper Value 1	Lower Value 2	Upper Value 2	Lower Value 3	Upper Value 3	~2\T

Record nos. to be searched

Start 1   Stop 170585

<F1> Proceed ■ <Esc> Exit

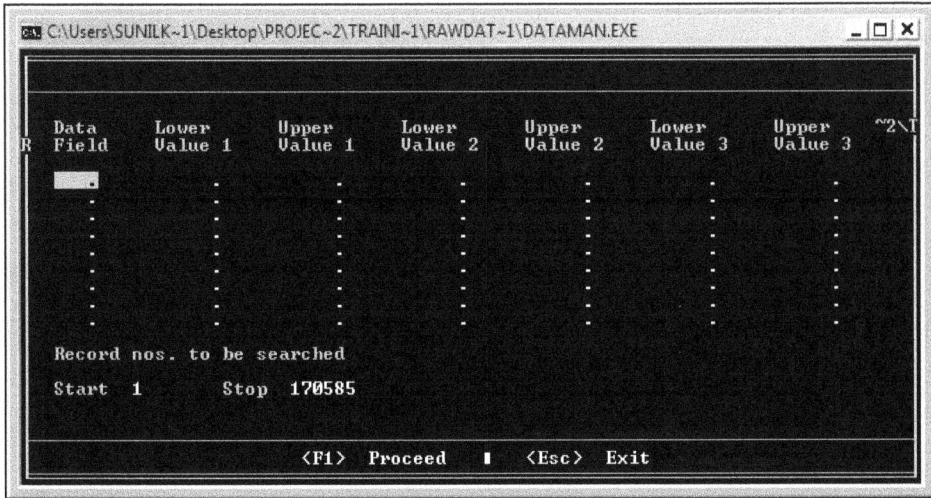

Snapshot 4: This wizard is used if wish to extract part of the data. Specify options and precede using F₁ command. Do nothing if wish to extract all RTs. Next step will produce output file in PRN format.

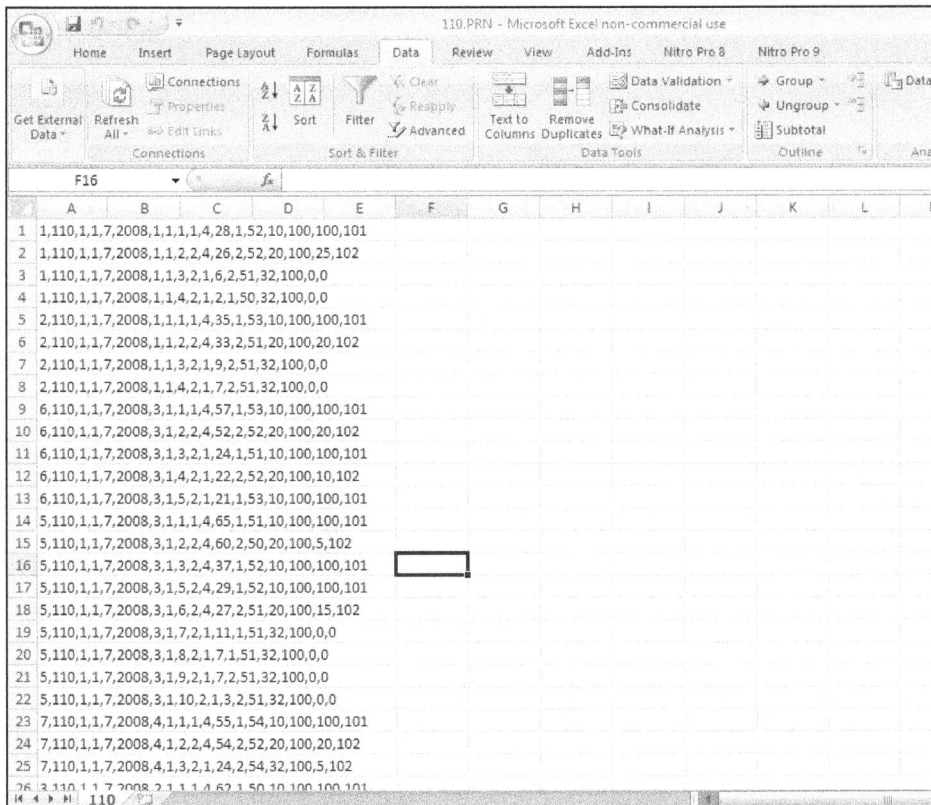

110.PRN - Microsoft Excel non-commercial use

Home Insert Page Layout Formulas Data Review View Add-Ins Nitro Pro 8 Nitro Pro 9

F16

	A
1	1,110,1,1,7,2008,1,1,1,1,4,28,1,52,10,100,100,101
2	1,110,1,1,7,2008,1,1,2,2,4,26,2,52,20,100,25,102
3	1,110,1,1,7,2008,1,1,3,2,1,6,2,51,32,100,0,0
4	1,110,1,1,7,2008,1,1,4,2,1,2,1,50,32,100,0,0
5	2,110,1,1,7,2008,1,1,1,1,4,35,1,53,10,100,100,101
6	2,110,1,1,7,2008,1,1,2,2,4,33,2,51,20,100,20,102
7	2,110,1,1,7,2008,1,1,3,2,1,9,2,51,32,100,0,0
8	2,110,1,1,7,2008,1,1,4,2,1,7,2,51,32,100,0,0
9	6,110,1,1,7,2008,3,1,1,1,4,57,1,53,10,100,100,101
10	6,110,1,1,7,2008,3,1,2,2,4,52,2,52,20,100,20,102
11	6,110,1,1,7,2008,3,1,3,2,1,24,1,51,10,100,100,101
12	6,110,1,1,7,2008,3,1,4,2,1,22,2,52,20,100,10,102
13	6,110,1,1,7,2008,3,1,5,2,1,21,1,53,10,100,100,101
14	5,110,1,1,7,2008,3,1,1,1,4,65,1,51,10,100,100,101
15	5,110,1,1,7,2008,3,1,2,2,4,60,2,50,20,100,5,102
16	5,110,1,1,7,2008,3,1,3,2,4,37,1,52,10,100,100,101
17	5,110,1,1,7,2008,3,1,5,2,4,29,1,52,10,100,100,101
18	5,110,1,1,7,2008,3,1,6,2,4,27,2,51,20,100,15,102
19	5,110,1,1,7,2008,3,1,7,2,1,11,1,51,32,100,0,0
20	5,110,1,1,7,2008,3,1,8,2,1,7,1,51,32,100,0,0
21	5,110,1,1,7,2008,3,1,9,2,1,7,2,51,32,100,0,0
22	5,110,1,1,7,2008,3,1,10,2,1,3,2,51,32,100,0,0
23	7,110,1,1,7,2008,4,1,1,1,4,55,1,54,10,100,100,101
24	7,110,1,1,7,2008,4,1,2,2,4,54,2,52,20,100,20,102
25	7,110,1,1,7,2008,4,1,3,2,1,24,2,54,32,100,5,102
26	3,110,1,1,7,2008,2,1,1,1,4,62,1,50,10,100,100,101

110

Snapshot 5. If opening file in Excel, data will look like this. The file includes data for all 40 RTs and underlying variables in PRN format.

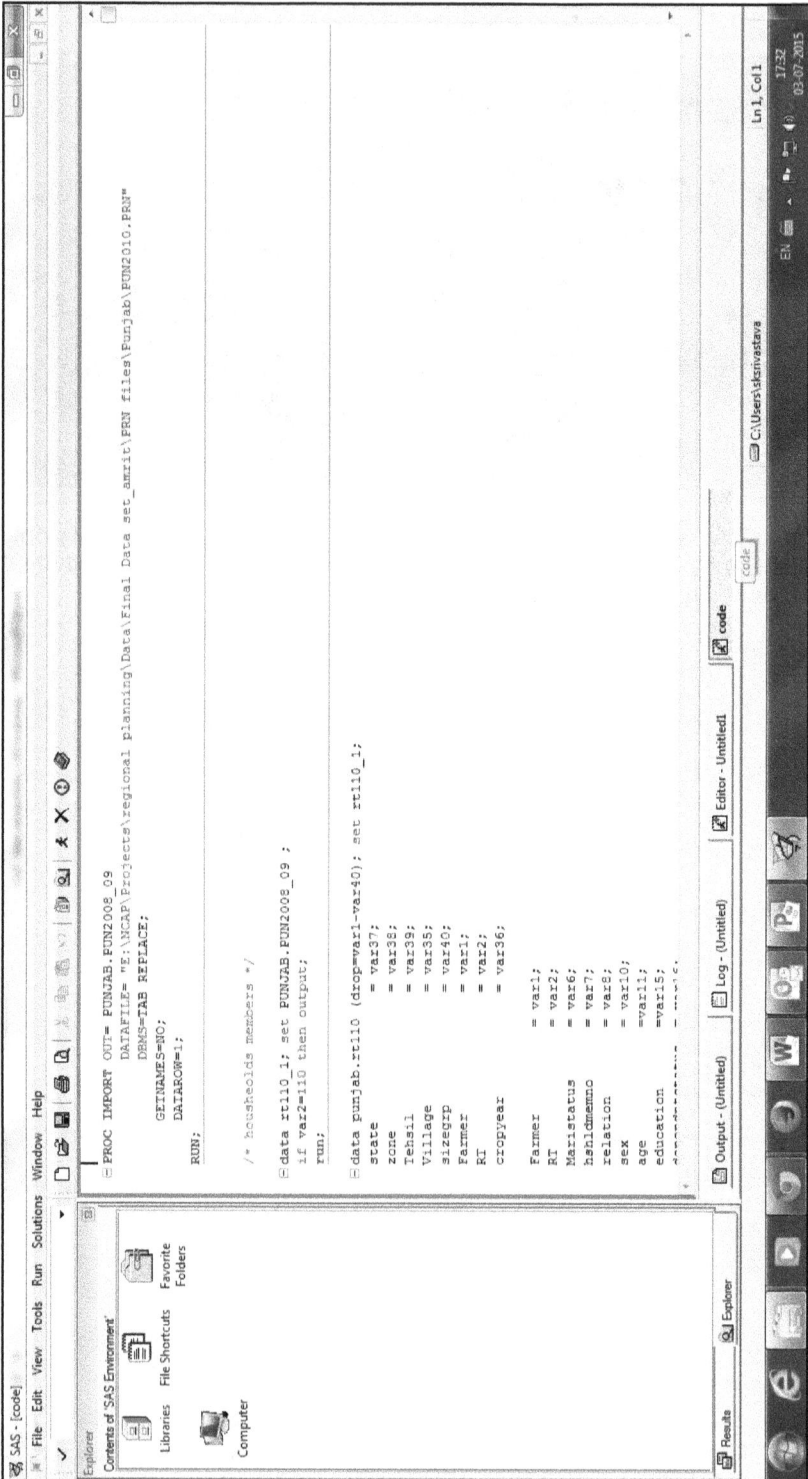

Sanpshot 6. Use SAS for importing the PRN file and data extraction and retrieving from each RT.

Index

www.ingramcontent.com/pod-product-compliance
Lightning Source LLC
Chambersburg PA
CBHW050522190326
41458CB00005B/1630